Ascites, Hyponatremia and Hepatorenal Syndrome: Progress in Treatment

Frontiers of Gastrointestinal Research

Vol. 28

Series Editor

Markus M. Lerch Greifswald

Ascites, Hyponatremia and Hepatorenal Syndrome: Progress in Treatment

Volume Editor

Alexander L. Gerbes Munich

23 figures and 31 tables, 2011

KARGER

Basel · Freiburg · Paris · London · New York · Bangalore · Bangkok · Shanghai · Singapore · Tokyo · Sydney

Frontiers of Gastrointestinal Research
Founded 1975 by L. van der Reis, San Francisco, Calif.

Alexander L. Gerbes
Klinikum München-Grosshadern
Liver Center Munich
Ludwig Maximilian University of Munich
Munich, Germany

Library of Congress Cataloging-in-Publication Data

Ascites, hyponatremia, and hepatorenal syndrome : progress in treatment / volume editor, Alexander L. Gerbes Munich.
p. ; cm. -- (Frontiers of gastrointestinal research, ISSN 0302-0665 ; v. 28)
Includes bibliographical references and indexes.
ISBN 978-3-8055-9591-9 (hard cover : alk. paper) -- ISBN 978-3-8055-9592-6 (e-ISBN)
1. Liver--Cirrhosis--Complications--Treatment. I. Gerbes, A. L. (Alexander L.) II. Series: Frontiers of gastrointestinal research ; v. 28. 0302-0665
[DNLM: 1. Liver Cirrhosis--complications. 2. Liver Cirrhosis--therapy. 3. Ascites--therapy. 4. Hepatorenal Syndrome--therapy. 5. Hyponatremia--therapy. W1 FR946E v.28 2011 / WI 725]
RC848.C5A83 2011
616.3'624--dc22

2010032384

Bibliographic Indices. This publication is listed in bibliographic services, including Current Contents®.

www.karger.com
Printed in Switzerland on acid-free and non-aging paper (ISO 9706) by Reinhardt Druck, Basel
ISSN 0302–0665
ISBN 978–3–8055–9591–9
e-ISBN 978–3–8055–9592–6

Contents

VII **Preface**
Gerbes, A.L. (Munich)

1 **Differential Diagnosis of Ascites**
Appenrodt, B. (Bonn)

11 **Current Treatment Strategies: Diuretics**
Bernardi, M. (Bologna)

23 **Paracentesis**
Sanyal, A.J.; Bajaj, J.S.; Shaw, J. (Richmond, Va.)

32 **Large-Volume Paracentesis: Which Plasma Expander?**
Terg, R.A. (Buenos Aires)

40 **Albumin: Not Just a Plasma Expander**
Davies, N.A.; Garcia, R.; Proven, A.; Jalan, R. (London)

52 **Transjugular Intrahepatic Portosystemic Shunt for Ascites: Which Patients Will Benefit?**
Salerno, F.; Cazzaniga, M. (San Donato Milanese)

65 **Spontaneous Bacterial Peritonitis – Prophylaxis and Treatment**
Wiest, R. (Regensburg); Garcia-Tsao, G. (New Haven, Conn./West Haven, Conn.)

83 **Clinical Implications of Hyponatremia in Cirrhosis**
Heuman, D.M. (Richmond, Va.)

91 **Vaptans for Ascites – Chances and Risks**
Wong, F. (Toronto, Ont.)

102 **Cardiorenal Syndrome – A New Entity?**
Møller, S.; Krag, A. (Hvidovre)

112 **Renal Failure in Cirrhosis**
Gustot, T. (Brussels/Clichy/Paris); Moreau, R. (Clichy/Paris)

122 **Novel Definition of Hepatorenal Syndrome: Clinical Consequences**
Fernandez, J.; Arroyo, V. (Barcelona)

130 **Role of Infections in Hepatorenal Syndrome**
Wiest, R. (Regensburg)

142 **TIPS for HRS**
Sauerbruch, T.; Appenrodt, B. (Bonn)

149 **Vasoconstrictor Therapy for Hepatorenal Syndrome**
Yeo, C.-M. (New Haven, Conn.); Garcia-Tsao, G. (New Haven, Conn./West Haven, Conn.)

163 Terlipressin for Hepatorenal Syndrome: The US Experience
Musana, A.K.; Sanyal, A.J. (Richmond, Va.)

172 Terlipressin for Hepatorenal Syndrome: Predictors of Response
Cárdenas, A.; Ginès, P. (Barcelona)

178 Safety of Terlipressin for Hepatorenal Syndrome
Krag, A.; Møller, S. (Hvidovre)

189 Terlipressin for Hepatorenal Syndrome: Novel Strategies and Future Perspectives
Angeli, P. (Padova)

198 Hepatorenal Syndrome and Liver Transplantation
Gonwa, T.A. (Jacksonville, Fla.)

208 Author Index

209 Subject Index

Preface

In patients with cirrhosis of the liver treatment focuses on the therapy of complications.

Ascites is the most frequent and hepatorenal syndrome the most lethal complication of liver cirrhosis. Fortunately, major progress has been made in recent years in providing effective treatment and thus reducing mortality in these patients. Therefore, the topics of ascites, hyponatremia and hepatorenal syndrome are very well suited to be presented as a book in the *Frontiers in Gastrointestinal Research* series.

Consequently, this project highlights and critically appraises recent achievements and novel advances. It also provides the background needed to grasp the novel concepts, but is not intended to represent an encyclopedic textbook. Contributions are provided by the most renowned experts at the forefront of clinical research. Their state of the art contributions provide up-to-date references and conclude with a bullet point summary.

Just to pick some of the hot topics that are elaborated in this book. The Transjugular Intrahepatic Portosystemic Shunt (TIPS) and paracentesis, respectively have been introduced into clinical routine, but several pitfalls need to be observed. Chapters deal with the most relevant issues of complications of paracentesis, the right choice of plasma expanders, and selection of patients who will experience survival benefit from TIPS. Beneficial effects of albumin infusion independent of its properties as a plasma expander are discussed.

There is a broad spectrum of acute kidney injury in cirrhosis. Hepatorenal syndrome was considered as a terminal renal failure in cirrhosis until recently. Now, drug treatment can improve renal function and prolong survival – a clinical breakthrough. However, important issues for clinical outcome are still under debate, such as predictors of response and ways to reduce the incidence of side effects of vasoconstrictor therapy. The role of combined kidney-liver transplantation versus conventional liver-only transplantation is considered.

Finally, hyponatremia, an indicator of poor prognosis in cirrhosis can now be addressed with vaptans, new pharmaceutical compounds. The role of vaptans for treating patients with ascites is still a matter of controversy.

I gladly accepted the invitation by Markus Lerch, the series editor, to design and organize this volume, and am very grateful that a highly selected group of international experts has contributed to this book. I do appreciate that despite their extremely busy agenda they took the time to share their knowledge and expertise. They come from the Americas and from Europe and thus provide a truly universal perspective.

It is my hope that this book provides practical advice for practitioners and clinicians who care for patients with cirrhosis. Furthermore, clinicians and scientists working in the field should find the latest data and inspiration for future research.

Alexander L. Gerbes
Munich, Germany

Gerbes AL (ed): Ascites, Hyponatremia and Hepatorenal Syndrome: Progress in Treatment.
Front Gastrointest Res. Basel, Karger, 2011, vol 28, pp 1–10

Differential Diagnosis of Ascites

B. Appenrodt

Department for Internal Medicine I, University of Bonn, Bonn, Germany

Abstract

Approximately 80–85% of causes of ascites are related to portal hypertension; however, malignancy-related ascites, cardiac failure and tuberculosis and other less common causes should always be considered. If ascites is suspected the patient should be carefully evaluated, including clinical history and physical examination. Diagnostic paracentesis should be performed routinely to determine the cause of ascites and spontaneous bacterial peritonitis. Basic tests include a cell count with differential and total protein concentration in ascitic fluid. Culture and other optional tests like the serum ascites albumin gradient can be performed based on clinical suspicion. New tests have been developed especially for the diagnosis of spontaneous bacterial peritonitis such as measurement of lactoferrin concentration in ascitic fluid or detection of bacterial DNA. These tests still need to be evaluated further.

Ascites is defined as accumulation of fluid in the peritoneal cavity. It is a common complication of cirrhosis, indicating portal hypertension which occurs in 80–85% of patients with ascites [1]. Nearly 60% of patients with compensated liver cirrhosis develop ascites within 10 years after onset of the liver disease. Once patients have developed ascites their prognosis is poor; nearly half of them die within 2–3 years [2]. However, other less common causes of ascites should be evaluated in the differential diagnosis of ascites. Other causes of ascites are, for example, malignancy (10%), cardiac failure (5%) and abdominal tuberculosis (2%) (table 1) [3].

Clinical Work-Up and Problems

In patients where cirrhosis is not the cause of ascites, a clinical work-up should be elicited for other causes of ascites. Furthermore, in approximately 5–10% of patients there is more than one cause of ascites [1].

Table 1. Causes of ascites

Cirrhosis Alcoholic hepatitis Partial nodular transformation Fulminant hepatic failure Hepatocellular carcinoma (usually with cirrhosis)

Cardiac disease
    Congestive heart failure
    Valvular disease
    Constrictive pericarditis
    Cardiomyopathy

Malignancy

Vascular disease
    Hepatic vein obstruction (Budd-Chiari syndrome)/sinusoidal obstruction syndrome
    Portal vein occlusion (thrombosis, tumor)

Peritoneal tuberculosis
Nephrotic syndrome
Ovarian disease (like Meigs syndrome, struma ovarii of ovarian overstimulation syndrome)

Pancreatic ascites
    Rupture of pseudocyst
    Leak from pancreatic duct

Bile ascites
    Gallbladder rupture
    Traumatic bile leak

Chylous ascites
    Rupture (traumatic, surgical) of abdominal lymphatics
    Obstructed lymphatics

Rare causes
    HIV-related ascites
    Peritoneal vasculitides
    Myxedema
    Whipple's disease
    Sarcoidosis
    Gynecologic lesions
    Malnutrition
    Hypoalbuminemia
    Protein-losing enteropathy

History and Physical Examination

Ascites is rarely the sole physical finding. Evidence of liver disease must be considered (jaundice, spider angiomata, palmar erythema, caput medusae, muscle wasting, splenomegaly, gynecomastia). Hepatomegaly may be absent if cirrhosis exists, possible causes of hepatomegaly with ascites include Budd-Chiari syndrome, cardiomyopathy with congestive heart failure or liver metastases. Edema of the lower extremities or significant proteinuria may suggest a nephrotic syndrome as the cause of ascites due to, for example, glomerulonephritis, collagen diseases or diabetes. Jugular venous distention, pathologic heart sound, pulmonary crackles, dyspnea and peripheral edema imply right-side heart failure. Clinical tests for ascites include inspection for bulging flanks and flank dullness and the fluid wave test. If the volume of ascites is low, these techniques are not helpful; 1,500 ml of fluid must be present before shifting dullness can be detected [4].

Diagnostic Imaging Techniques

Abdominal ultrasonography is a cost-effective technique to confirm ascites and to detect potential causes such as liver disease and should be performed first. It may help confirm the presence of ascites and differentiate it from other conditions such as pregnancy or ovarian cysts [4].

Small amounts of ascites (<100 ml) and the best possible location to perform paracentesis can be detected by ultrasound.

A CT scan of the abdomen should be performed to determine the presence of primary malignancy of the gastrointestinal tract or peritoneal carcinomatosis and other structures in the abdomen.

To rule out congestive heart failure, further cardiac work-up can be performed.

Diagnostic Paracentesis and Ascitic Fluid Analysis

A diagnostic paracentesis should be performed during the initial evaluation of ascites to determine its cause and to diagnose spontaneous bacterial peritonitis (SBP) [5].

It should be performed in (a) all patients with new onset of ascites, (b) patients who are admitted to hospital because of cirrhosis-related complications, and (c) in patients with clinical signs or laboratory abnormalities suggestive of infection [5].

For the diagnostic approach, 20–40 ml of ascitic fluid must be obtained.

In patients with new-onset ascites, the fluid should be evaluated for:

- macroscopic appearance
- cell count and differential
- total protein

- (optional) cultures
- (optional) ascitic and serum albumin for SAAG
- (optional) other parameters.

Macroscopic Appearance of Ascites

Ascitic fluid is transparent. In jaundiced patients it is slightly yellow due to the presence of bilirubin.

Ascitic fluid may be cloudy due to the presence of neutrophils >5,000/mm^3, while it appears pink due to red blood cells >10,000/mm^3. Bloody ascites is usually due to traumatic puncture. Causes of nontraumatic bloody ascitic fluid include peritoneal tuberculosis or malignancy. Approximately 20% of malignant ascites are bloody. The ascitic fluid of patients with cirrhosis and hepatocellular carcinoma is bloody in up to 50% of the cases [6].

Chylous or 'milky' ascites is often due to the presence of a high concentration of triglycerides (a triglyceride concentration >200 mg/dl establishes the diagnosis of chylous ascites) and is often found in malignancy-related ascites. However, in 20% of patients with cirrhosis ascites is chylous [7]. Another cause of chylous ascites is disruption of the lymphatic system due to abdominal surgery.

Diagnostic Tests for Ascites

Following diagnostic paracentesis of ascites, it has to be decided which tests should be performed and which parameters should be analyzed.

While many tests are available, it is neither useful nor cost effective to carry them all out. Further tests can be performed as indicated by the initial specimen (table 2).

As most patients with ascites have liver disease, exclusion of malignancy, tuberculosis or other less common causes is normally not required after the first paracentesis.

Cell Count

Cell count, as a mandatory test, may be performed in an EDTA tube using a small amount of fluid. The average normal total white blood cell count in patients with ascites due to liver disease is 100–500/mm^3. In bloody ascites, the white blood cell count could be misinterpreted: one PMN count per 250 red blood cells can be taken as contamination. In SBP, the total white blood cell count as well as the absolute PMN count are elevated. A PMN count >250/mm^3 is defined as spontaneous bacterial peritonitis (SBP) and indicates initiation of an empiric antibiotic regime [5].

Table 2. Ascitic tests

Mandatory	Optional	Rarely used
Cell count / differential	Albumin (ascitic and blood)	Bilirubin
Total protein	Cytology	Triglycerides
	Culture	Tumor markers
	Cholesterol	LDH
		Glucose
		Amylase

In tuberculous or malignant ascites, lymphocytes dominate in the ascitic fluid [6]. If malignant ascites is suspected, cytology should be performed. If tuberculosis is suspected, microbiological tests and a polymerase chain reaction-based method can be performed.

Cytology

Ascitic fluid cytology should be performed in suspected cases of malignancy-related ascites. The fluid should be examined rapidly after paracentesis – either fresh or fixed. The amount of ascitic fluid should be 50–100 ml.

Cell count is often elevated in malignant ascites. However, in patients with hepatocellular carcinoma ascitic cytology is positive in <10% [8].

Total Protein

Ascites used to be divided into exudative and transudative types using a cut-off value of 2.5 g/dl total protein [9]. Ascites due to secondary abdominal processes like malignancy or abdominal tuberculosis (50%) would be exudates (>2.5 g/dl), whereas ascites due to portal hypertension would be transudates (<2.5 g/dl). However, approximately 20% of cirrhotic patients have an ascitic total protein of >2.5 g/dl and would therefore be categorized incorrectly [10]. Furthermore, patients with cardiac ascites have a high total protein (>2.5 g/dl).

Serum Ascites Albumin Gradient

Calculation of the serum ascites albumin gradient (SAAG) may differentiate the causes of ascites into two groups. It helps determine whether or not ascites is related to portal hypertension. The gradient can be calculated by measuring the albumin concentration in blood and ascitic fluid and subtracting the ascitic from the serum value. If a patient has portal hypertension, there must be a high oncotic gradient, which means a high albumin gradient between blood and ascitic fluid.

If the SAAG is ≥1.1 g/dl, the cause of ascites is portal hypertension with a reliability of more than 90% [9], another cause could be cardiac disease with a high protein content in ascitic fluid.

While SAAG enables differentiation of ascites into one of two categories, it cannot replace further evaluation. A SAAG of <1.1 g/dl indicates that the patient does not have portal hypertension, but that a process such as peritoneal carcinomatosis, abdominal tuberculosis, pancreatic ascites, nephrotic syndrome, or biliary ascites may be present.

If the gradient has been determined at the initial paracentesis, it is not necessary to repeat this calculation.

Microbiological Culture and Gram Stain

Ascites culture is negative in approximately 40% of patients with SBP [11]. The cultures should be collected at the bedside, including aerobic and anaerobic media with a minimum amount of 10 ml ascitic fluid. Ascitic fluid Gram stain is generally a useless investigation due to the low concentration of bacteria in patients with SBP. Furthermore, an ascites smear for diagnosis of tuberculosis is also not helpful [12]. The sensitivity of fluid culture of mycobacteria is approximately 50%.

Other Ascitic Fluid Tests

Cholesterol

No laboratory test completely distinguishes malignant ascites from ascites associated with cirrhosis. It has been suggested that a fraction of the cholesterol could be derived from a malignant cell [14]. Measurement of total ascitic cholesterol concentration seems to be a rapid and cost-effective diagnostic test for discrimination between ascites of malignant and benign origin. A cholesterol concentration of >45 mg/dl is suspicious for malignant ascites. A cytologic examination should follow [14, 15].

Lactate Dehydrogenase

Lactate dehydrogenase (LDH) as a diagnostic test has little clinical relevance in delineating the cause of ascites. An elevation of LDH is common in SBP, tuberculous peritonitis or secondary bacterial peritonitis with a fluid:serum LDH ratio >0.5, a ratio >1.0 is suspicious of abdominal tuberculosis [16].

Glucose

The ascitic glucose concentration does not fall during intraperitoneal infection. Gut perforation seems to be one exception. Low levels of glucose in ascitic fluid – compared to serum glucose levels – could indicate secondary bacterial peritonitis [17].

Amylase

Ascitic amylase is increased if amylase is released into ascitic fluid, e.g. due to pancreatitis or gut perforation. In pancreatic ascites, the amylase concentration is often higher than that found in gut perforation [18].

Tumor Markers

Measurement of tumor markers in ascitic fluid like carcinoembryonic antigen has been suggested as an aid in the diagnosis of malignancy-related ascites. However, this has achieved only little clinical relevance because of its low sensitivity [19].

Some Common Causes of Ascites

Malignant Ascites

Approximately 50% of all malignant ascites are due to peritoneal carcinomatosis [6]. In patients with malignancy-related ascites, SAAG is usually low in up to 80–85% of the cases and ascites may be bloody. The ascitic cell count is generally high with normal glucose, normal LDH and elevated cholesterol levels. Cytological investigation is specific with a low sensitivity of <70% [14].

Cardiac Ascites

Ascites due to heart failure may be difficult to distinguish from ascites due to cirrhosis. Common causes are ischemic heart disease, cardiomyopathy, valvular and restrictive lung disease and constrictive pericarditis. The characteristics of cardiac ascitic fluid are high SAAG (≥1.1 g/dl) with a high total protein level (>2.5 g/dl). Sometimes it is necessary to carry out a more invasive testing procedure such as measurement of the hepatic venous pressure gradient [20].

Tuberculous Peritonitis

The mechanism of formation of ascites is exudation of fluid from the peritoneal surface affected by the disease. The SAAG and protein is variable, the SAAG is often <1.1 g/dl and the protein value >2.5 g/dl.

The ascitic cell count is elevated between 1,000 and 3,000/mm^3 with a predominance of lymphocytes. The red blood cell count in ascites could be mildly elevated. Glucose values are usually within the normal limits, and LDH levels could be high. Fluid culture and polymerase chain reaction-based analysis should be performed. A direct smear is not recommended because of a low sensitivity [12, 13].

Novel Aspects and Future Developments

New Tests for the Diagnosis of Ascitic Infection: Urinary Reagent Strips, Lactoferrin and Bacterial DNA in Ascitic Fluid

Using Urinary Reagent Strips
As an alternative test for a more rapid diagnosis of SBP, the use of urinary reagent strips was proposed to achieve a rapid bedside diagnosis of SBP. The first studies reported enthusiastic results with a sensitivity and specificity between 90 and 100% [21]. However, when this method was evaluated several years later in a study with a larger population, the promising results of the previous study could not be confirmed and the poor sensitivity (45%) of this test was revealed [22].

Measurement of Lactoferrin
Measurement of lactoferrin in ascitic fluid may offer an alternative to the PMN count for the diagnosis of SBP. Lactoferrin is released by leukocytes upon activation of these cells and its presence in body fluids is proportional to the flux of neutrophils. The data available on the diagnostic value of the measurement of lactoferrin in ascitic fluid for SBP diagnosis are limited to a single study. In this study, in which ascitic fluid lactoferrin was measured in a total of 218 samples, the specificity and sensitivity for SBP diagnosis was 95 and 97%, respectively [23]. However, the quantitative lactoferrin assay used is not available commercially.

It must be stressed that urinary reagent strips and ascitic lactoferrin tests are qualitative methods and need to be further confirmed for use in the diagnosis of SBP.

Detection of Bacterial DNA in Ascitic Fluid
In patients with cirrhosis, bacterial translocation from the intestinal lumen is thought to precede the development of SBP. Once microbes reach the ascitic fluid, SBP may develop. According to this hypothesis, it should be possible to detect bacteria in the ascitic fluid. However, the major part of the culture obtained is negative. In 2002, bacterial DNA could be detected in culture-negative ascites using the polymerase chain reaction-based method [24]. Such et al. [24] detected bacterial DNA in ascites and postulated bacterial DNA as a surrogate marker for bacterial translocation, which needs to be further evaluated for use in the diagnosis of SBP.

Key Messages

- The most common cause of ascites is portal hypertension in 80–85% of the cases; malignancy, cardiac failure, abdominal tuberculosis and others are less common causes.
- A diagnostic paracentesis should be performed in the initial evaluation of ascites to determine the cause of ascites and to make the diagnosis of SBP. The fluid should be evaluated for cell count and differential and total protein. Optional parameters could be determined based on clinical suspicion.
- There are promising new diagnostic ascitic tests like measurement of lactoferrin concentration in ascitic fluid or detection of bacterial DNA which have to be evaluated and tested further.

References

1 Ginés P, Quintero E, Arroyo V, Terés J, Bruguera M, Rimola A, Caballería J, Rodés J, Rozman C: Compensated cirrhosis: natural history and prognostic factors. Compensated cirrhosis: natural history and prognostic factors. Hepatology 1987;7: 122–128.

2 D'Amico G, Morabito A, Pagliaro L, Marubini E: Survival and prognostic indicators in compensated and decompensated cirrhosis. Dig Dis Sci. 1986;31: 468–475.

3 Cattau EL, Benjamin SB, Knuff TE, Castell DO: The accuracy of the physical examination in the diagnosis of suspected ascites. JAMA 1982;247: 1164.

4 Goldberg BB, Goodman GA, Clearfield HR: Evaluation of ascites by ultrasound. Radiology 1970; 96:15–22.

5 Gerbes AL, Gülberg V, Wiest R, Sauerbruch T, et al: S3-guideline 'Diagnosis and treatment of ascites, spontaneous bacterial peritonitis, and hepatorenal syndrome in cirrhosis' of the German Society for Digestive and Metabolic Diseases (DGVS). 2010;in preparation.

6 Runyon BA, Hoefs JC, Morgan TR. Ascitic fluid analysis in malignancy-related ascites. Hepatology 1988;8:1104–1109.

7 Rector WG Jr: Spontaneous chylous ascites of cirrhosis. J Clin Gastroenterol 1984;6:369–372.

8 Gulyás M, Kaposi AD, Elek G, Szollár LG, Hjerpe A: Value of carcinoembryonic antigen (CEA) and cholesterol assays of ascitic fluid in cases of inconclusive cytology. J Clin Pathol 2001;54:831–835.

9 Rector WG Jr, Reynolds TB: Superiority of the serum-ascites albumin difference over the ascites total protein concentration in separation of 'transudative' and 'exudative' ascites. Am J Med 1984;77: 83–85.

10 Sampliner RE, Iber FL: High protein ascites in patients with uncomplicated hepatic cirrhosis. Am J Med Sci 1974;267:275–279.

11 Runyon BA, Canawati HN, Akriviadis EA: Optimization of ascitic fluid culture technique. Gastroenterology 1988;95:1351–1355.

12 Singh MM, Bhargava AN, Jain KP: Tuberculous peritonitis: an evaluation of pathogenetic mechanisms, diagnostic procedures and therapeutic measures. N Engl J Med 1969;281:1091–1094.

13 Chow KM, Chow VC, Hung LC, Wong SM, Szeto CC: Tuberculous peritonitis-associated mortality is high among patients waiting for the results of mycobacterial cultures of ascitic fluid samples. Clin Infect Dis 2002;35:409–413.

14 Gerbes AL, Jüngst D, Xie YN, Permanetter W, Paumgartner G: Ascitic fluid analysis for the differentiation of malignancy-related and nonmalignant ascites: proposal of a diagnostic sequence. Cancer 1991;68:1808–1814.

15 Jüngst D, Gerbes AL, Martin R, Paumgartner G: Value of ascitic lipids in the differentiation between cirrhotic and malignant ascites. Hepatology 1986;6: 239–243.

16 Sevinc A, Sari R, Fadillioglu E: The utility of lactate dehydrogenase isoenzyme pattern in the diagnostic evaluation of malignant and nonmalignant ascites. J Natl Med Assoc 2005;97:79–84.

17 Runyon BA, Hoefs JC: Ascitic fluid analysis in the differentiation of spontaneous bacterial peritonitis from gastrointestinal tract perforation into ascitic fluid. Hepatology 1984;4:447–450.

18 Runyon BA: Amylase levels in ascitic fluid. J Clin Gastroenterol 1987;9:172–174.

19 Archimandritis A, Kapsalas D, Douvara M, Tjivras M, Tsirantonaki M, Fertakis A: Value of ascitic fibronectin and cholesterol concentration in the differentiation between malignancy-related and nonmalignant ascites. Ann Med Interne 1996;147:145–150.

20 Myers RP, Cerini R, Sayegh R, Moreau R, Degott C, Lebrec D, Lee SS: Cardiac hepatopathy: clinical, hemodynamic, and histologic characteristics and correlations. Hepatology 2003;37:393–400.

21 Castellote J, López C, Gornals J, Tremosa G, Fariña ER, Baliellas C, Domingo A, Xiol X: Rapid diagnosis of spontaneous bacterial peritonitis by use of reagent strips. Hepatology 2003;37:893–896.

22 Nousbaum JB, Cadranel JF, Nahon P, et al: Diagnostic accuracy of the Multistix 8 SG reagent strip in diagnosis of spontaneous bacterial peritonitis. Hepatology 2007;45:1275–1281.

23 Parsi MA, Saadeh SN, Zein NN, Davis GL, Lopez R, Boone J, Lepe MR, Guo L, Ashfaq M, Klintmalm G, McCullough AJ: Ascitic fluid lactoferrin for diagnosis of spontaneous bacterial peritonitis. Gastroenterology 2008;135:803–807.

24 Such J, Francés R, Muñoz C, Zapater P, Casellas JA, Cifuentes A, Rodríguez-Valera F, Pascual S, Sola-Vera J, Carnicer F, Uceda F, Palazón JM, Pérez-Mateo M: Detection and identification of bacterial DNA in patients with cirrhosis and culture-negative, nonneutrocytic ascites. Hepatology 2002;36:135–141.

Beate Appenrodt
Department for Internal Medicine I, University of Bonn
Sigmund-Freud-Strasse 25
DE–53115 Bonn (Germany)
Tel. +49 228 28715507, Fax +49 228 28719718, E-Mail beate.appenrodt@ukb.uni-bonn.de

Gerbes AL (ed): Ascites, Hyponatremia and Hepatorenal Syndrome: Progress in Treatment.
Front Gastrointest Res. Basel, Karger, 2011, vol 28, pp 11–22

Current Treatment Strategies: Diuretics

Mauro Bernardi

Dipartimento di Medicina Clinica, Alma Mater Studiorum – University of Bologna, Semeiotica Medica – Policlinico S. Orsola-Malpighi, Bologna, Italy

Abstract

Diuretics are needed to counteract renal sodium retention in decompensated cirrhosis, which is responsible for ascites and edema formation. As secondary hyperaldosteronism is a major pathogenetic mechanism, aldosterone antagonists should always be administered at a dose of up to 400 mg/day. They have a very long elimination half-life and can be given once a day. Their main side effects are hyperkalemia and painful gynecomastia. When the glomerular filtration rate declines, as occurs in advanced stages of the disease, excessive sodium reabsorption by the proximal tubule becomes the main cause of sodium retention. In such cases, loop diuretics should be associated. These very potent and short-acting drugs should be given with caution because of their potential side effects: renal impairment, hyponatremia, hypokalemia, hypochloremic alkalosis and hepatic encephalopathy. The maximum recommended dosage for furosemide is 160 mg/day, which is seldom reached in clinical practice because of the adverse side effects at lower doses. Treatment can be sequential, i.e. starting with aldosterone antagonist monotherapy at increasing doses, with the eventual addition of a loop diuretic in case of failure, or combined, i.e. starting with the association straight away. Controlled clinical trials suggest that sequential treatment is to be preferred in patients with ascites at their first presentation, and a well-preserved glomerular filtration rate, where natriuresis can be achieved in more than 90% of the cases, and dose adjustments are less common. Patients with long-standing recidivant ascites would benefit from the combined treatment, which induces natriuresis more rapidly with a lower incidence of hyperkalemia.

Renal sodium retention is the pathogenetic mechanism that promotes extracellular fluid expansion in cirrhosis [1]. The fluid overload is then compartmentalized as ascites because of postsinusoidal portal hypertension and edema. Therefore, the medical treatment of ascites aims to establish a negative sodium balance, and diuretics represent the mainstay of therapy to achieve this goal in uncomplicated ascites, i.e. neither infected nor associated with hepatorenal syndrome [2]. Complicated ascites is characterized by either refractoriness to treatment or ascitic fluid infection, renal failure or severe hyponatremia and requires different approaches that are described elsewhere in this book.

A rational choice of diuretics cannot overlook the mechanisms responsible for sodium retention or the nephron sites where this occurs. Briefly, the fundamental afferent factor is reduced effective volemia, mostly due to peripheral arterial vasodilation, that evokes the compensatory activation of systems devoted to extracellular fluid defense such as the renin-angiotensin-aldosterone axis, the sympathetic nervous system and the secretion of arginine vasopressin [3]. Among these efferent factors, secondary hyperaldosteronism plays a major role. Indeed, excessive sodium reabsorption mainly takes place at the distal nephron, even though the proximal convoluted tubule, under the effects of angiotensin II and sympathoadrenergic drive, also plays a role [1]. Progression of cirrhosis is associated with a worsening of effective volemia, which ultimately impairs the glomerular filtration rate (GFR) thereby further enhancing proximal sodium reabsorption, which becomes prevalent when GFR is severely depressed. Thus, both distal and proximal sodium reabsorption are enhanced in advanced cirrhosis due to secondary hyperaldosteronism and reduced renal perfusion, respectively [4] (fig. 1a, b).

Given this pathophysiological background, aldosterone antagonists represent the first-choice treatment, but when proximal reabsorption is also enhanced, other diuretics should be associated. Unfortunately, only carbonic anhydrase inhibitors counteract sodium reabsorption at the proximal tubule, but their side effects and scarce effectiveness once GFR is depressed prevent their use in this setting. Thus, the potent loop diuretics are employed even though Henle's loop, their site of action, does not seem to play a major role in the renal sodium handling abnormalities of cirrhosis.

Aldosterone Antagonists

Aldosterone exerts its action on the epithelial cells of the late distal and collecting ducts by binding the cytosolic mineralocorticoid receptor. The aldosterone-receptor complex migrates into the nucleus where it enhances both the synthesis of a long-lasting protein that facilitates sodium transport from the tubular lumen through the amiloride-sensitive sodium channel (ASSC) and de novo synthesis of channel proteins (ASSC, Na-K-ATPase) [5]. As a result, more sodium crosses the luminal membrane through ASSC and leaves the tubular cell through the Na-K-ATPase transporter located at the basolateral membrane. Antagonists compete with aldosterone at the mineralocorticoid receptor, thus blocking its actions on gene expression [6] (fig. 2). This mechanism implies clinically relevant consequences: (a) the drug dosage to achieve full antagonism is proportional to the degree of hyperaldosteronism [7], and (b) the effect of antagonists has a latency of at least 48 h from their administration. Thus, making a decision about their efficacy and/or increasing dosage earlier is not rational.

Spironolactone is a 17-spirolactone steroid with high selectivity and efficacy, and is the most widely used aldosterone antagonist in clinical practice. This lipophylic

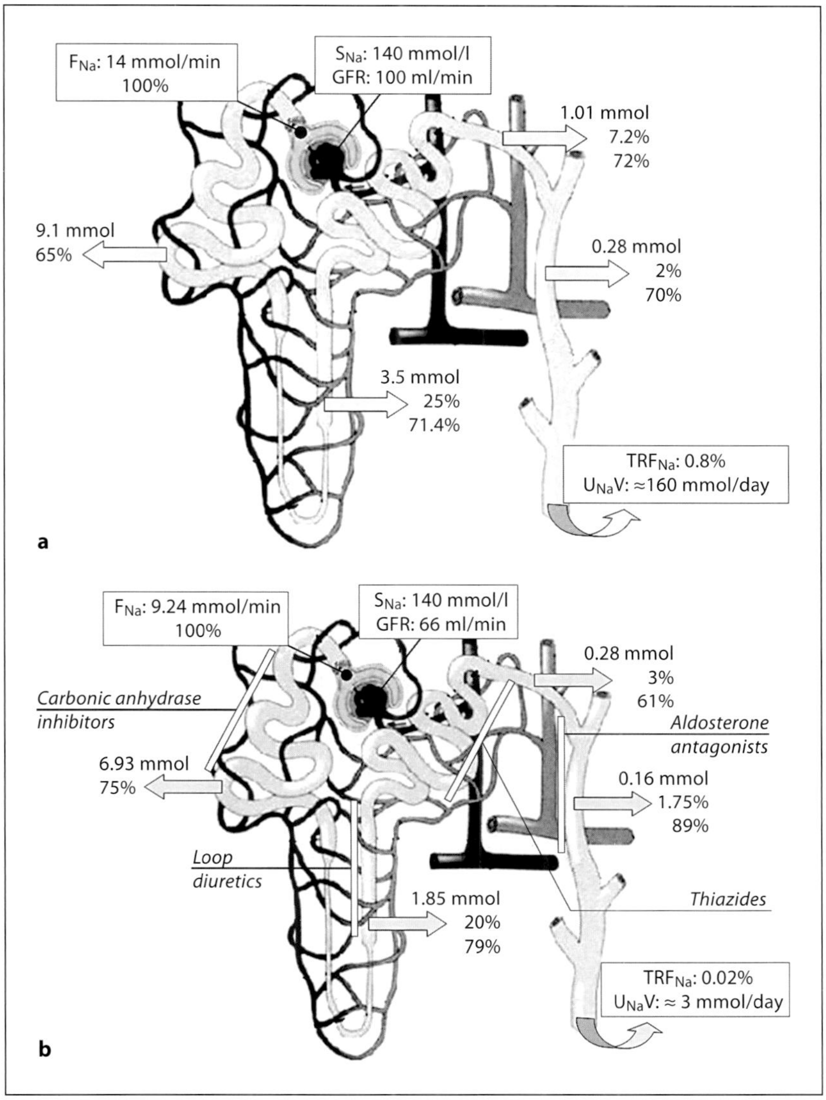

Fig. 1. a Renal sodium reabsorption at the different nephron sites in normal conditions. Calculations were made assuming: serum sodium concentration (S_{Na}) = 140 mmol/l; GFR = 100 ml/min. Data represent rough estimates. F_{Na} = Filtered load of sodium; TRF_{Na} = tubular rejection fraction of sodium; $U_{Na}V$ = urine sodium excretion. Each box reports absolute amount of sodium reabsorbed (mmol/min), relative amount of sodium reabsorbed with respect to the F_{Na}, and relative amount of sodium reabsorbed with respect to the amount delivered to that segment. **b** Renal sodium reabsorption at the different nephron sites in cirrhosis with avid renal sodium retention. Calculations were made assuming serum sodium concentration (S_{Na}) = 140 mmol/l and GFR = 66 ml/min. Abbreviations and reported data as in **a**. Note the increase in the relative sodium reabsorption by the proximal convoluted tubule (from 65 to 75%) as a consequence of GFR reduction, and the striking increase in the relative amount of sodium reabsorbed by the aldosterone-sensitive distal nephron (from 70 to 89%). The sites of action of diuretics are also indicated.

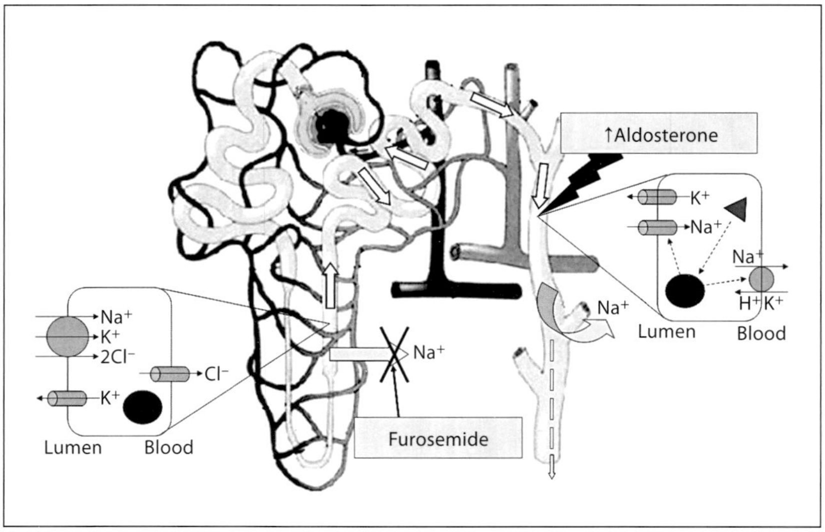

Fig. 2. Mechanism leading to failure of the natriuretic effect of loop diuretics in patients with severe hyperaldosteronism. Furosemide blocks the reabsorption of sodium at the thick ascending limb of Henle's loop by inhibiting the $Na^+2Cl^-K^+$ symporter. As a result, the distal delivery of sodium increases (white arrows). However, unopposed hyperaldosteronism leads to avid sodium reabsorption at the mineralocorticoid-sensitive segments of the nephron. The natriuretic response to furosemide is greatly attenuated or even abolished. Some mechanisms leading to sodium reabsorption by tubular cells are also illustrated. In the epithelial cells lining the thick ascending limb of Henle's loop (left) sodium is reabsorbed by the $Na^+2Cl^-K^+$ symporter located in the luminal membrane; this transport is counteracted by loop diuretics. In the epithelial cells lining, the aldosterone-sensitive cortical collecting duct (right) and the aldosterone-mineralocorticoid receptor complex (grey triangle) migrate into the nucleus (black circle), where they enhance both the synthesis of a long-lasting protein that facilitates sodium transport from the tubular lumen through the amiloride-sensitive sodium channel located in the luminal membrane and de novo synthesis of channel proteins (amiloride-sensitive sodium channel; Na-K-ATPase, located in the basolateral membrane). Antagonists compete with aldosterone at the mineralocorticoid receptor, thus blocking its actions on gene expression.

molecule undergoes an almost complete first-pass effect in the liver, so that its action is promoted by its metabolite canrenone that contributes to, but does not fully account for the biological activity of spironolactone [5]. In fact, spironolactone metabolism produces a number of further and still active molecules. This, along with their reduced clearance in cirrhosis [8], explains the persistent anti-mineralocorticoid effect after withdrawal lasting up to a week or more. Canrenoate, a hydrophilic molecule that can be administered i.v., derives from a modification of the canrenone lateral chain. It has no intrinsic activity, but exerts biological effects by virtue of its interconversion with canrenone in the plasma, thus avoiding the hepatic first-pass effect [9]. The epoxy derivative of aldosterone eplerenone has a more selective binding affinity for the mineralocorticoid receptor. It has been widely used for treating hypertension and heart failure [10], but no controlled studies in advanced cirrhosis and ascites are available.

Aldosterone antagonists undergo a ready and almost complete intestinal absorption (bioavailability 75–95%) facilitated by the presence of food. Their elimination half-life is prolonged (up to 24 h), and they can be administered once daily.

Spironolactone exerts anti-androgenic effects, leading to painful gynecomastia and impotence through different mechanisms: decreased testosterone production in the adrenal gland, secondary to microsomal cytochrome P450 (CP450) depletion and inhibition of the CP450-dependent enzymes 17α-hydroxylase and desmolase, and competitive inhibition of dihydrotestosterone-receptor binding, which interferes with its nuclear translocation [11]. K-canrenoate metabolism has much less impact on CP450, and its anti-androgenic effects are substantially attenuated [11]. Protection from such effects also derives from a more selective binding affinity for the mineralocorticoid receptor, as reported with epleronone [12].

Aldosterone antagonists favor bicarbonate and reduce hydrogen ion excretions, potentially leading to metabolic acidosis, but this seldom becomes clinically significant [13]. Instead, hyperkalemia may be severe, but this usually occurs in patients with an impaired GFR. Otherwise, if aldosterone antagonist administration is followed by natriuresis, hyperkalemia does not develop even with high dosages [4].

The recommended starting dosage of spironolactone or other antagonists (canrenone, K-canrenoate) is 100–200 mg/day, which should be increased by 100 (200) mg/day every third day [2, 14, 15]. Provided the GFR is fairly well preserved [7], dosages should theoretically be increased up to complete aldosterone antagonism, which could be assessed by transtubular potassium gradient (urine K × serum K^{-1}/urine osmolality × plasma $osmolality^{-1}$; values <3 suggest aldosterone blockade). However, a controlled clinical trial [4] showed that the response rate obtained by K-canrenoate up to 600 mg/day was about 80%, and about 70% with 400 mg/day. Thus, doses higher than 400 mg/day do not substantially increase the success rate and need time to achieve and favor the occurrence of side effects. Therefore, all guidelines indicate 400 mg/day as the maximal recommended dose for spironolactone [2, 14, 15], which can be extended to canrenone and K-canrenoate.

Other 'Potassium-Sparing' Diuretics

Triamterene and amiloride also act at the distal nephron, somehow mimicking the effect of aldosterone antagonists by blocking the ASSC. There are no controlled clinical trials devoted to the use of triamterene in cirrhosis. The only randomized study comparing amiloride (20–60 mg/day) versus K-canrenoate (150–500 mg/day) reported a lower effectiveness [16]. Thus, these drugs are seldom used in clinical practice.

Loop Diuretics

These organic acids are secreted into the tubular fluid by the proximal tubule and inhibit the $Na^+2Cl^-K^+$ symporter located in the luminal membrane of epithelial cells lining the thick ascending limb of Henle's loop [17] (fig. 2). This nephron segment reabsorbs up to 25% of the filtered sodium load. Therefore, loop diuretics can exert an intense diuretic action as the distal nephron does not have the reabsorptive capacity to compensate for this increased load; cirrhosis, however, may represent an exception, as will be discussed later. Part of the loop diuretic effect is mediated by prostaglandin E_2 synthesis, and nonsteroidal anti-inflammatory agents impair their efficacy [18].

Loop diuretics are rapidly absorbed by the gut (30 min to 2 h); their bioavailability is variable, ranging from about 80% for bumetanide and torasemide to 40–60% for furosemide. Their action occurs promptly: it starts within 30 min after oral administration, peaks within 1–2 h, and ends in 3–4 h [17]. Whether furosemide pharmacokinetics are altered in cirrhosis is debated: some authors reported a reduced bioavailability [19], but others did not [20]. In any case, there appear to be no major alterations.

The most widely employed loop diuretic is furosemide. Guidelines indicate an initial oral dose of 20–40 mg/day, to be progressively increased every other day up to 160 mg/day [2, 14, 15]. However, such a dosage can seldom be reached because of the occurrence of even severe side effects at lower doses. Similar indications can be followed for other loop diuretics, taking into account that 40 mg of furosemide is equivalent to about 1 mg of bumetanide, 30 mg of torasemide and 50 mg of ethacrynic acid.

Otoxicity is a potential side effect of loop diuretics, namely ethacrynic acid that has been almost abandoned for this reason. Other side effects are somehow exacerbated by the peculiar pathophysiological context of advanced cirrhosis. (1) Their brisk and potent action can induce a sudden blood volume contraction that cannot be compensated by vasoconstriction because of the blunted cardiovascular responsiveness to vasoconstrictors [21]. Thus, effective volemia deteriorates and worsens hyperaldosteronism, impairs GFR and increases arginine-vasopressin secretion, ultimately leading to renal failure and hyponatremia. (2) Potassium, magnesium and calcium depletions are exacerbated by secondary hyperaldosteronism if an adequate aldosterone blockade is not achieved. (3) The inhibition of sodium and chloride reabsorption at Henle's loop impairs free water clearance and favors hyponatremia (see also point 1). (4) Because of hydrogen ion, chloride and potassium depletions, along with plasma volume contraction, hypochloremic alkalosis can ensue. Alkalosis favors hydrogen ion entry into the tubular cells, where it enhances ammonia generation, and augments blood-brain barrier permeability to ammonia. Hypovolemia, alkalosis and increased ammonia production can worsen or precipitate hepatic encephalopathy [22], a phenomenon that is amplified by concomitant hyponatremia.

There is no scientific evidence for preferring one loop diuretic to another. The main problem with this class of diuretics is related to their violent action, and a drug exerting a longer-term effect could be better tolerated. This may be the case of torasemide, but available data do not suggest a substantial advantage over furosemide [23]. Under appropriate clinical conditions, continuous furosemide infusion could maximize its diuretic action and minimize untoward hemodynamic effects. This practice has been extensively studied in other contexts, such as heart failure [24], but no controlled data are available in cirrhosis. Studies addressing this issue are warranted.

Diuretic Treatment Strategies in Decompensated Cirrhosis

Extent of Diuretic-Induced Negative Fluid Balance

Diuretics invariably lower blood volume, the expansion of which represents an important compensatory mechanism against effective hypovolemia due to vasodilation. Diuretic-induced negative fluid balance can be monitored simply by body weight assessment and should not exceed 700–800 ml/day, an amount that can be replaced by ascites mobilization to minimize its impact on effective volemia. As peripheral edema can be more easily mobilized than ascites, it allows a daily weight reduction of up to 1.5 kg [25]. Failure to comply with these limitations can result in diuretic-induced renal failure and/or hyponatremia.

Importance of Aldosterone Antagonism

Secondary hyperaldosteronism is always present in decompensated cirrhosis, and can be severe. Thus, aldosterone antagonists, whose efficacy has been clearly demonstrated by several controlled clinical trials [4, 26], should be always administered. Spironolactone proved to be more effective than furosemide in uncomplicated ascites [26], even though this may appear paradoxical, as furosemide is endowed with a far greater natriuretic potency. Indeed, the amount of sodium not reabsorbed in Henle's loop under furosemide action is reabsorbed in the distal nephron by the unopposed effect of aldosterone (fig. 2). However, when GFR is severely depressed (<60 ml/min), sodium reabsorption at the proximal tubule reduces its delivery to the distal nephron, the site of action of aldosterone antagonists, thereby cancelling out their effect. These patients cannot be treated with aldosterone antagonists alone, and loop diuretics should be added.

Sequential versus Combined Treatment

The sequential or 'stepped care' treatment of ascites is widely popular: an aldosterone antagonist is given at a starting dose of 100 mg/day and is progressively increased to the highest recommended dose if no response is achieved. Loop diuretics are eventually associated in those patients who still fail to develop natriuresis.

The starting dose of furosemide is 20–40 mg and is increased every other day up to the maximum recommended dose. Sequential treatment is effective in up to 90–95% of patients with fairly-well-preserved GFR [4]. However, reaching high dosages of aldosterone antagonists is time consuming and may favor the occurrence of side effects.

Combined treatment begins with both an aldosterone antagonist (100 mg/day) and furosemide (40 mg/day), with parallel increases in dosages every third day, if needed, up to the respective maximum dosages. This therapy has been recommended by some guidelines since 1994 [27], even though evidence favoring combined treatment had not emerged from the few clinical studies available [28]. Data from two more recent controlled clinical trials are apparently conflicting. The first study did not find significant differences between sequential and combined treatments (spironolactone and furosemide) in terms of response rate, rapidity of ascites mobilization and incidence of diuretic-induced complications. However, sequential therapy was deemed more suitable for outpatients, because it needs less-frequent dose adjustments (34 vs. 68% of cases) [29]. The second study found that the combined treatment (K-canrenoate and furosemide) was superior because of the shorter time to achieve natriuresis (15 vs. 21 days) and lower incidence of side effects, chiefly hyperkalemia [30]. These discrepancies likely rely on the different patient populations enrolled. Most patients in the first study [29] had their first decompensation and mild hyperaldosteronism, and all had normal GFRs. A high rate of response to spironolactone, at even low doses, could be anticipated: 91% developed natriuresis and 72% responded to 200 mg/day. In contrast, most patients in the second study [30] had recidivant ascites and severe hyperaldosteronism. In addition, many even had a substantially reduced GFR. A low efficacy of K-canrenoate monotherapy had to be expected in such patients: 41% responded to the highest dose and 26% needed furosemide administration.

Thus, patients at the first decompensation, with preserved GFR, could be given aldosterone antagonists alone as natriuresis will likely occur at relatively low doses and side effects will be unlikely. Those with a long history of ascites, recidivant effusions and impaired GFR will likely benefit from the combined regimen, which will induce natriuresis more rapidly and reduce the risk of hyperkalemia [31].

Monitoring and Counteracting Side Effects

Up to a third of patients develop significant diuretic-induced side effects. Therefore, thorough clinical and laboratory monitoring is needed. Patients should be weighed regularly and instructed to monitor their weight at home to avoid excessive fluid loss. Should this occur, dosage of the diuretic should be reduced, starting with the loop diuretics if given. As renal impairment up to renal failure and/or dilutional hyponatremia can occur in about 20% of cases, serum electrolytes and creatinine should be assessed regularly. These complications require early recognition, and usually resolve by stopping treatment and, if needed, plasma volume expansion. Both hyper- and

Table 1. Definition and diagnostic criteria of refractory ascites

Definition		
Refractory ascites: ascites that cannot be mobilized or the early recurrence of which (i.e. after therapeutic paracentesis) cannot be satisfactorily prevented by medical therapy		
It can be divided into		
1		Diuretic-resistant ascites: ascites that cannot be mobilized or the early recurrence of which cannot be prevented because of a lack of response to dietary sodium restriction and intensive diuretic treatment
2		Diuretic-intractable ascites: ascites that cannot be mobilized or the early recurrence of which cannot be prevented because of the development of diuretic-induced complications that preclude the use of an effective diuretic dosage
Diagnostic criteria		
1		Treatment duration: patients must be on intensive diuretic therapy (spironolactone 400 mg/day and furosemide 160 mg/day) for at least 1 week and on a salt-restricted diet of <90 mmol/day or 5.2 g salt/day.
2		Lack of response: mean weight loss of <0.8 kg over 4 days and urinary sodium output less than the sodium intake
3		Early ascites recurrence: reappearance of grade 2 or 3 ascites within 4 weeks of initial mobilization
4		Diuretic-induced complications
	a	Diuretic-induced hepatic encephalopathy: development of encephalopathy in the absence of any other precipitating factor
	b	Diuretic-induced renal impairment: increase of serum creatinine by >100% to a value >2 mg/dl in patients with ascites responding to treatment
	c	Diuretic-induced hyponatremia: decrease of serum sodium by >10 mmol/l to a serum sodium of <125 mmol/l
	d	Diuretic induced hypo- or hyperkalemia: change in serum potassium to <3 mmol/l or >6 mmol/l despite appropriate measures.

Grade 1 ascites is mild ascites only detectable by ultrasound examination. Grade 2 ascites or moderate ascites is manifest by moderate symmetrical distension of the abdomen. Grade 3 ascites is large or gross ascites with marked abdominal distension.

hypokalemia can occur. Hypokalemia obviously requires supplementation, whereas hyperkalemia needs dosage reduction or temporary withdrawal of aldosterone antagonists. Cation-exchange resins should be given in severe cases to allow treatment with these drugs to be continued. Painful gynecomastia under spironolactone can benefit from the shift to K-canrenoate, if available. The pathophysiology of muscle cramps remains unsettled, but they appear to be related to hypovolemia and benefit from human albumin infusion [32]. Lastly, hepatic encephalopathy should be recognized promptly, concomitant (e.g. hyponatremia) or alternative causes excluded and specific treatment instituted; diuretic withdrawal may be required.

Recognizing Refractory Ascites

The diagnosis of refractory ascites has been defined stringently [2] and relies on the response to diuretics (table 1). Diuretic resistance, which is associated with GFR impairment up to renal failure, can be related to insufficient sodium delivery to the nephron segments where either loop diuretics or aldosterone antagonists act because of the reduced filtered load and increased proximal reabsorption (fig. 1). Diuretic intractability mainly reflects hemodynamic instability and the failure to compensate diuretic-induced hypovolemia.

Diuretics themselves, however, can induce reversible refractoriness, which should be recognized as it implies a different prognosis and treatment. Diuretic-induced renal failure and/or hyponatremia due to excessive diuresis can be reverted by diuretic withdrawal and plasma volume expansion, while the adjustment of diuretic therapy can resolve apparent refractoriness due to monotherapy with loop diuretics or low-dose aldosterone antagonists in patients with severe hyperaldosteronism, or monotherapy with aldosterone antagonists in patients with impaired GFR. Reversible refractoriness to diuretics can also be induced by excessive dietary sodium intake or non-steroidal anti-inflammatory drugs. These conditions should be identified as they can easily be resolved.

Key Messages

- Renal retention of sodium in cirrhosis occurs both at the proximal convoluted tubule and the aldosterone-sensitive collecting duct. Aldosterone antagonists represent the first-choice treatment, and loop diuretics are also needed when proximal reabsorption is substantial.
- The effect of aldosterone antagonists has a latency of at least 48 h and their dose should be proportional to actual hyperaldosteronism. Painful gynecomastia and hyperkalemia are the most important side effects.
- Loop diuretics are very potent and fast-acting, so that their side effects (renal impairment, hyponatremia, and hypochloremic alkalosis) are favored by the hemodynamic background of cirrhosis. They can also precipitate hepatic encephalopathy.
- The negative fluid balance induced by diuretic treatment should not be greater than 700 ml/day. This limit can be exceeded in the presence of edema.
- Sequential treatment should be preferred in patients with ascites of recent onset and well-preserved GFR. Combined treatment seems to be more beneficial to patients with long-standing ascites and impaired GFR.
- Refractory ascites needs to be carefully diagnosed. Mechanisms leading to transient refractoriness, including inappropriate diuretic treatment, should be identified and corrected.

References

1 Bernardi M, Trevisani F, Gasbarrini A, Gasbarrini G: Hepatorenal disorders: the role of renin-angiotensin-aldosterone system. Semin Liver Dis 1994;14:23–34.

2 Moore KP, Wong F, Gines P, Bernardi M, Ochs A, Salerno F, Angeli P, Porayko M, Moreau R, Garcia-Tsao G, Jimenez W, Planas R, Arroyo V: The management of ascites in cirrhosis: report on the consensus conference of the International Ascites Club. Hepatology 2003;38:258–266.

3 Schrier RW, Arroyo V, Bernardi M, Epstein M, Henriksen JH, Rodés J: Peripheral arterial vasodilation hypothesis: a proposal for the initiation of renal sodium and water retention in cirrhosis. Hepatology 1988;8:1151–1158.

4 Bernardi M, Laffi G, Salvagnini M, Azzena G, Bonato S, Marra F, Trevisani F, Gasbarrini G, Naccarato R, Gentilini P: Efficacy and safety of the stepped care medical treatment of ascites in liver cirrhosis: a randomized controlled clinical trial comparing two diets with different sodium content. Liver 1993;13:156–162.

5 Agarwal MK, Mirshahi M: General overview of mineralocorticoid hormone action. Pharmacol Ther 1999;84:273–326.

6 Karim A: Spironolactone metabolism in man revisited; in Brunner HR (ed): Contemporary Trends in Diuretic Therapy. Amsterdam, Excerpta Medica, 1986, pp 22–37.

7 Bernardi M, Servadei D, Trevisani F, Rusticali AG, Gasbarrini G: Importance of plasma aldosterone concentration on the natriuretic effect of spironolactone in patients with liver cirrhosis and ascites. Digestion 1985;31:189–193.

8 Sungaila I, Bartle WR, Walker SE, DeAngelis C, Uetrecht J, Pappas C, Vidins E: Spironolactone pharmacokinetics and pharmacodynamics in patients with cirrhotic ascites. Gastroenterology 1992;102:1680–1685.

9 Parthasarathy HK, MacDonald TM: Mineralocorticoid receptor antagonists. Curr Hypertens Rep 2007;9:45–52.

10 McManus F, McInnes GT, Connell JM: Drug insight: eplerenone, a mineralocorticoid-receptor antagonist. Nat Clin Pract Endocrinol Metab 2008;4:44–52.

11 Andriulli A, Arrigoni A, Gindro T, Karbowiak I, Buzzetti G, Armanini D: Canrenone and androgen receptor-active materials in plasma of cirrhotic patients during long-term K-canrenoate or spironolactone therapy. Digestion 1989;44:155–162.

12 Mimidis K, Papadopoulos V, Kartalis G: Eplerenone relieves spironolactone-induced painful gynaecomastia in patients with decompensated hepatitis B-related cirrhosis. Scand J Gastroenterol 2007;42:1516–1517.

13 Gabow PA, Moore S, Schrier RW: Spironolactone-induced hyperchloremic acidosis in cirrhosis. Ann Intern Med 1979;90:338–340.

14 Runyon BA, AASLD Practice Guidelines Committee: Management of adult patients with ascites due to cirrhosis: an update. Hepatology 2009;49:2087–2107.

15 EASL Clinical Practice Guidelines on the management of ascites, spontaneous bacterial peritonitis, and hepatorenal syndrome in cirrhosis. J Hepatol 2010;53:397–417.

16 Angeli P, Dalla Pria, M, De Bei E, Albino G, Caregaro L, Merkel C, Ceolotto G, Gatta A: Randomized clinical study of the efficacy of amiloride and potassium canrenoate in nonazotemic cirrhotic patients with ascites. Hepatology 1994;19:71–79.

17 Suki WN, Stinebaugh BJ, Frommer JP, Eknoyan G: Physiology of diuretic action; in Seldin DW, Giebish G (eds): The Kidney Physiology and Pathophysiology. New York, Raven Press, 1985, pp 2127–2162.

18 Planas R, Arroyo V, Rimola A, Pérez-Ayuso RM, Rodés J: Acetylsalicylic acid suppresses the renal hemodynamic effect and reduces the diuretic action of furosemide in cirrhosis with ascites. Gastroenterology 1983;84:247–252.

19 Pinzani M, Daskalopoulos G, Laffi G, Gentilini P, Zipser RD: Altered furosemide pharmacokinetics in chronic alcoholic liver disease with ascites contributes to diuretic resistance. Gastroenterology 1987;92:294–298.

20 Sawhney VK, Gregory PB, Swezey SE, Blaschke TF: Furosemide disposition in cirrhotic patients. Gastroenterology 1981;81:1012–1016.

21 Ryan J, Sudhir K, Jennings G, Esler M, Dudley F: Impaired reactivity of the peripheral vasculature to pressor agents in alcoholic cirrhosis. Gastroenterology 1993;105:1167–1172.

22 Córdoba J, Mínguez B: Hepatic encephalopathy. Semin Liver Dis 2008;28:70–80.

23 Gerbes AL, Bertheau-Reith U, Falkner C, Jüngst D, Paumgartner G: Advantages of the new loop diuretic torasemide over furosemide in patients with cirrhosis and ascites: a randomized, double blind cross-over trial. J Hepatol 1993;17:353–358.

24 Thomson MR, Nappi JM, Dunn SP, Hollis IB, Rodgers JE, Van Bakel AB: Continuous versus intermittent infusion of furosemide in acute decompensated heart failure. J Cardiac Fail 2010;16:188–193.

25 Shear LS, Ching S, Gabuzda GJ: Compartmentalization of ascites and edema in patients with cirrhosis. N Engl J Med 1970;282:1391–1395.

26 Pérez-Ayuso RM, Arroyo V, Planas R, Gaya J, Bory F, Rimola A, Rivera F, Rodés J: Randomized comparative study of efficacy of furosemide versus spironolactone in patients with liver cirrhosis and ascites. Gastroenterology 1983;84:961–968.

27 Runyon BA: Care of patients with ascites. N Engl J Med 1994;30:337–342.

28 Fogel MR, Sawhney VK, Neal EA, Miller RG, Knauer CM, Gregory PB: Diuresis in the ascitic patient: a randomized controlled trial of three regimens. J Clin Gastroenterol 1981;3(suppl 1):73–80.

29 Santos J, Planas R, Pardo A, Durández R, Cabré E, Morillas RM, Granada ML, Jiménez JA, Quintero E, Gassull MA: Spironolactone alone or in combination with furosemide in the treatment of moderate ascites in nonazotemic cirrhosis: a randomized comparative study of efficacy and safety. J Hepatol 2003;39:187–192.

30 Angeli P, Fasolato S, Mazza E, Okolicsanyi L, Maresio G, Velo E, Galioto A, Salinas F, D'Aquino M, Sticca A, Gatta A: Combined versus sequential diuretic treatment of ascites in non-azotaemic patients with cirrhosis: results of an open randomised clinical trial. Gut 2010;59:98–104.

31 Bernardi M: Optimum use of diuretics in managing ascites in patients with cirrhosis. Gut 2010;59:10–11.

32 Angeli P, Albino G, Carraro P, Dalla Pria M, Merkel C, Caregaro L, De Bei E, Bortoluzzi A, Plebani M, Gatta A: Cirrhosis and muscle cramps: evidence of a causal relationship. Hepatology 1996;23:264–273.

Prof. Mauro Bernardi
Semeiotica Medica, Policlinico S. Orsola-Malpighi
Via Albertoni, 15
IT–40138 Bologna (Italy)
Tel. + 39 051 391 549, Fax +39 051 636 2930, E-Mail mauro.bernardi@unibo.it

Gerbes AL (ed): Ascites, Hyponatremia and Hepatorenal Syndrome: Progress in Treatment.
Front Gastrointest Res. Basel, Karger, 2011, vol 28, pp 23–31

Paracentesis

Arun J. Sanyal[a] · Jasmohan S. Bajaj[a,b] · Jawaid Shaw[c]

[a]Division of Gastroenterology, Hepatology and Nutrition, Department of Internal Medicine, Virginia Commonwealth University Medical Center, [b]Division of Gastroenterology, and [c]Department of Internal Medicine, Hunter Holmes VA Medical Center, Richmond, Va., USA

Abstract

Ascites is one of the most prevalent complications of cirrhosis. Ascites can hamper the patients' quality of life as well as predispose them to develop spontaneous bacterial peritonitis. Paracentesis is often used for diagnostic as well as therapeutic purposes in the management of cirrhotics with ascites. It is often performed as an outpatient procedure with or without the aid of ultrasound marking and the preferred site is the left lower quadrant. Diagnostic paracentesis is needed to ascertain the etiology of ascites as well as to exclude spontaneous bacterial peritonitis. Therapeutic paracentesis, total or large volume, is employed to relieve patient discomfort in cases refractory or resistant to diuretics. While coagulopathy is common in cirrhosis, it is not a contraindication to paracentesis, unless there is evidence of hyperfibrinolysis. Post-paracentesis circulatory dysfunction can occur in 20% of patients after therapeutic paracentesis and should be prevented by using albumin infusion during the procedure. Paracentesis, both diagnostic and therapeutic, is an essential and safe procedure for the management of end-stage liver disease and cirrhosis.

Chronic liver disease in the United States is mainly caused by hepatitis C and alcohol. Cirrhosis which represents the end stage of any chronic liver disease (CLD) is the twelfth leading cause of death in the US [1]. Ascites is not only the most common complication of decompensated liver disease but also the most common cause of hospital admissions [2]. Further on, development of ascites in a cirrhotic patient confers poor prognosis with around 44% dying within 5 years [3]. Appropriate management of ascites thus forms the cornerstone in the overall care of a cirrhotic patient.

Nomenclature Used in Assessment of Ascites

The International Ascites Club has broadly divided ascites into uncomplicated and refractory ascites. The former has been graded according to severity from mild to severe as 1, 2 and 3. The latter group has been subdivided into diuretic-resistant and

Table 1. Classification of ascites according to severity and response to diuretics

Uncomplicated ascites	Refractory ascites	
No infection		
No hepatorenal syndrome	diuretic-resistant	diuretic-intractable
Grade 1 (mild)		
Ascites diagnosed on USG only		
Grade 2 (moderate) Clinically appreciated with moderate distention	ascites unresponsive to low sodium diet and maximal diuretic dose	the effective diuretic dosage cannot be used due to side effects
Grade 3 (large)		
Clinically marked or tense distention		

diuretic-intractable category according to response to diuretic treatment (table 1) [4, 5].

Confirmation and Ascitic Fluid Analysis

For confirmation of ascites, abdominal paracentesis followed by relevant analysis of fluid to figure out the etiology and complications is considered a safe as well as informative procedure [5]. Paracentesis is a vital skill for the internists, especially those taking care of patients with liver diseases.

Indications of Abdominal Paracentesis

Indications can be broadly divided into diagnostic when a limited amount of ascitic fluid is used to aid in diagnosis versus therapeutic aimed at relieving pressure symptoms in a patient with tense ascites (table 2).

Contraindications

Other than frank evidence of fibrinolysis or disseminated intravascular coagulation there are no absolute contraindications to abdominal paracentesis [6]. Though there are certain special situations like pregnancy, in patients with massive organomegaly or bowel obstruction use of USG may reduce the risk of injury to the patient during the procedure. To minimize the complications, use commonsense precautions like catheterization of distended urinary bladder, nasogastric decompression in case of

Table 2. Indication for paracentesis in a patient with ascites

Diagnostic	Therapeutic
With new onset ascites to detect etiology	To relieve respiratory distress/abdominal pain in tense ascites
With pre-existing ascites when SBP is suspected clinically or on laboratory parameters	Serial large-volume paracentesis in refractory cases
Hospitalized patients with ascites	Prior to TIPS and USG for better procedural success and visualization
	To prevent impending rupture of umbilical hernia

bowel obstruction, avoiding sites such as areas of infection, abdominal wall hematomas, surgical scars, visibly engorged vessels and the anatomic location of the inferior epigastric arteries for paracentesis [7].

Paracentesis Techniques

Various hospitals use different pre-packaged kits for paracentesis. The operator should be familiar with the type of kit being used in his hospital. Nevertheless, the principles of abdominal paracentesis remain the same regardless of the kit being used. After discussing the procedure with the patient, written consent should be obtained. The patient should be placed in a comfortable position which is usually supine.

In the past, the infraumblical midline site 2 cm below the umbilicus was used – a preferred site in the belief that this region had no blood vessels [5]. This approach has been abandoned now as one laparoscopic study found that in patients with portal hypertension there are collaterals in the midline which can rupture during paracentesis [8]. Amongst the lateral approach, either right or left lower quadrant (2–4 cm medial and cephalad to the anterior superior iliac spine), the left lower quadrant is the preferred position. This is because a study using USG found that the abdominal wall in the left lower quadrant is significantly thinner with a larger pool of ascitic fluid in this location as compared to the midline infraumblical location [9]. As the prevalence of obesity rises, this becomes particularly relevant. There is also a minor risk of perforating a dilated cecum (especially if the patient is on lactulose) if the right lower quadrant is used [6].

Paracentesis should be performed using standard sterile precautions. The entry site and the deeper tissues in the anticipated tract of the needle along with the pain-sensitive parietal peritoneum should be numbed with a local anesthetic (5–10 ml of 1 or 2% lidocaine). A small puncture with either a scalpel or a large-bore needle (gauge 18) is made at the entry site to facilitate entry of the paracentesis needle [7].

Usually, various needle sizes are chosen depending upon whether the patient is thin or obese (1.5–3.5 inch, 22-gauge needle). Many experts prefer to use steel needles as compared to plastic-sheathed cannulas because of problems in draining the fluid due to kinking and obstruction of flow after the cannula is removed [10]. One of the most common complications of paracentesis is the leakage of fluid from the puncture site described as 5% in one study [11]. To prevent this special needle insertion, special techniques (namely angular insertion and Z-tract technique) are employed [12]. In the former, 45° angulation of the needle is used all along its tract from the epidermis into the peritoneal cavity while in the latter the skin is pulled 2 cm downwards before insertion of the needle and is then let go only after ascitic fluid is seen to be flowing. With these techniques, the needle tract gets sealed as the skin resumes its normal shape. The key to a successful outcome is to advance the needle in slow increments (approximately 5 mm) with the dominant hand while using the other hand to guide the needle path and intermittently aspirating on the needle. When the ascitic fluid is seen, the advancement of the needle should be stopped and the catheter guided over the needle while the needle is withdrawn. Further on, depending on the indication of paracentesis (if for diagnostics around 30–60 ml fluid is withdrawn using a syringe and if the intent is therapeutic), attaching vaccumized containers via high pressure connection tubing is performed. A sterile dressing is placed over the paracentesis site as the procedure is completed.

Large-Volume Paracentesis

Approximately 10% of patients with cirrhosis develop ascites refractory to medical treatment alone [13] and hence need serial therapeutic paracentesis. In large-volume paracentesis (LVP) more than 5 liters of ascitic fluid is drained. Other indications for LVP may include tense ascites, respiratory distress, and impending rupture of the umbilical hernia prior to adequate USG examination of liver and transjugular intrahepatic portosystemic shunt (TIPS) placement [14].

The role of plasma expanders in LVP has been dealt with in another chapter of this book. It is sufficient to mention here that if albumin is the plasma expander being infused, using 6–8 g/l is appropriate if greater than 5 liters of ascitic fluid is removed [3]. This is useful since in about 20% of patients LVP gets complicated by postparacentesis circulatory dysfunction (PPCD) [14]. As opposed to LVP, in total volume paracentesis (TVP) all the ascitic fluid is drained and this can be performed safely when albumin has been used [14]. Both LVP and TVP are associated with immediate symptomatic relief but this is short lived as there is recurrence of ascites. Hence, repeated procedures are involved without a significant increase in survival [15].

Transjugular intrahepatic portosystemic shunt (TIPS) is yet another modality of treatment available for the treatment of refractory ascites. TIPS is a side-to-side portocaval shunt aimed at correcting the portal hypertension [16]. It is hence effective in not only controlling ascites but also in preventing its re-accumulation. In a recently published meta-analysis of 4 large-scale published trails comparing the effect of TIPS versus LVP in cirrhotics with refractory ascites, it was concluded that TIPS was significantly better than LVP in transplant-free survival but encephalopathy occurred more in the former group as compared to the latter [17]. TIPS improved the quality of life in all patients apart from those who developed encephalopathy. Of the above trials, The North American Study of Treatment of Refractory Ascites (NASTRA) had the largest number of patients in each group and this trial clearly demonstrated that, similar to LVP, TIPS did not improve patients' survival [18]. The authors concluded that TIPS should be considered as a second-line therapy or a bridge to liver transplantation (LT). Referral to a LT center should be hastened in these patients as LT is considered to be the only treatment which improves the morbidity and mortality in these patients.

Ascitic Fluid Analysis

If clinically uncomplicated ascites is suspected, the baseline laboratory parameters to be ordered include: total cell count with differentials, albumin, total protein concentration, and calculation of serum-ascites albumin gradient (SAAG), which is calculated by subtracting the ascitic fluid albumin level from concurrently tested serum albumin level. The clinical utility of SAAG is that it can predict that ascites is due to portal hypertension with 97% accuracy if the value of SAAG is equal to or greater than 1.1 g/dl [19].

Appropriate specimen tubes (EDTA-treated tube for cell counts and differentials and a plain tube for albumin) for collection of aspirated fluid should be used for prompt delivery to the laboratory. In those patients who get serial LVP in an outpatient setting, ordering total and differential cell counts is sufficient if they appear to be clinically stable [6].

A genuine concern in the evaluation of a patient with ascites is to determine whether the fluid is infected either spontaneously or secondarily. A polymorphonuclear cell (PMN) count of ≥250 cells/mm^3 along with a positive fluid culture without an obvious intra-abdominal source points towards spontaneous bacterial peritonitis (SBP) [20]. SBP, unlike secondary bacterial peritonitis, is usually a mono-microbial infection, therefore >1 organism on culture should raise the suspicion of secondary peritonitis. Further tests to help differentiate between SBP and secondary peritonitis include lactate dehydrogenase, glucose and total proteins [21]. Gram stain of ascitic fluid has a low yield (7–10%) in early SBP but it may be helpful in secondary bacterial peritonitis. The causes of hemorrhagic ascites (due to ascitic red blood cells >50,000/

mm^3) include traumatic tap, cirrhosis (2%), malignancy, peritoneal carcinomatosis and congestive heart failure [22]. Appropriate correction to PMN cell counts should be applied in this scenario.

Specific tests should be ordered in response to a particular clinical scenario like ordering ascitic fluid triglyceride level if chylous ascites is drained, carcinoembroyonic antigen or alkaline phosphatase level if gut perforation is suspected, checking ascitic fluid amylase if pancreatic etiology is suspected, and tubercular cultures if tubercular peritonitis is suspected. Ascitic fluid cytology is an expensive test and should only be ordered if peritoneal carcinomatosis is a diagnostic consideration.

Coagulopathy in Liver Disease

In patients with liver disease, the hemostatic balance is maintained by multiple and often opposing variables which are in a dynamic state [23]. There is a delicate balance between the pro-thrombotic and anti-thrombotic forces which sometimes gets further challenged by additional factors like infections, thrombocytopenia and severity of underlying liver disease. While bacterial infections in cirrhotic patients have been shown to predispose to bleeding (due to heparin-like effect) nonalcoholic fatty liver disease and the metabolic syndrome is associated with a prothrombotic state [24]. From a simplistic view, this state can be likened to a 'see-saw' with the net clinical status of the patient being determined by which forces dominate. To further complicate this picture, the global tests of coagulation prothrombin time and international normalized ratio (PT-INR) do not reflect the changes in the anticoagulants and, hence, may not accurately predict bleeding risks [25]. There is no data-supported evidence to use coagulation parameters to assess bleeding risk in a patient with liver disease undergoing potentially hemorrhagic procedure like liver biopsy or paracentesis. Hence, no cut-off values for PT exist beyond which paracentesis should be avoided [5].

Patients with hyperfibrinolysis clinically present with mucocutaneous bleeding or hematoma formation which is diagnosed using euglobin clot lysis time (ELT) <120 min [26]. Some experts recommend using EACA in patients with hyperfibrinolysis after documenting the same using ELT and performing paracentesis only after ELT improves [6].

In a prospective study (163 patients and 410 paracentesis) conducted in an emergency room setting under ultrasound guidance, the pre-procedure INR for PT was more than 1.5 in 142 paracentesis with platelet count <50,000 cells/mm^3. A minor complication rate of only 0.5% was reported. They concluded that bleeding complications are uncommon and mild even if they occur and that routine correction and checking of elevated INR or platelets is not desired [27].

Till the time that better tests for measuring coagulopathy in liver disease become available, it is advisable to use clinical judgment not only to assess risk of bleeding in an individual but also as a guide to using agents such as platelets, blood factors and or antifibrinolytics.

Complications

The fear about serious complications of abdominal paracentesis including death stems from the older literature when trocars were used. Currently, paracentesis is considered a safe procedure [6]. The complications of diagnostic paracentesis may be divided into bleeding complications, perforation of intra-abdominal organs, introduction of local or peritoneal infection and post-paracentesis persistent leakage of ascitic fluid. The bleeding complications present themselves either as abdominal wall hematoma, hemorrhage into the peritoneal cavity or bleeding related to direct puncture of the inferior epigastric artery.

In a large retrospective study (4,729 procedures), 9 patients (0.19%) were identified to have developed severe hemorrhage: all of these patients were in hospital and had significantly impaired renal function [28]. The mortality following bleeding complications in 0.02% of all paracentesis occurred in those patients who were hospitalized with severe thrombocytopenia and/or elevated INR. A prospective study (628 patients/1100 LVP) carried out in an outpatient setting reported no major complications: the preprocedure platelet counts ranged from 19,000 to 341,000 cells/mm^3 and INRs for PT ranged from 0.9 to 8.7. They also reported a very low incidence of persistent leakage from the paracentesis site (0.36%) which responded to local measures [29]. Another retrospective study did not find any increased bleeding in patients who had PT/PTT even up to twice the normal or platelet count of 50,000–99,000 cells/mm^3. The overall transfusion-requiring events were very low at 0.2%, which led the authors to conclude that prophylactic treatment with blood products is not necessary [30]. A more recent prospective study (171 patients/515 paracentesis) observed complications in 10.5% which were mostly minor (8.9%). Local bleeding was observed in 2.3% of the cases and overflow of ascitic fluid from the puncture site in 5% of the cases. The major complications accounting for 1.6% included 2 patients with major hematoma, 3 cases with intraperitoneal bleeding and 3 cases with infectious complications. Technical problems were observed in 5.6% of the cases which included repeating the puncture due to flow interruption, repositioning of the catheter, and no ascites at the first attempt. Major complications were significantly associated with therapeutic procedures. In this study, a plastic sheath was used which could have accounted for the increased rate of complications [11].

Iatrogenic infection of the ascitic fluid is a concern. An earlier prospective study [5] did not report this complication while a more recent study observed infectious complications in 0.6% of the patients [11].

On review of the literature there seems to be no convincing evidence about coagulopathy or thrombocytopenia precluding abdominal paracentesis, either diagnostic or therapeutic, and if hemorrhagic complications occur at all they are minor and easily controlled. Major hemorrhagic complications occur mainly in severely sick patients with comorbid illnesses like renal failure. It seems that LVP as compared to diagnostic paracentesis does not seem to be have increased complication rates [5].

In about 20% of the patients, LVP gets complicated by postparacentesis circulatory dysfunction which is a complication unique to LVP [7]. This is characterized pathophysiologically as worsening of vasodilatation manifesting as hypotension, hyponatremia and increased catecholamine and renin levels. This state peaks at around 24–48 h and can lead to renal failure and even death [14].

Key Messages

- Abdominal paracentesis for acquisition of ascitic fluid for diagnostic or therapeutic considerations is a quick, common and safe procedure.
- There are no absolute contraindications for paracentesis except hyperfibrinolysis.
- Using sterile precautions, proper tools and techniques along with the safest site, i.e. left lower abdominal quadrant, for paracentesis will help minimize the complications.
- The bleeding complications even in patients with deranged currently used parameters for coagulopathy in liver diseases and low platelet counts are rarely seen.
- Large-volume paracentesis effectively relieves pressure symptoms in patients with tense refractory ascites but can get complicated by postparacentesis circulatory dysfunction.

References

1 Minino AM, Heron MP, Smith BL: Deaths: preliminary data for 2004. Natl Vital Stat Rep 2006;54:1–49.

2 Lucena MI, Andrade RJ, Tognoni G, Hidalgo R, De La Cuesta FS: Multicenter hospital study on prescribing patterns for prophylaxis and treatment of complications of cirrhosis. Eur J Clin Pharmacol 2002;58:435–440.

3 Planas R, Montoliu S, Balleste B, et al: Natural history of patients hospitalized for management of cirrhotic ascites. Clin Gastroenterol Hepatol 2006;4:1385–1394.

4 Arroyo V, Gines P, Gerbes AL, et al: Definition and diagnostic criteria of refractory ascites and hepatorenal syndrome in cirrhosis. International Ascites Club. Hepatology 1996;23:164–176.

5 Runyon BA: Paracentesis of ascitic fluid: a safe procedure. Arch Intern Med 1986;146:2259–2261.

6 Runyon BA: Management of adult patients with ascites due to cirrhosis: an update. Hepatology 2009;49:2087–2107.

7 Thomsen TW, Shaffer, Robert W, White B, Setnik GS: Paracentesis. NEJM 2006:19.

8 Oelsner DH, Caldwell SH, Coles M, Driscoll CJ: Subumbilical midline vascularity of the abdominal wall in portal hypertension observed at laparoscopy. Gastrointest Endosc 1998;47:388–390.

9 Sakai H, Sheer TA, Mendler MH, Runyon BA: Choosing the location for non-image guided abdominal paracentesis. Liver Int 2005;25:984–986.

10 Runyon BA: Ascites and spontaneous bacterial peritonitis; in Feldman M (ed): Sleissenger and Fordtran's Gastrointestinal and Liver Disease. Philadelphia, Saunders, 2006.

11 De Gottardi A, Thevenot T, Spahr L, et al: Risk of complications after abdominal paracentesis in cirrhotic patients: a prospective study. Clin Gastroenterol Hepatol 2009;7:906–909.

12 Promes SB: Paracentesis; in: Reichman EF, Simon RR: Emergency medicine procedures. New York, McGraw-Hill, 2004, pp 467–477.

13 Perez-Ayuso RM, Arroyo V, Planas R, et al: Randomized comparative study of efficacy of furosemide versus spironolactone in nonazotemic cirrhosis with ascites: relationship between the diuretic response and the activity of the renin-aldosterone system. Gastroenterology 1983;84:961–968.

14 Sandhu BS, Sanyal AJ: Management of ascites in cirrhosis. Clin Liver Dis 2005;9:715–732, viii.
15 Hou W, Sanyal AJ: Ascites: diagnosis and management. Med Clin North Am 2009;93:801–817, vii.
16 Ochs A, Rossle M, Haag K, et al: The transjugular intrahepatic portosystemic stent-shunt procedure for refractory ascites. N Engl J Med 1995;332:1192–1197.
17 Salerno F, Camma C, Enea M, Rossle M, Wong F: Transjugular intrahepatic portosystemic shunt for refractory ascites: a meta-analysis of individual patient data. Gastroenterology 2007;133:825–834.
18 Sanyal AJ, Genning C, Reddy KR, et al: The North American Study for the Treatment of Refractory Ascites. Gastroenterology 2003;124:634–641.
19 Runyon BA, Montano AA, Akriviadis EA, Antillon MR, Irving MA, McHutchison JG: The serum-ascites albumin gradient is superior to the exudate-transudate concept in the differential diagnosis of ascites. Ann Intern Med 1992;117:215–220.
20 Hoefs JC, Canawati HN, Sapico FL, Hopkins RR, Weiner J, Montgomerie JZ: Spontaneous bacterial peritonitis. Hepatology 1982;2:399–407.
21 Akriviadis EA, Runyon BA: Utility of an algorithm in differentiating spontaneous from secondary bacterial peritonitis. Gastroenterology 1990;98:127–133.
22 DeSitter L, Rector WG Jr: The significance of bloody ascites in patients with cirrhosis. Am J Gastroenterol 1984;79:136–138.
23 Caldwell SH, Hoffman M, Lisman T, et al: Coagulation disorders and hemostasis in liver disease: pathophysiology and critical assessment of current management. Hepatology 2006;44:1039–1046.
24 Montalto P, Vlachogiannakos J, Cox DJ, Pastacaldi S, Patch D, Burroughs AK: Bacterial infection in cirrhosis impairs coagulation by a heparin effect: a prospective study. J Hepatol 2002;37:463–470.
25 Tripodi A, Caldwell SH, Hoffman M, Trotter JF, Sanyal AJ: Review article: the prothrombin time test as a measure of bleeding risk and prognosis in liver disease. Aliment Pharmacol Ther 2007;26:141–148.
26 Gunawan B, Runyon B: The efficacy and safety of epsilon-aminocaproic acid treatment in patients with cirrhosis and hyperfibrinolysis. Aliment Pharmacol Ther 2006;23:115–120.
27 Lin CH, Shih FY, Ma MH, Chiang WC, Yang CW, Ko PC: Should bleeding tendency deter abdominal paracentesis? Dig Liver Dis 2005;37:946–951.
28 Pache I, Bilodeau M: Severe haemorrhage following abdominal paracentesis for ascites in patients with liver disease. Aliment Pharmacol Ther 2005;21:525–529.
29 Grabau CM, Crago SF, Hoff LK, et al: Performance standards for therapeutic abdominal paracentesis. Hepatology 2004;40:484–488.
30 McVay PA, Toy PT: Lack of increased bleeding after paracentesis and thoracentesis in patients with mild coagulation abnormalities. Transfusion 1991;31:164–171.

Arun J. Sanyal, MBBS, MD
Pharmacology and Pathology
MCV Box 980341
Richmond, VA 23298 (USA)
Tel. +1 804 828 6314, Fax +1 804 828 4945, E-Mail ajsanyal@vcu.edu

Gerbes AL (ed): Ascites, Hyponatremia and Hepatorenal Syndrome: Progress in Treatment.
Front Gastrointest Res. Basel, Karger, 2011, vol 28, pp 32–39

Large-Volume Paracentesis: Which Plasma Expander?

Ruben Alberto Terg

Hospital de Gastroenterología Bonorino Udaondo, Buenos Aires, Argentina

Abstract

Large-volume paracentesis without plasma volume expansion is associated with a significant increase in plasma renin activity in 70% of the cases, and is known as paracentesis-induced circulatory dysfunction (PICD). Patients with this complication are more likely to be hospitalized, need diuretics, and have a shorter survival time. In contrast, albumin administration at doses of 6–8 g/l of ascites removed can prevent the occurrence of this circulatory dysfunction. The efficacy of other plasma expanders, less expensive than albumin, in the prevention of this complication has been studied in several randomized controlled trials. In several small studies, dextran 70 and polygeline have been shown to be as safe as albumin. A large randomized, controlled trial, however, demonstrated that albumin infusion is more effective than dextran or polygeline. The incidence of PICD in patients treated with albumin was 18%, compared with 35 and 40% in patients receiving either dextran 70 or polygeline, respectively. Only when the volume of removed ascites is lower than 5 liters was dextran 70 or polygeline shown to have a similar effect as albumin. Albumin's longer half-life may account for its superior effect, but recent data suggest a direct endothelial mechanism for the efficacy. Further, the cost-benefit of replacing albumin volume expansion with vasoconstrictors in patients with large-volume paracentesis has not been proven. **Conclusion:** Albumin is the safest plasma expander in cirrhotic patients treated with paracentesis >5 liters.

Large-Volume Paracentesis in Clinical Practice

Since the reintroduction of therapeutic paracentesis accompanied with intravenous albumin infusion in 1985, several studies have demonstrated that this procedure should be considered as the treatment of choice for cirrhotic patients with tense ascites and potentially in the management of cirrhotic patients with refractory ascites. These studies showed that the risks of complications such as renal impairment, hyponatremia, and hepatic encephalopathy were lower in cirrhotic patients with tense ascites treated with large-volume paracentesis than in patients treated with diuretics [1–4].

In patients with refractory ascites, 5 randomized controlled clinical trials compared large-volume paracentesis with transjugular intrahepatic portosystemic stents-shunts (TIPS) [5–9] and showed TIPS to be much more effective than paracentesis to control ascites, but at the expense of more frequent episodes of encephalopathy. Moreover, a recent meta-analysis showed that TIPS does not improve survival compared with repeated large-volume paracentesis [10].

Rationale for Using Plasma Volume Expansion

Without plasma volume expansion, hemodynamic and hormonal changes after large-volume paracentesis have been extensively reported in previous studies [11–14]. Immediately after the mobilization of a large amount of ascites, a significant reduction in intra-abdominal pressure occurs, leading to decreased intrathoracic pressure and increased transmural pressure, venous return, heart volume, and cardiac performance. As a consequence of the increased cardiac output, systemic vascular resistance is reduced to accommodate the higher blood volume in systemic circulation. Endothelial vasodilators such as nitric oxide, sensitive to shear stress, vasodilator peptides and carbon monoxide are all probable mediators in the pathogenesis of the drop in systemic vascular resistance.

However, these beneficial effects, secondary to improved effective blood volume, are rapidly reversed if the large-volume paracentesis is not accompanied by plasma volume expansion. After 12 h of paracentesis, cardiac output and systemic vascular resistance fall below baseline, and renin, aldosterone and norepinephrine increase progressively to compensate the aggravation of arteriolar vasodilation. Finally, the persistence and magnitude of vasoconstriction system activation may lead to renal impairment due to significantly decreased renal perfusion and glomerular filtration rate.

Unchanged plasma volume following large-volume paracentesis [15, 16] can lead to paracentesis-induced circulatory dysfunction (PICD), defined as an increase in plasma renin activity by more than 50% from the pretreatment level to a level greater than 4 ng/ml/h on the sixth day after paracentesis. It is predominantly associated with aggravated arteriolar vasodilation already present in untreated cirrhotic patients with ascites. The mechanism of PICD is not yet completely understood, but available evidence suggests that the acute reduction of a high intra-abdominal pressure after paracentesis promotes the accentuation of arteriolar vasodilation and results in PICD. Patients with a severe decrease in intra-abdominal pressure, which can be measured by abdominal inferior vena cava catheterization, have a greater reduction in systemic vascular resistance [17].

The only large, randomized, controlled trial comparing therapeutic paracentesis with or without intravenous albumin administration showed that paracentesis plus albumin did not induce significant changes in plasma renin activity, plasma aldosterone concentration, and renal function test [11]. In comparison, therapeutic paracentesis without albumin was followed by a significant increase in blood urea nitrogen, marked elevations in plasma renin activity and aldosterone concentration, and a significant reduction in serum sodium concentration.

Evidence Supporting the Use of Albumin for Plasma Expansion

Since albumin is derived from human plasma and the cost is relatively high, its availability in many countries is limited. A number of randomized clinical trials have investigated whether albumin can be substituted by less-expensive plasma expanders in therapeutic paracentesis.

Dextran 70 was evaluated in at least two randomized studies. In the first study by Planas et al. [18], 88 patients with tense ascites and treated with total paracentesis were randomized to receive either intravenous albumin or dextran 70 at a dose of 8 g/l ascitic fluid removed. Neither treatment group showed significant changes in renal and serum electrolytes. The rate of survival and causes of death were similar between the two groups of patients. However, a significant increase in plasma renin activity and aldosterone concentration was observed in 51% of patients treated with dextran 70, compared with only 15% of those treated with albumin. The author concluded that although dextran 70 is less efficacious than albumin to prevent effective hypovolemia, it appears to prevent renal and electrolyte complications induced by paracentesis.

A second study by Fassio et al. [19] compared dextran 70 with albumin in 41 patients who were treated with 5-liter paracentesis daily until the resolution of ascites. Patients were given dextran 70 or albumin at a dose of 6 g/l of ascites evacuated. The results showed no significant changes in renal function, serum electrolytes, and plasma renin activity at 1 and 4 days after the final paracentesis. The probability of survival was similar in both groups during follow-up. The authors suggested that paracentesis with dextran 70 may be considered the treatment of choice in cirrhotic patients with tense ascites because of its lower cost.

Hemaccel was studied in a randomized, controlled trial conducted by Salerno et al. [20] in patients with refractory ascites. Twenty-seven patients received 6 g of intravenous albumin and 27 patients received an intravenous infusion of 150 ml of hemaccel per liter of ascites removed with total paracentesis. No significant changes in renal function, serum electrolytes, and plasma renin activity and aldosterone concentration were observed at 1, 3 and 6 days after the paracentesis. In addition, the rate of survival during follow-up was similar in the two groups.

Finally, dextran 40 and intravenous saline infusion were evaluated noncomparatively with albumin in patients treated with total paracentesis.

Solá et al. [21] gave 49 patients with tense ascites total paracentesis plus intravenous dextran 40 or diuretic treatment. Plasma renin activity and plasma aldosterone concentration increased significantly in 70% of the cases. Cabrera et al. [22] performed a pilot study of 14 patients with tense ascites treated with paracentesis and intravenous saline infusion.

The results of the above-described studies with dextran 70 or hemaccel are insufficient to conclude that the less-expensive plasma expanders can replace albumin in patients treated with large-volume paracentesis. For dextran 70 use [18], plasma renin activity had increased significantly in one but not in the other study [19]; total paracentesis was performed in one study and repeated paracentesis up to 5 liters was performed in the other. The hemaccel study included a small number of patients (n = 27), and PICD was a spontaneous reversible complication. Finally, patients who received dextran 40 had a negative outcome, and saline infusion was only used in a very small pilot study.

A large randomized trial investigated whether dextran 70 or hemaccel can prevent PICD and the impact of PICD on morbidity and mortality [23]. A total of 289 cirrhotic patients with ascites were randomized to receive total paracentesis plus intravenous albumin (n = 97), dextran 70 (n = 93), or polygeline (n = 99). PCID occurred significantly more frequently in patients treated with dextran 70 (34.4%) and polygeline (37.8%) than in those treated with albumin (18.5%). Arterial pressure decreased in all three groups, and hematocrit did not change in any group. Serum creatinine and plasma renin activity increased and serum sodium decreased significantly in patients treated with either dextran 70 or polygeline, but not in those treated with albumin. The total number and types of complications, including hyponatremia, renal impairment, hepatic encephalopathy, and death during hospitalization, were similar among all three groups. In addition, no difference was seen among the groups in the number of patients requiring re-admission, cause of re-admission, and number of deaths.

The study also showed that, in patients with PICD, the initial increase in plasma renin activity persisted 1 and 6 months after discharge from the hospital, patients had a significantly higher probability of being re-admitted to the hospital for ascites, and were more likely to require diuretics. More importantly, PICD was associated with a shorter length of survival (fig. 1). In the univariate analysis, only serum sodium, Child-Pugh score, serum creatinine and PICD were significantly related to survival. It confirmed other evidence of portal pressure increase in patients with PICD and a marked activation of the renin-angiotensin and the sympathetic nervous systems [24].

A second important finding of the study was that only volume of ascites removed and type of the plasma expanders had predictive value for the risk of developing PICD, but when the paracentesis volume was 5 liters or less, the incidence of PICD in patients receiving albumin was similar to that in patients receiving other expanders (14.2 vs. 15.4%). However, when the volume of ascites removed was greater than 5 liters, the incidence of PICD in patients treated with dextran 70 or polygeline rose to 31% when the paracentesis volume was 5–9 liters, and 55.7% when the volume removed was more than 9 liters (fig. 2).

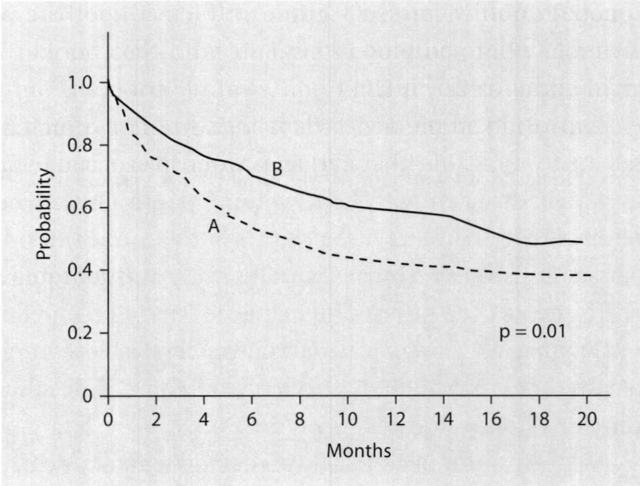

Fig. 1. Probability of survival after entry into the study in the patients who (A) did and (B) did not develop postparacentesis circulatory dysfunction. Reproduced with permission from Ginés et al. [27].

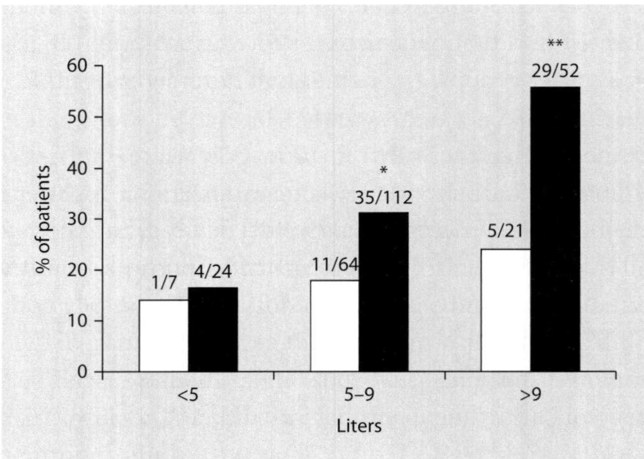

Fig. 2. Incidence of postparacentesis circulatory dysfunction according to the plasma expander used (albumin □, dextran 70 or polygeline ■) and the volume of ascitic fluid removed. * p = 0.04 and ** p = 0.02 with respect to the incidence in patients receiving albumin. Reproduced with permission from Ginés et al. [27].

Although the advantage of albumin appears to be related to plasma volume expansion due to its long half-life (about 21 days), recent data suggest that the prolonged improvement in circulatory function with albumin infusion can be attributed to its direct effect on the microcirculation. In patients with spontaneous bacterial peritonitis (SBP), albumin administration improved the systemic hemodynamics due to a decrease in arterial vasodilation and improving cardiac function. In addition, in patients with SBP, albumin administration, but not hydroxyethyl starch, was associated with a significant decrease in the plasma levels of factor VIII and von Willebrand-related antigen, indicating that albumin decreases endothelial activation [25, 26].

To date, no other study has been performed to change the conclusions of the Ginés et al. [27] study, which supports the advantage of albumin over less-expensive plasma expanders with therapeutic paracentesis. However, other approaches to managing cirrhotic patients treated with paracentesis can be explored. First, the dose of albumin at 6–8 g/l of ascites removed is arbitrary. It is unknown if lower amounts of albumin can be utilized with the same efficacy. Large controlled studies comparing recommended doses of albumin versus low doses are needed.

In addition, if the main cause of PICD is the aggravation of vasodilation, the use of vasoconstrictors instead of plasma expanders may be effective. Terlipressin has been compared with albumin in patients with cirrhosis treated with paracentesis [28, 29]. In a pilot study, Moreau et al. [28] randomized 20 patients to receive either terlipressin 3 mg or albumin 8 g/l of removed ascites on the day of paracentesis. No changes were seen at 4–6 days after paracentesis in plasma renin aldosterone, serum creatinine, or serum sodium levels between the two groups. Three months after the paracentesis, the survival rate was similar in both groups. The cost of terlipressin is slightly less than that of intravenous albumin. The authors concluded that terlipressin may be as effective as intravenous albumin in preventing a decrease in effective arterial blood volume in patients with cirrhosis treated with large-volume paracentesis. The second randomized pilot study also compared albumin and terlipressin with therapeutic paracentesis. Plasma renin activity and plasma aldosterone at 4–6 days after treatment did not differ between the two groups. Similar to the previous study, the authors concluded that terlipressin may be as effective as albumin in preventing PICD in patients with cirrhosis after therapeutic paracentesis [29].

Midodrine, an oral α-adrenoceptor agonist, was also compared with albumin in cirrhotic patients with tense ascites for the prevention of PICD [30]. Twenty-four patients were randomized to receive either midodrine 12.5 mg three times per day over 2 days or albumin 8 g/l of removed ascites. PICD developed in 60% of the patients in the midodrine group and in 31% of the patients in the albumin group. The authors decided that midodrine is not as effective as albumin in preventing paracentesis-induced circulatory dysfunction.

In conclusion, on the basis of available data in the literature, albumin is the recommended plasma volume expander in cirrhotic patients with more than 5 liters of ascites removed by paracentesis. Dextran 70 or polygeline may safely substitute albumin only in patients treated with paracentesis of no more than 5 liters. There is insufficient evidence to recommend terlipressin as a substitute for albumin accompanying large paracentesis because of its similar cost to albumin.

Key Message

- On the basis of these data, it is strongly recommended that large-volume paracentesis should be performed along with plasma volume expansion.

References

1 Ginés, Arroyo V, Quinteros E, et al: Comparison of paracentesis and diuretics in the treatment of cirrhotics with tense ascites: results of a randomized study. Gastroenterology 1987;93:234–241.

2 Salerno F, Badalamenti S, Incerti P, et al: Repeated paracentesis and i.v. albumin infusion to treat 'tense' ascites in cirrhotic patients: a safe alternative therapy. J Hepatol 1987;5:102–108.

3 Acharya S, Balwinder S, Padee A, et al: Large volume paracentesis and intravenous dextran to treat tense ascites. J Clin Gastroenterol 1992;14:31–35.

4 Hagege H, Ink O, Ducreaux M, et al: Traitment de l´ascite chez les maladie atteints de cirrhose sans hyponatremie ni insuffisance rénale: résultats d'une étude randomisée comparant les diurétiques et les ponctions compensées par l'albumine. Gastroenterol Clin Biol 1992;16:751–755.

5 Lebrec D, Giuily N, Hadenque A, et al: Transjugular intrahepatic porto-systemic shunt – comparison with paracentesis in patients with cirrhosis and refractory ascites: a randomized trial. J Hepatol 1996;25:135–144.

6 Rossle M, Ochs A, Gulberg V, Siegerstetter V, et al: A comparison of paracentesis and transjugular intrahepatic porto systemic shunting in patients with ascites. N Engl J Med 2000;342:1701–1707.

7 Sanyal A, Gennings C, Reddy K, et al: A randomized controlled study of TIPS versus large volume paracentesis in the treatment of refractory ascites. Gastroenterology 2003;124:634–643.

8 Ginés P, Uriz J, Calahorra B, et al: Transjugular intrahepatic porto systemic shunt versus repeated paracentesis plus intravenous albumin for refractory ascites in cirrhosis: a multicenter randomized comparative study. Gastroenterology 2002;123:1839–1847.

9 Salerno F, Merli M, Riggio O, et al: Randomized controlled study of TIPS vs. paracentesis with albumin in cirrhosis with refractory ascites. Hepatology 2004;40:629–635.

10 D'Amico G, Luca A, Morabito A, et al: Uncovered transjugular intrahepatic porto systemic shunt for refractory ascites: a meta-analysis. Gastroenterology 2005;129:1282–1293.

11 Ginés P, Titó L, Arroyo V, et al: Randomized comparative study of therapeutic paracentesis with and without intravenous albumin in cirrhosis. Gastroenterology 1988;94:1493–1502.

12 García-Compeán D, Villareal J, Cuevas H, et al: Total therapeutic paracentesis (TTP) with and without intravenous albumin in the treatment of cirrhotic tense ascites: a randomized controlled trial. Liver 1993;13:233–238.

13 Simon D, McCain J, Bonkovsky H, et al: Effects of therapeutic paracentesis on systemic and hepatic hemodynamics and on renal and hormonal function. Hepatology 1987;7:423–429.

14 Pozzi M, Osculati G, Boari G, et al: Time course of circulatory and humoral effects of rapid total paracentesis in cirrhotic patients with tense, refractory ascites. Gastroenterology 1994:106:709–719.

15 Kao H, Rakov N, Savage E, et al: The effects of large volume paracentesis on plasma volume: a cause of hypovolemia? Hepatology 1985;5:403–407.

16 Saló J, Ginés P, Piera C, et al: Effects of therapeutic paracentesis on plasma volume and transvascular escape rate of albumin in patients with cirrhosis. J Hepatol 1997;27:645–653.

17 Monescillo A, Urman J, Gonzalez M, et al: Influencia de la presión intrabdominal en el desarrollo de la disfunción circulatoria post paracentesis. Gastroenterol Hepatol 1999;22(suppl 1):52.

18 Planas R, Ginés P, Arroyo V, et al: Dextran 70 versus albumin as plasma expanders in cirrhotic patients with tense ascites treated with total paracentesis: results of a randomized study. Gastroenterology 1990;99:1736–1744.

19 Fassio E, Terg R, Landeira G, et al: Paracentesis with dextran 70 vs paracentesis with albumin in cirrhosis with tense ascites. J Hepatol 1992;14:310–316.

20 Salerno F, Badalamenti S, Lorenzano E, et al: Randomized comparative study of hemaccel versus albumin infusion after total paracentesis in cirrhotic patients with refractory ascites. Hepatology 1991;13: 707–713.

21 Solá R, Vila C, Andreu M, et al: Total paracentesis with dextran 40 vs diuretics in the treatment of ascites in cirrhosis: a randomized controlled trial. J Hepatol 1994;20:282–288.

22 Cabrera J, IngladaL, Quintero E, et al: Large-volume paracentesis and intravenous saline: effects on the renin-angiotensin system. Hepatology 1991;14: 1025–1028.

23 Ginés A, Fernandez-Esparrach G, Monescillo A, et al: randomized trial comparing albumin, dextran 70 and polygeline in cirrhotic patients with ascites treated by paracentesis. Gastroenterology 1996;111: 1002–1010.

24 Ruiz del Arbol L, Monescillo A, Jimenez W, et al: Paracentesis-induced circulatory dysfunction: mechanism and effect on hepatic and hemodynamics in cirrhosis. Gastroenterology 1997;113:579–586.

25 Fernandez J, Navasa M, García-Pagan J, et al: Effects of intravenous albumin on systemic and hepatic hemodynamics and vasoactive neurohormonal systems in patients with cirrosis and spontaneous bacterial peritonitis. J Hepatol 2004;41:384–390.
26 Fernandez J, Monteagudo J, Bargallo X, et al: A randomized unblinded pilot study comparing albumin versus hydroxyethyl starch in spontaneous bacterial peritonitis. Hepatology 2005;42:627–634.
27 Ginés A, Fernandez-Esparrach G, Monescillo A, et al: Randomized trial comparing albumin, dextran 70 and polygeline in cirrhotic patients with ascites treated with paracentesis. Gastroenterology 1996;111:1002–1010.
28 Moreau R, Asselah T, Condat B, et al: Comparison of the effect of terlipressin and albumin on arterial blood volume in patients with cirrhosis and tense ascites treated by paracentesis: a randomized pilot study. Gut 2002;50:90–94.
29 Singh V, Kumar R, Nain C, et al: Terlipressin versus albumin in paracentesis-induced circulatory dysfunction in cirrhosis: a randomized study. J Gastroenterol Hepatol 2006;21:303–307.
30 Appenrodt B, Wolf A, Grunhage F, et al: Prevention of paracentesis-induced circulatory dysfunction: midodrine vs. albumin: a randomized pilot study. Liver Int 2008;28:1019–1025.

Ruben Alberto Terg
Hospital de Gastroenterología Bonorino Udaondo
Av. Caseros 2061 (1264)
Buenos Aires (Argentina)
Tel. +54 11 4247 2904, E-Mail rterg@intramed.net

Gerbes AL (ed): Ascites, Hyponatremia and Hepatorenal Syndrome: Progress in Treatment.
Front Gastrointest Res. Basel, Karger, 2011, vol 28, pp 40–51

Albumin: Not Just a Plasma Expander

Nathan A. Davies · Rita Garcia · Andrew Proven · Rajiv Jalan

UCL Institute of Hepatology, UCL Medical School, Royal Free Campus, London, UK

Abstract

Human serum albumin is important for health and normal metabolic function. It comprises over half of the extracellular protein in blood and is the main regulator of plasma oncotic pressure. Traditionally, its main use has been as a volume expansion agent. Albumin undertakes a wide variety of transport functions and is essential for carrying metabolic products to the liver for metabolism and excretion. Due to its redox-active properties, it also acts as a first line of defence against pro-oxidant and free radical injury. In subjects with liver disease its concentration is reduced, an effect that is further compounded by studies that demonstrate that the remaining protein is functionally impaired. This lack of metabolic function most likely contributes to exacerbation of the disease processes. Administration of albumin to both patients with liver disease, and for a wide variety of other indications, shows beneficial effects that go far beyond simple fluid resuscitation.

Human serum albumin (HSA) comprises over half of the plasma extracellular protein (40–50 g/l in healthy individuals) and is responsible for approximately 75% of plasma colloid oncotic pressure. It is produced exclusively in the liver (9–12 g/day), and, as would be expected, there is a significant decrease in its serum concentration as a consequence of liver disease (see figure 1).

In addition to its role as a plasma volume regulator, albumin undertakes a variety of transport functions through a variety of designated binding sites formed within its tertiary structure. Albumin has the capacity to bind an extraordinarily diverse range of molecules (including drugs) and actively transports metabolic products including long-chain fatty acids, bilirubin, anions, bile acids and metals [1]. It also plays an enzymatic role in the metabolism of endogenous lipids and eicosanoids [2].

HSA is a relatively small (67 kDa) globular protein comprised of 609 amino acids, 35 of which are cysteine residues forming 17 disulphide bridges which stabilize the configuration of the molecule, a heart shaped tertiary structure with a high α-helical content (see figure 2). The remaining cysteine (cys-34) residue accounts for the single free redox-active thiol (–SH) moiety of the molecule, capable of thiolation and nitrosylation. Due to the amount of HSA in the circulation and the reactive capacity of the

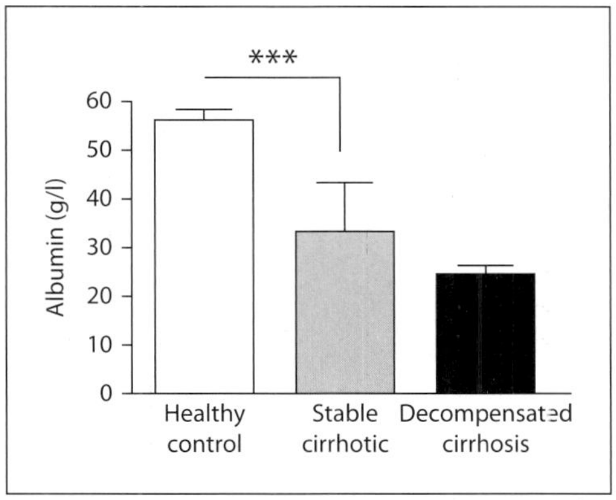

Fig. 1. Bar graph showing plasma concentrations of albumin from healthy volunteers (n = 10), stable outpatients with confirmed cirrhosis (n = 12) and patients admitted to hospital with decompensated liver disease (n = 20). A significant decrease in the albumin level is observed in subjects with liver disease (*** $p < 0.001$).

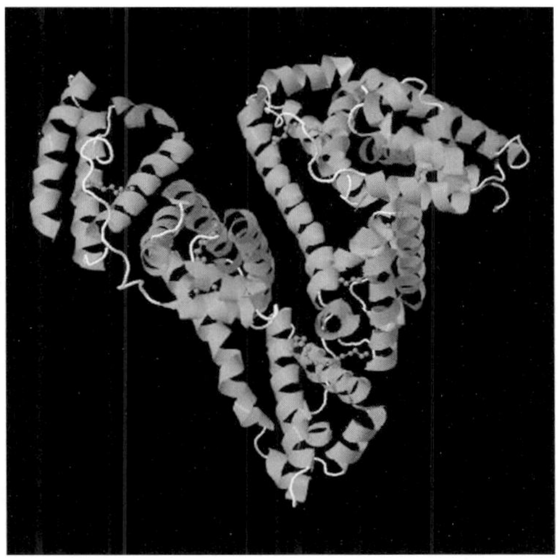

Fig. 2. Representation of the structure of the albumin molecule, displaying the distinctive heart shape established from X-ray crystallography.

cys-34 thiol group as a scavenger of harmful reactive oxygen and nitrogen species, this provides the body's main front line extracellular defence against free radical injury.

Albumin in Liver Disease

Liver failure is the all too common result of progressive chronic liver diseases, resulting from the impairment in liver function and the subsequent accumulation of metabolic toxins. The culmination of the disease process usually involves multiple organs and their function decreases accordingly with the severity of the liver condition.

Patients with cirrhosis develop portal hypertension which results in splanchnic arterial vasodilatation, consequently leading to high cardiac output, increased heart rate, a reduced peripheral vascular resistance and arterial pressure. This particular cardiovascular scenario is known as circulatory dysfunction that deteriorates with the development of liver failure and leads to a progressive reduction in individual organ perfusion. Indeed, liver failure causes high morbidity and its mortality without liver transplantation (the only curative treatment but limited to a selected population) remains disturbingly high.

Albumin was introduced as a treatment in the management of cirrhotic patients with hypoalbuminaemia and ascites in the 1950s. Initially, it was thought that its benefits were limited to its oncotic properties and its capacity to expand intravascular volume. In subsequent years, better understanding of the pathophysiology of liver failure and its complications, in combination with the determination of the structure and physiological properties of albumin, have altered this opinion. In recent years, improvements in the management of cirrhotic patients have led to increases in survival and quality of life. This clinical approach now includes established indications for albumin infusion:

- Spontaneous bacterial peritonitis (SBP) is a frequent infection in cirrhotic patients with ascites that can be complicated with systemic inflammatory response. This trigger can cause deterioration in liver and hemodynamic functions and subsequently progress to multiorgan failure, in spite of sterilization of the ascitic fluid with antibiotics. Studies have evaluated the effect of albumin infusion during an episode of SBP and found that its administration together with antibiotics reduced mortality and improved outcome in these patients [3] (table 1), and are now part of the AASLD management guidelines for patients with SBP [4].
- Hepatorenal syndrome (HRS) develops from an extreme form of circulatory dysfunction. The splanchnic arterial vasodilatation results in severe underfilling of the systemic vascular territory with renal hypoperfusion ultimately leading to renal failure. Several studies have demonstrated that a combination strategy of albumin infusion with vasoconstrictors has a significant survival benefit in patients with this condition [5–8] (table 2).
- In addition, albumin infusion has also been shown to have a positive effect in preventing patient deterioration. Paracentesis-induced circulatory dysfunction (PICD) consists of an exacerbation of arteriolar vasodilatation leading to a large volume paracentesis. This syndrome develops in 80% of patients after a large-volume paracentesis and can cause acute renal failure with a high associated mortality rate. Albumin infusion has been widely evaluated in the prevention of this syndrome (table 3). Evidence suggests that albumin appears to be the most effective drug in the prevention of humoral, hemodynamic, and clinical effects associated with this syndrome, consequently showing a significant improvement in morbidity and mortality [9–16].

Recent studies have suggested that albumin infusion benefits are not limited to its plasma oncotic properties. Fernandez et al. [17] studied 12 patients with SBP treated with albumin infusion plus antibiotic therapy, examining both the humoral (plasma

Table 1. Clinical studies that evaluated albumin infusion in spontaneous bacterial peritonitis in cirrhosis

Author, year	Design	Treatment	Control group	Number of subjects	Aim	Effect
Sort, 1999	randomised	cefotaxime+ albumin	albumin	126 (63/63)	renal failure and 90 days mortality	reduction in renal failure and mortality
Fernandez, 2004	cohorts	ceftriaxone+ albumin	no	12	systemic and splanchnic hemodynamics	improvement
Choi, 2005	randomised	large paracentesis+ albumin	diuretics + albumin	42 (21/21)	effectiveness and safety at 90 days in SBP	same benefit
Fernandez, 2005	randomised	albumin+ antibiotic	hydroxyethyl starch 200/0.5 + antibiotic	20 (10/10)	systemic haemodynamics	superiority of treatment
Sigal, 2007	cohorts	albumin+ antibiotic (high -risk patients)	antibiotic (low-risk patients)	36 (21/15)	renal impairment	no benefits of albumin in low-risk patients
Chen, 2009	randomised	albumin + antibiotic	antibiotic	30 (15/15)	Systemic and ascetic endotoxin and cytokines	decrease of inflammatory mediators

renin activity, nitric oxide, interleukin-6) and hemodynamic (systemic and splanchnic) changes. The resolution of infection was associated with an improvement in cardiac function, but also indicated an increased peripheral vascular resistance. This study suggests that albumin provides a beneficial effect in addition to its role as a volume expander.

A clinical study carried out in patients with acute diuretic-induced hepatic encephalopathy compared the effects of either a 4.5% albumin or colloid infusion. It was found that an improvement in systemic hemodynamic measures with a complementary reduction in plasma ammonia occurred in both groups. However, a significantly more marked improvement in hepatic encephalopathy together with a reduction in oxidative stress markers was found in the albumin-treated patients. These results suggest that the beneficial effects in the albumin group are not related to the haemodynamic improvement or the decrease in ammonia and could be related to the antioxidant effects of albumin [18].

In a randomised controlled study performed in patients with severe hepatic encephalopathy (HE grades 3 or 4 in the West-Haven scale), an improvement in HE grade was reached faster and more frequently in patients receiving standard

Table 2. Clinical studies that evaluated the effectiveness of albumin infusion in hepatorenal syndrome

Author, year	Design	Treatment	Control group	Number of subjects	Aim	Effect
Guevara, 1998	prospective, open label	ornipresin+ albumin (3 days)	ornipresin+ albumin (15 days)	16 (8/8)	resolution HRS	effective in prolonged arm
Ortega, 2002	prospective, open label	terlipresin+ albumin	terlipresin	21 (13/8)	resolution HRS, 3 months' survival	superiority of treatment
Pomier-Layrargues, 2003	randomised, cross-over	octreotido+ albumin	placebo+ albumin	14 (6/8)	Improvement renal function	no benefits
Alessandria, 2007	randomised, unblinded	noradrenaline+ albumin	terlipresin+ albumin	22 (10/12)	resolution HRS	same effect
Testro, 2008	retrospective	terlipresin+ albumin	no	69	survival free-transplant	recurrence type 1 HRS decrease survival
Neri, 2008	randomised	terlipresin+ albumin	albumin	52 (26/26)	improvement renal function, 3 months' survival	superiority of treatment
Sanyal, 2008	randomised	terlipresin+ albumin	placebo+ albumin	112 (56/56)	resolution HRS	superiority of treatment
Marti-Llahi, 2008	randomised	terlipresin+ albumin	albumin	46 (23/23)	improvement renal function, 3 months' survival	superiority in renal function, same survival
Sharma, 2008	randomised, open label	noradrenaline + albumin	terlipresin + albumin	40 (20/20)	resolution HRS	same effect
von Kalckreuth, 2009	retrospective	terlipresin+ albumin	no	30	predictors of response	short treatment and high dose in responders
Skagen, 2009	cohorts	midodrine + octreotide + albumin	no treatment	162 (75/87)	renal function, survival free of transplant	improvement of treatment

medical therapy plus albumin dialysis than in those who received standard medical therapy alone [19]. In this study, the patient's blood was dialysed against albumin across a high-flux membrane. This allows the removal of albumin-bound and water-soluble toxins, though it prevents albumin exchange. This study indicates that the observed effect cannot be related to the albumin oncotic properties but rather

Table 3. Clinical studies that evaluated efficacy of albumin infusion in the prevention of paracentesis-induced circulatory dysfunction

Author, year	Design	Treatment	Control group	Number of subjects	Aim	Effect
Gines, 1988	randomised	albumin	no treatment	105 (52/53)	prevention of PICD	effective
Planas, 1990	randomised	albumin	dextran 70	88 (43/45)	prevention of PICD	same renal effects, higher humoral changes
Salerno, 1991	randomised	albumin	hemaccel	54 (27/27)	prevention of PICD	same effect
Fasio, 1992	randomised	albumin	dextran 70	41 (21/20)	prevention of PICD	same effect
Bruno, 1992	randomised	albumin	ascites filtration and reinfusion	35 (18/17)	prevention of PICD	same efficacy, high safety
Garcia Compean, 1993	randomised	albumin	no treatment	35 (17/18)	prevention of PICD	effective
Luca, 1995	randomised	albumin	no treatment	18 (9/9)	prevention of humoral and haemodynamic changes	effective
Hernandez Perez, 1995	randomised	albumin	dextrano 70	16 (8/8)	prevention of PICD	same effect
Gines, 1996	randomised	albumin	dextran 70 or polygeline	289 (97/93/99)	prevention of PICD and survival	superiority
Altman, 1998	randomised	albumin	hydroxyethyl starch	60 (33/27)	prevention of PICD	same effect
Zhao, 2000	randomised	albumin	mannitolum 20%	68 (36/32)	prevention of PICD	same effect
Garcia-Compean, 2002	randomised	albumin	dextran 40	96 (48/48)	prevention of PICD	superiority
Moreau, 2002	randomised	albumin	terlipresin	20 (10/10)	prevention of PICD	same effect
Sola-Vera, 2003	randomised, cross-over	albumin	saline	72 (37/35)	prevention of PICD	superiority
Singh, 2006	randomised	albumin	terlipressin	40 (20/20)	prevention of PICD	same effect
Singh, 2006	randomised	albumin	noradrenaline	40 (20/20)	prevention of PICD	same effect
Lata, 2007	randomised	albumin	terlipressin	49	prevention of PICD	same effect

Table 3. Continued

Author, year	Design	Treatment	Control group	Number of subjects	Aim	Effect
Appenrodt, 2008	randomised	albumin	midodrine	23 (13/11)	prevention of PICD	superiority in humoral changes
Umgelter, 2008	prospective, uncontrolled	albumin (in critically ill with HRS)	no	19	prevention worsening in renal function	effective and safe
Schneditz, 2008	prospective, uncontrolled	albumin	no	11	prevention haemodynamic changes 2 h post-paracentesis	failed
Singh, 2008	randomised	albumin	midodrine	40 (20/20)	prevention of PICD	same effect

suggests that the detoxification properties of albumin have a therapeutic benefit in this condition.

The beneficial effects derived from the detoxification properties of albumin were also demonstrated in a clinical trial comparing 15 patients with SBP who received albumin infusion plus antibiotics with 15 receiving antibiotics alone. In the albumin-treated arm, a significant decrease in TNF-α and interleukin-6 in plasma and ascitic fluid occurred together with a decrease in ascitic endotoxin levels [20]. These actions on bacterial products and inflammatory mediators are thought to be linked to the anti-inflammatory properties of albumin. In a separate study, neutrophil dysfunction induced by incubating normal healthy neutrophils with the plasma from a patient with alcoholic hepatitis is completely ameliorated when additional albumin is added during the incubation process [21]. In addition, other studies have shown increasing evidence of the potential benefits attributed to the capacity of albumin to bind many endogenous and exogenous compounds [22].

These new data highlight the role of albumin function in liver diseases and provide us with a better knowledge of the physiological basis of its therapeutic properties.

Albumin in Non-Liver Disease

There has been much debate regarding the use of human albumin solution for volume expansion in the treatment of circulatory support, much of which has centred on cost/benefit analysis.

In 1998, a Cochrane group meta-analysis of 30 randomised controlled trials including 1,419 randomised patients that were critically ill with hypovolaemia, burns, or hypoalbuminaemia, stated that there was a strong suggestion that albumin may increase mortality [23]. They went on to suggest that it should not be used except in blind randomised controlled clinical trials. Following this publication, the use of HSA decreased worldwide.

These findings were heavily disputed. Wilkes and Navickis [24] subsequently performed a second meta-analysis, this time incorporating 55 trials. Their study contained many of the same trials included in the Cochrane report, but crucially they found that albumin use when compared to crystalloid use had no significant difference regarding mortality. Their findings supported the safety of albumin and suggested a need for further well-designed clinical trials. In 2004, the SAFE (saline vs. albumin fluid evaluation) study was published in the *New England Journal of Medicine* [25]. Patients were randomly assigned to receive either 4% albumin or normal saline following admission to the ICU for intravascular fluid resuscitation during the 28 days from admission. Of the 6,997 patients in the trial, approximately 20% died in both groups, with secondary outcomes also very similar between the two study arms. It was observed that a subset of trauma patients with head injury showed an increase in mortality with the use of HAS, possibly due to an increase in interstitial albumin in the brain increasing brain water/ICP.

Contrary to this finding, it has been reported that serum albumin is inversely correlated with mortality in stoke victims [26]. In the Bergen stroke study, patients had a greater chance of survival when admitted with a higher serum albumin. Other studies have supported the use of albumin infusion in stroke patients post-infarction suggesting an effect greater than that restricted to colloid osmotic pressure changes [27–29]. In the ALIAS trial, a dose-dependent beneficial effect of albumin infusion to stroke patients was found, with patients at the higher dose levels showing improved recovery and lower long-term morbidity [29]. Another possible neurological benefit lies in the use of albumin in the treatment of cerebral malaria from *Plasmodium falciparum* infection [30] although there is some contention regarding the trial methods and interpretation of the results.

In a cardiac surgery study using discharge data from 19,578 patients undergoing coronary artery bypass, Sedrakyan et al. [31] suggested a lower incidence of morbidity and mortality than those given non-protein colloids (41.3% received albumin as a plasma expander).

It is interesting to note that a low serum albumin concentration is a strong predictor of mortality after cardiac surgery [32, 33] with the use of albumin reported as having a protective effect [34] showing a 25% lower odds ratio using multivariable analysis for mortality rates in these patient groups.

Fluid resuscitation is a major aspect of treatment following admission to the burns unit. The Parklands formula allows calculation of appropriate fluid volume (normally Ringer's solution), but in approximately 20% of patients 'fluid creep' ensues leading to an increased risk of further morbidity. This is ameliorated using albumin in conjunction with the crystalloid [35]. Interestingly, with the concomitant use of an iNOS inhibitor in a rat model of burns, albumin significantly reduces bacterial translocation compared to rats given an iNOS inhibitor alone [36].

Serum albumin in the elderly is, as with many other pathologies, a marker for survival following admission to hospital. Low albumin levels are associated with reduced appendicular muscle mass [37] notwithstanding nutritional and physical activity and inflammatory status. Visser et al. [37] showed a weak correlation with lean body mass and a significant finding that low serum albumin leads to sarcopenia, after controlling for confounding factors. There may also be an anti-inflammatory effect of albumin following infusion in the elderly, possibly due its anti-oxidant properties.

Functional Characteristics in Liver Disease and Failure – Albumin Is Dysfunctional, Why?

Recently, our group has described an impairment in the functional capacity of albumin in cirrhotic patients [38]. In this study, the functional capacity of albumin was assessed with two different techniques: electron paramagnetic resonance spectroscopy analyzed the capacity of albumin to bind and transport fatty acids and ischaemia-modified albumin measured the ability of albumin to bind metals (cobalt). This study showed a reduced functional ability in patients' albumin closely correlated to the degree of liver insufficiency. Moreover, the ratio ischaemia-modified albumin/total serum albumin correlated with severity of liver disease and was significantly higher in non-surviving patients with acute-on-chronic liver failure. MARS therapy showed a reduction in albumin-bound metabolites (bilirubin), but crucially did not restore the functional ability of the albumin in the 12 patients submitted to this treatment.

The origin of the dysfunction remains unclear. The fact that a poorer liver function, and a more advanced disease state, correlates with albumin dysfunction suggests that toxin accumulation may physically change albumin structure and cause prevention of normal function. Or it is possible that the albumin structure has been chemically modified in such a way that either the binding sites are altered and/or there is a change in the tertiary structure. It is also not currently known whether hepatocytes of the cirrhotic liver are capable of producing normal, functional albumin.

Due to the fact that the cirrhotic liver displays a marked inability to effectively filter and remove metabolic toxins, there is an accumulation of endogenous substances that could have a pathogenic role in cirrhosis' complications (i.e. short-chain fatty acids, bilirubin and metals). Furthermore, as cirrhotic patients typically display hypoalbuminaemia together with dysfunction of the albumin present leads to a severe disturbance in the transport, metabolism and excretion of metabolic by-products, effectively contributing to systemic toxin overload. The results of these processes are alterations in other systems habitually influenced by a normal albumin function (redox balance, oxidative stress, microvasculature permeability, coagulation, inflammation) [1, 39].

In summary, liver diseases leads to a decrease in systemic albumin functional capacity, contributed to by both reduced albumin levels and impaired function of the protein present. This effectively reduces the ability of the body to transport metabolic products and causes an impairment in the sequestration of bacterial endotoxins with an associated increase in inflammation. Albumin infusion has been shown improve outcome in these patients. The beneficial properties seem not to be limited to the colloid oncotic effect of volume expansion but, instead, work through a combination of improved metabolic function and anti-inflammatory and anti-oxidant properties.

Key Messages

- Albumin is decreased in liver disease, both in plasma concentration and functional ability, thereby limiting metabolism.
- Administration of albumin has been demonstrated to have a number of positive benefits in a range of conditions in addition to liver dysfunction, which far exceed its traditional role as a volume expansion agent.
- The anti-oxidant, anti-inflammatory and metabolic properties of albumin indicate that it should be considered as a therapeutic agent rather than a simple fluid for infusion.

References

1 Evans TW: Albumin as a drug – biological effects of albumin unrelated to oncotic pressure. Aliment Pharmacol Ther 2002;16(suppl 5):6–11.
2 Peters T: All About Albumin: Biochemistry, Genetics, and Medical Applications. San Diego, Academic Press, 1996.
3 Sort P, Navasa M, Arroyo V, et al: Effect of intravenous albumin on renal impairment and mortality in patients with cirrhosis and spontaneous bacterial peritonitis. N Engl J Med 1999;341:403–409.
4 Runyon BA: Management of adult patients with ascites due to cirrhosis. Hepatology 2004;39:841–856.
5 Ortega R, Gines P, Uriz J, Cardenas A, et al: Terlipressin therapy with and without albumin for patients with hepatorenal syndrome: results of a prospective, nonrandomized study. Hepatology 2002;36:941–948.
6 Neri S, Pulvirenti D, Malaguarnera M, et al: Terlipressin and albumin in patients with cirrhosis and type I hepatorenal syndrome. Dig Dis Sci 2008;53:830–835.
7 Sanyal AJ, Boyer T, Garcia-Tsao G, et al: A randomized, prospective, double-blind, placebo-controlled trial of terlipressin for type 1 hepatorenal syndrome. Gastroenterology 2008;134:1360–1368.
8 Martin-Llahi M, Pepin MN, Guevara M, et al: Terlipressin and albumin vs. albumin in patients with cirrhosis and hepatorenal syndrome: a randomized study. Gastroenterology 2008;134:1352–1359.
9 Gines P, Tito L, Arroyo V, et al: Randomized comparative study of therapeutic paracentesis with and without intravenous albumin in cirrhosis. Gastroenterology 1988;94:1493–1502.
10 Planas R, Gines P, Arroyo V, et al: Dextran-70 versus albumin as plasma expanders in cirrhotic patients with tense ascites treated with total paracentesis. Results of a randomized study. Gastroenterology 1990;99:1736–1744.
11 Garcia-Compean D, Blanc P, Larrey D, et al: Treatment of cirrhotic tense ascites with Dextran-40 versus albumin associated with large volume paracentesis: a randomized controlled trial. Ann Hepatol 2002;1:29–35.

12 Luca A, Garcia-Pagan JC, Bosch J, et al: Beneficial effects of intravenous albumin infusion on the hemodynamic and humoral changes after total paracentesis. Hepatology 1995;22:753–758.
13 Gines A, Fernandez-Esparrach G, Monescillo A, et al: Randomized trial comparing albumin, dextran 70, and polygeline in cirrhotic patients with ascites treated by paracentesis. Gastroenterology 1996;111:1002–1010.
14 Sola-Vera J, Minana J, Ricart E, et al: Randomized trial comparing albumin and saline in the prevention of paracentesis-induced circulatory dysfunction in cirrhotic patients with ascites. Hepatology 2003;37:1147–1153.
15 Appenrodt B, Wolf A, Grunhage F, et al: Prevention of paracentesis-induced circulatory dysfunction: midodrine vs. albumin – a randomized pilot study. Liver Int 2008;28:1019–1025.
16 Umgelter A, Reindl W, Wagner KS, et al: Effects of plasma expansion with albumin and paracentesis on haemodynamics and kidney function in critically ill cirrhotic patients with tense ascites and hepatorenal syndrome: a prospective uncontrolled trial. Crit Care 2008;12:R4.
17 Fernandez J, Navasa M, Garcia-Pagan JC, et al: Effect of intravenous albumin on systemic and hepatic hemodynamics and vasoactive neurohormonal systems in patients with cirrhosis and spontaneous bacterial peritonitis. J Hepatol 2004;41:384–390.
18 Jalan R, Kapoor D: Reversal of diuretic-induced hepatic encephalopathy with infusion of albumin but not colloid. Clin Sci (Lond) 2004;106:467–474.
19 Hassanein TI, Tofteng F, Brown RS Jr, et al: Randomized controlled study of extracorporeal albumin dialysis for hepatic encephalopathy in advanced cirrhosis. Hepatology 2007;46:1853–1862.
20 Chen TA, Tsao YC, Chen A, et al: Effect of intravenous albumin on endotoxin removal, cytokines, and nitric oxide production in patients with cirrhosis and spontaneous bacterial peritonitis. Scand J Gastroenterol 2009;44:619–625.
21 Stadlbauer V, Mookerjee RP, Wright GA, et al: Role of Toll-like receptors 2, 4, and 9 in mediating neutrophil dysfunction in alcoholic hepatitis. Am J Physiol Gastrointest Liver Physiol 2009;296:G15–G22.
22 Sen S, Mookerjee RP, Cheshire LM, Davies NA, Williams R, Jalan R: Albumin dialysis reduces portal pressure acutely in patients with severe alcoholic hepatitis. J Hepatol 2005;43:142–148.
23 Cochrane Injuries Group Albumin Reviewers: Human albumin administration in critically ill patients: systematic review of randomised controlled trials. BMJ 1998;317:235–240.
24 Wilkes MM, Navickis RJ: Patient survival after human albumin administration: a meta-analysis of randomized, controlled trials. Ann Intern Med 2001;135:149–164.
25 Finfer S, Bellomo R, Boyce N, French J, Myburgh J, Norton R: A comparison of albumin and saline for fluid resuscitation in the intensive care unit. N Engl J Med 2004;350:2247–2256.
26 Idicula TT, Waje-Andreassen U, Brogger J, Naess H, Thomassen L: Serum albumin in ischemic stroke patients: the higher the better. The Bergen Stroke Study. Cerebrovasc Dis 2009;28:13–17.
27 Belayev L, Liu Y, Zhao W, Busto R, Ginsberg MD: Human albumin therapy of acute ischemic stroke: marked neuroprotective efficacy at moderate doses and with a broad therapeutic window. Stroke 2001;32:553–560.
28 Koch S, Concha M, Wazzan T, Romano JG, Forteza A: High dose human serum albumin for the treatment of acute ischemic stroke: a safety study. Neurocrit Care 2004;1:335–341.
29 Palesch YY, Hill MD, Ryckborst KJ, Tamariz D, Ginsberg MD: The ALIAS Pilot Trial: a dose-escalation and safety study of albumin therapy for acute ischemic stroke. II. Neurologic outcome and efficacy analysis. Stroke 2006;37:2107–2114.
30 Maitland K, Pamba A, English M, et al: Randomized trial of volume expansion with albumin or saline in children with severe malaria: preliminary evidence of albumin benefit. Clin Infect Dis 2005;40:538–545.
31 Sedrakyan A, Gondek K, Paltiel D, Elefteriades JA: Volume expansion with albumin decreases mortality after coronary artery bypass graft surgery. Chest 2003;123:1853–1857.
32 Engelman DT, Adams DH, Byrne JG, et al: Impact of body mass index and albumin on morbidity and mortality after cardiac surgery. J Thorac Cardiovasc Surg 1999;118:866–873.
33 Magovern JA, Sakert T, Magovern GJ, et al: A model that predicts morbidity and mortality after coronary artery bypass graft surgery. J Am Coll Cardiol 1996;28:1147–1153.
34 Goldwasser P, Feldman J: Association of serum albumin and mortality risk. J Clin Epidemiol 1997;50:693–703.
35 Lawrence A, Faraklas I, Watkins H, et al: Colloid administration normalizes resuscitation ratio and ameliorates 'fluid creep'. J Burn Care Res 2010;31:40–47.
36 Chen LW, Wang JS, Hwang B, Chen JS, Hsu CM: Reversal of the effect of albumin on gut barrier function in burn by the inhibition of inducible isoform of nitric oxide synthase. Arch Surg 2003;138:1219–1225.

37 Visser M, Kritchevsky SB, Newman AB, et al: Lower serum albumin concentration and change in muscle mass: the Health, Aging and Body Composition Study. Am J Clin Nutr 2005;82:531–537.
38 Jalan R, Schnurr K, Mookerjee RP, et al: Alterations in the functional capacity of albumin in patients with decompensated cirrhosis is associated with increased mortality. Hepatology 2009;50:555–564.
39 Quinlan GJ, Martin GS, Evans TW: Albumin: biochemical properties and therapeutic potential. Hepatology 2005;41:1211–1219.

Prof. Rajiv Jalan
UCL Institute of Hepatology
UCL Medical School, Royal Free Campus
London, NW3 2PF (UK)
Tel. +44 207 433 2795, E-Mail r.jalan@ucl.ac.uk

Gerbes AL (ed): Ascites, Hyponatremia and Hepatorenal Syndrome: Progress in Treatment.
Front Gastrointest Res. Basel, Karger, 2011, vol 28, pp 52–64

Transjugular Intrahepatic Portosystemic Shunt for Ascites: Which Patients Will Benefit?

Francesco Salerno · Massimo Cazzaniga

Internal Medicine, Policlinico IRCCS San Donato, School of Medicine of the University of Milan, San Donato Milanese, Italy

Abstract

Transjugular intrahepatic portosystemic shunt (TIPS) is a radiological interventional procedure useful in portal hypertension-related complications. It is able to resolve variceal bleeding and refractory ascites. However, it can lead to serious side effects such as refractory encephalopathy, cardiac failure, and end-stage liver failure. Patients with refractory ascites represent the most frequent indication for TIPS. Clinicians are challenged by the necessity to select the best candidates for TIPS, so that the procedure can be successful as far as both efficacy and survival are concerned. The correct process to select TIPS for cirrhotic patients with ascites includes different steps: first, patients with absolute contraindications, such cardiopulmonary dysfunction or too severe liver failure, should be excluded, and second, criteria to predict post-TIPS survival should be considered. The most effective predictors of survival are serum creatinine, serum bilirubin, serum sodium, age and MELD or Child-Pugh scores. According to an arbitrary choice of two thresholds of different risks for each variable, we propose a simple estimation of the whole risk after TIPS placement.

Transjugular intrahepatic portosystemic shunt (TIPS) is a radiologic interventional procedure which lowers high portal pressure. Therefore, it represents an important therapeutic resource in order to treat or prevent complications of portal hypertension.

Historically, the concept of TIPS was developed in the late 1960s, when the initial attempts to connect a hepatic vein with an intrahepatic branch of the portal vein using nonexpandable tubing in experimental animals failed because of shunt obstruction [1, 2].

The TIPS technique was improved in 1982 by Colapinto et al. [3] who used a 9-mm catheter in men. However, only after the introduction of an expandable flexible metal shunt prosthesis originally designed for the biliary tract could a stable shunt patency be achieved [4, 5].

These pioneering experiences stimulated the interest of hepatologists and interventional radiologists, and many centers have experimented with TIPS during the last 20 years refining the technique and the materials. The most recent improvement has been the introduction of a polytetrafluoroethylene (PTFE)-covered stent which markedly decreased the rate of stent stenosis [6, 7]. Nowadays, TIPS has almost completely replaced the surgical portacaval shunt in the management of complications of portal hypertension [8].

From a functional point of view, TIPS effectively functions as a side-to-side portocaval shunt because it is able to decompress the intrahepatic sinusoidal circulation [9, 10]. Therefore, in suitably selected patients, TIPS is particularly effective in the treatment of refractory or recidivant ascites, so that these currently represent the first indication for TIPS insertion. Other indications are the emergency treatment of variceal bleeding refractory to other therapeutic strategies, such as endoscopic variceal banding and vasoconstrictors, or the prevention of variceal rebleeding in patients where prophylaxis with nonselective beta-blockers and/or endoscopic variceal banding has failed [11]. Less-frequent indications are Budd-Chiari syndrome [12] and cirrhotic hydrothorax [13].

Indications and contraindications to the use of TIPS, as recently defined by the American Association for the Study of Liver Disease (AASLD) [14], are reported in table 1.

Treatment of Ascites

The success of TIPS in treating cirrhotic ascites has been ascribed to two main effects. The first is the reduction of sinusoidal hydrostatic pressure, which reduces fluid leakage into the interstitial space and the lymphatic vessels. The second is the increase of the venous blood return to the right heart that increases cardiac preload and, consequently, cardiac output. These hemodynamic effects improve the central blood volume with a reduction of the release of vasoconstrictors (renin and norepinephrine) and increased renal blood perfusion [15, 16]. Additionally, it was demonstrated that a functional TIPS is able to deafferentiate a hypothetical hepato-renal reflex [17]. The final result of this chain of events is an increase in the glomerular filtration rate and the urinary sodium excretion rate [18].

Some uncontrolled studies showed the improvement of renal function in cirrhotic patients treated with TIPS and found a concomitant improvement in the capacity of diuretic medications to reduce peritoneal fluid accumulation [19–22].

The efficacy of TIPS in correcting refractory or recidivant ascites has been confirmed by 5 randomized controlled trials (RCTs) which compared TIPS and large-volume paracentesis (LVP) [23–27]. Four of these RCTs showed a superiority of TIPS in resolving severe ascites, but they did not agree on the effect of TIPS on survival. Traditional meta-analysis showed a marginal advantage of TIPS in regard

Table 1. Indications and contraindications to the use of TIPS in cirrhotic patients (adapted from the American Association for the Study of the Liver Diseases [14])

Absolute contraindications	Relative contraindications	Indications
Primary prevention of variceal bleeding	Hepatoma, especially if central	Secondary prevention of variceal bleeding
Congestive heart failure	Obstruction of all hepatic veins	Refractory ascites
Multiple hepatic cysts	Portal vein thrombosis	Refractory variceal bleeding
Uncontrolled systemic infection or sepsis	Severe coagulopathy (INR=5)	Portal hypertensive gastropathy
Unrelieved biliary obstruction	Thrombocytopenia of <20,000/cm^3	Bleeding gastric varices
Severe pulmonary hypertension	Moderate pulmonary hypertension	Gastric antral vascular ectasia[1]
		Refractory hepatic hydrothorax
		Hepatorenal syndrome (type 1 or type 2)[1]
		Budd-Chiari syndrome
		Veno-occlusive disease[1]
		Hepatopulmonary syndrome

[1] Indications that are based on uncontrolled studies or are controversial.

to survival [28, 29]. A meta-analysis on individual patient data collected by the four RCTs unequivocally showed an improved survival of patients treated with TIPS [30].

Nonetheless, TIPS can also cause important side effects: first hepatic encephalopathy, second stent malfunction because of stenosis or thrombosis, followed by a series of less-frequent but serious complications such as stent dislocation, hemolytic anemia, cardiac failure when the increase of preload exceeds the ability of the heart to increase its contractility, and the most feared complication – irreversible liver failure.

Hepatic encephalopathy occurs after TIPS in about 40% of the cases and cannot be prevented [31]. In most cases, however, the episode of encephalopathy is treated successfully by standard therapy with nonabsorbable antibiotics or disaccharides. However, in a few cases, reduction of the stent size or its occlusion is necessary to restore normal neurological function [32].

Accordingly, to obtain the best clinical benefit with the use of TIPS, it is mandatory to perform a good selection of the candidates in order to minimize the risk of side-effects and identify patients who will experience an improvement of symptoms, quality of life and, possibly, survival. A precaution to reduce the risk of encephalopathy is obtained with a portosystemic pressure gradient reduction to a final value not lower than 10 mm Hg or equal to 50% of the pre-TIPS value.

To exclude patients with a considerable risk of invalidating or lethal complications, it is necessary to carry out a careful pre-TIPS evaluation of the cardiopulmonary and liver functions. The first evaluation is necessary because TIPS causes an abrupt blood shift from the periphery to the central circulation that cannot be tolerated by patients with cardiac dysfunctions. The latter is necessary because TIPS causes an abrupt reduction of hepatic parenchymal venous blood perfusion. In most cases, this blood flow reduction is compensated by a concomitant hepatic arterial overflow (buffer effect), but this mechanism could be insufficient in patients with too advanced cirrhosis [33, 34].

There is wide consensus that TIPS should be excluded in patients with organic cardiac disorders, such as systolic and diastolic cardiac failure, severe arrhythmias, severe valve incompetence, high right atrial pressure, and pulmonary hypertension (>50 mm Hg). Thus, the candidate patient should be investigated with clinical history, examination, electrocardiography, and echocardiography. In some cases, also cardiac magnetic resonance imaging or cardiac catheterization are useful.

In contrast, to prevent cases of terminal liver failure, it is advisable exclude patients with too-advanced liver failure as can be indicated by high Child-Pugh or MELD (Model for End-Stage Liver Disease) scores or simply by high bilirubin levels.

Many investigations have been addressed to identify predictors of various post-TIPS outcomes, such as clinical efficacy, survival and development of complications (mainly hepatic encephalopathy) (table 2).

Some of these investigations created prognostic models based on the statistical association between pre-TIPS variables and post-TIPS events. Most of these models were obtained in populations of cirrhotic patients who were treated with TIPS either to prevent rebleeding or to treat severe ascites.

Prediction of Post-TIPS Survival

The most famous predictor of survival is the model of end-stage liver disease or MELD. This model consists of a formula based on the determinations of three simple biochemical variables, i.e. bilirubin, creatinine and prothrombin time expressed as international normalized ratio [35]. MELD was shown to predict short-term post-TIPS survival, and was also shown to predict survival in cirrhotic patients not treated with a portosystemic shunt. Accordingly, since 2002 it is used in United States to prioritize patients on the liver transplant waiting list. A new score including serum sodium into the original formula of MELD (the so-called MELD-Na) improved the prognostic performance in patients waiting for liver transplantation, especially in those with a relatively low MELD score [36]. MELD-Na has been shown to predict mortality also after TIPS [37].

Table 2. Studies which investigated factors predicting survival or other outcomes in patients undergoing TIPS

Study	Sample size	TIPS indications	Type of stent	Type of study
Harrod-Kim et al. [41]	99	refractory ascites	uncovered/covered	retrospective
Riggio et al. [44]	78	prevention of variceal bleeding, refractory ascites, refractory hydrothorax	covered	prospective
Guy et al. [37]	148	refractory ascites recurrent variceal bleeding	uncovered/covered	retrospective
Angermayr et al. [45]	566	elective TIPS, refractory ascites prevention of recurrent variceal bleeding	uncovered vs. covered	retrospective
Thalheimer et al. [40]	61	refractory ascites	uncovered	retrospective
Malinchoc et al. [35]	231	elective TIPS, refractory ascites prevention of recurrent variceal bleeding	uncovered	retrospective
Chalasani et al. [46]	129	variceal bleeding, refractory ascites, hepatic hydrothorax	uncovered	retrospective
Rabie et al. [39]	101	elective TIPS, refractory ascites, prevention of recurrent variceal bleeding	uncovered/covered	retrospective
Cazzaniga et al. [38]	32	elective TIPS, refractory ascites, prevention of recurrent variceal bleeding	uncovered/covered	prospective
Lebrec et al. [23]	25 (13 patients treated with TIPS)	refractory ascites	uncovered	RCT

Predictors of survival	Predictors of PSE	Predictors of QOL	Predictors of efficacy on ascites clearance
MELD>25 Child-Pugh C class portosystemic gradient after TIPS <8 mm Hg			
	age (HR 1.08) creatinine (HR 1.51) albumin (HR 0.35) sodium (HR 0.92)		
MELDNa (HR 1.09) MELD (HR 1.08)			
type of stent (HR 2.24) age (HR 1.038) Child-Pugh score (HR 1.21)			
creatinine (HR 1.02) Child-Pugh score (HR 2.03) encephalopathy (HR 3.01) platelet count (HR 1.04)	age		none
creatinine (HR 0.957) INR (HR 1.12) bilirubin (HR 0.378) cause of cirrhosis (HR 0.64)			
emergent TIPS ALT (>100) bilirubin (>3 mg/dl) pre-TIPS encephalopathy			
MELD (HR 1.1) E/A ratio <1 (HR 4.7)			age (HR 0.93) E/A ratio <1(HR 7.3)
1-month post-TIPS E/A ratio <1 (HR 8.9)			

Table 2. Continued

Study	Sample size	TIPS indications	Type of stent	Type of study
Rossle et al. [24]	60 (31 patients treated with TIPS)	refractory ascites	uncovered	RCT
Gines et al. [25]	70 (35 patients treated with TIPS)	refractory ascites	uncovered	RCT
Sanyal et al. [26]	109 (52 patients treated with TIPS)	refractory ascites	uncovered	RCT
Salerno et al. [27]	66 (33 patients treated with TIPS)	refractory ascites	uncovered	RCT
Salerno et al. [30]	149 patients treated with TIPS	refractory ascites	uncovered	meta-analysis of 4 RCTs
Campbell et al. [43]	106 (49 patients treated with TIPS)	refractory ascites	uncovered/covered	RCT
Ochs et al. [47]	50	refractory ascites	uncovered	prospective
Somberg et al. [20]	77			retrospective

Predictors of survival	Predictors of PSE	Predictors of QOL	Predictors of efficacy on ascites clearance
treatment with LVP age >60 gender bilirubin >3 sodium <125			
Child-Pugh class BUN levels	treatment with TIPS BUN levels		
treatment with LVP MELD			
age (>60) bilirubin (>3 mg/dl) sodium (<130)			
		physical component scale: baseline PCS (–0.53) 3 or more LVP (–5.1) confusion (–4.1) mental component scale: baseline MCS (–0.57) randomization to TIPS (5.29)	
age response to TIPS organic kidney disease bilirubin >1.3			
	etiology of liver disease other than alcohol female gender hypoalbuminemia		

Another means to predict post-TIPS survival was based on the evaluation of the cardiac and peripheral hemodynamics either pre- or post-TIPS. Accordingly, Cazzaniga et al. [38], studying an Italian population of cirrhotic patients treated with TIPS either to prevent variceal rebleeding either to treat refractory ascites, found that an echocardiography measurement of diastolic function, the E/A ratio, recorded 30 days after TIPS insertion strongly predicts patients' survival . This study was followed by new and more numerous investigations which showed that the pre-TIPS E/A ratio is also correlated with post-TIPS survival [39]. The association of the E/A ratio and TIPS outcome can be explained in two ways. First, a low E/A ratio indicates diastolic dysfunction and can then predict cardiac inability to manage with the post-TIPS hemodynamic re-setting. Second, it is conceivable that a low E/A ratio is a feature of patients with more advanced cirrhosis and then it is associated with a risk of rapid evolution to end-stage liver failure post-TIPS. This second hypothesis was supported by a close correlation between the E/A ratio and MELD score [38].

However, all these predictions of post-TIPS survival were obtained in populations with mixed indications for TIPS. This does not ensure that the same variables maintain their predictive value when tested in a population of patients with unique indications for TIPS. Accordingly, predictors have also been evaluated in studies that included only patients undergoing TIPS because of refractory or recidivant ascites. In a retrospective analysis, Thalheimer et al. [40] found that high Child-Pugh score, high serum creatinine, low platelet count and a history of encephalopathy were independent predictors of death in patients undergoing TIPS for ascites. Harrod-Kim et al. [41] retrospectively analyzed 99 patients who underwent successful TIPS insertion for refractory ascites and found that Child-Pugh class C, a MELD score greater than 25, and a portosystemic pressure gradient reduction below 8 mm Hg were independent predictors of post-TIPS mortality. Finally, the meta-analysis which included the individual data from 149 patients treated with TIPS compared to 156 patients treated with LVP clearly identified 3 different predictors of mortality, which are age greater than 60 years, serum bilirubin greater than 3 mg/dl, and serum sodium lower than 130 mEq/l, together with a high MELD score [30].

Predictors of Efficacy

Only one study found two predictors of efficacy (ascites clearance): younger age and a normal baseline E/A ratio [39].

Post-TIPS Quality of Life

Gulberg et al. [42] assessed the effect of TIPS on quality of life in cirrhotic patients with refractory or recidivant ascites and demonstrated that the quality of life index

Table 3. Variables predicting post-TIPS outcomes: thresholds for different risks in cirrhotic patients with refractory ascites[1]

Variables	Risk		
	low	intermediate	high
Serum bilirubin, mg/dl	<3	3–5	>5
Serum sodium, mEq/l[2]	>135	125–135	<125
Age, years	<60	60–70	>70
MELD score	<15	15–21	>21
Child-Pugh score	<10	10–11	>11

[1]Biochemical variables should be measured in stable conditions (no bleeding, no fever, etc.).
[2]Serum sodium should be measured with diuretics off.

significantly increased from 6.9 to 8.6 ($p < 0.001$). Specifically, the improvement of quality of life was more pronounced in patients with a complete response to TIPS.

Campbell et al. [43] investigated the quality of life after TIPS or LVP performed for refractory ascites and found that TIPS, baseline lack of confusion, less hospitalizations and improved ascites were independently associated with an improved quality of life.

Post-TIPS Hepatic Encephalopathy

In the meta-analysis on RCTs performed to compare TIPS and LVP [27] post-TIPS encephalopathy was significantly and independently predicted by baseline low blood pressure, baseline high MELD score and post-TIPS low portosystemic pressure gradient. Riggio et al. [44] studying 78 patients treated with PTFE-covered TIPS observed episodes of encephalopathy in 35 patients. Older age, high creatinine levels, low serum sodium and low albumin values were shown to be independent predictors of encephalopathy. Additionally, high creatinine levels strongly predicted cases of refractory encephalopathy.

In conclusion, taking into account the variability of the populations studied and of the results obtained by different studies, it is recommended to select candidates according to a stepwise path to achieve the best result with TIPS in patients with refractory or recidivant ascites.

First of all, it is important to exclude patients with absolute contraindications to TIPS (table 1). About 40% of cirrhotic patients with refractory ascites have one or more absolute contraindication to TIPS. The most important are cardiac failure, severe pulmonary dysfunctions, pulmonary hypertension, multiple liver cysts, biliary dilatation, and sepsis. Second, patients who are suspected of developing a relative failure of cardiac contractility (patients with a E/A ratio <1) should be evaluated by a deep evaluation of cardiac-related risks. Third, patients without absolute contraindications should be carefully evaluated for their chance to improve after TIPS and their probability for long-term survival. To do this, it is useful to take into account those variables that have been found to predict outcomes, mainly survival, but also encephalopathy and quality of life. The four most important predictors of post-TIPS survival are age, serum bilirubin, serum sodium, and MELD or Child-Pugh scores. Table 3 reports a tentative classification of the risks according to different thresholds for each variable.

Key Messages

- To obtain the best benefit from TIPS, cirrhotic patients with refractory ascites should be carefully evaluated for exclusion criteria. About 40% of such patients have one or more absolute contraindications to TIPS such as cardiac failure, severe pulmonary dysfunction or pulmonary hypertension, multiple liver cysts, biliary duct dilatation, and sepsis.
- Further evaluation in patients without contraindications to TIPS and their probability to achieve a beneficial effect from TIPS should include objective predictive factors and prognostic scores.
- The most relevant predictors of post-TIPS survival in patients with refractory ascites are age, serum bilirubin, serum sodium, and MELD or Child-Pugh scores.

References

1 Rosch J, Hanafee WN, Snow H: Transjugular portal venography and radiologic portacaval shunt: an experimental study. Radiology 1969;92:1112–1114.
2 Rosch J, Hanafee W, Snow H, Barenfus M, Gray R: Transjugular intrahepatic portacaval shunt: an experimental work. Am J Surg 1971;121:588–592.
3 Colapinto RF, Stronell RD, Birch SJ, et al: Creation of an intrahepatic portosystemic shunt with a Gruntzig balloon catheter. Can Med Assoc J 1982; 126:267–268.
4 Palmaz JC, Sibbitt RR, Reuter SR, Garcia F, Tio FO: Expandable intrahepatic portacaval shunt stents: early experience in the dog. Am J Roentgenol 1985; 145:821–825.
5 Rössle M, Richter GM, Nöldge G, et al: New nonoperative treatment for variceal haemorrhage. Lancet 1989;ii:153.
6 Bureau C, Pagan JC, Layrargues GP, et al: Patency of stents covered with polytetrafluoroethylene in patients treated by transjugular intrahepatic portosystemic shunts: long-term results of a randomized multicentre study. Liver Int 2007;27:742–747.
7 Jung HS, Kalva SP, Green field AJ, et al: TIPS: comparison of shunt patency and clinical outcomes between bare stents and expanded polytetrafluoroethylene stent-grafts. J Vasc Inerven Radiol 2009;20: 180–185.
8 Rössle M, Gerbes AL: TIPS for ascites – a critical appraisal. Gut 2010;in press.
9 Castells A, Saló J, Planas R, et al: Impact of shunt surgery for variceal bleeding in the natural history of ascites in cirrhosis: a retrospective study. Hepatology 1994;20:584–591.
10 Morali GA, Sniderman KW, Deitel KM, et al: Is sinusoidal portal hypertension a necessary factor for the development of hepatic ascites? J Hepatol 1992;16:249–250.
11 Banares R, Casado M, Rodriguez-Laiz JM, et al: Urgent transjugular intrahepatic portosystemic shunt for control of acute variceal bleeding. Am J Gastroenterol 1998;93:75–79.

12 Michl P, Bilzer M, Waggershauser T, et al: Successful treatment of chronic Budd-Chiari syndrome with a transjugular intrahepatic portosysemic shunt. J Hepatol 2000;32:516–520.
13 Gordon FD, Anastopoulos HT, Crenshaw W, et al: The successful treatment of symptomatic, refractory hepatic hydrothorax with transjugular intrahepatic portosystemic shunt. Hepatology 1997;25:1366–1369.
14 Boyer TD, Haskal ZJ: The role of transjugular intrahepatic portosystemic shunt in the management of portal hypertension. Hepatology 2005;41:386–400.
15 Salerno F, Cazzaniga M, Pagnozzi G, et al: Humoral and cardiac effects of TIPS in cirrhotic patients with different 'effective' blood volume. Hepatology 2003; 38:1370–1377.
16 Stanlej AJ, Redhead DN, Bouchier IAD, et al: Acute effects of the transjugular intrahepatic stent-shunt (TIPSS) on renal blood flow and cardiopulmonary haemodynamics in cirrhosis. Am J Gastroenterol 1998;93:2463–2468.
17 Lang F, Tschernko E, Schulze E, et al: Hepatorenal reflex regulating kidney function. Hepatology 1991; 14:590–598.
18 Wong F, Sniderman K, Liu P, et al: Transjugular intrahepatic portosystemic stent shunt: effects on hemodynamics and sodium homeostasis in cirrhosis and refractory ascites. Ann Intern Med 1995;122: 816–822.
19 Ferral H, Bjarnason H, Wegryn SA, et al: Refractory ascites: early experience in treatment with transjugular intrahepatic portosystemic shunt. Radiology 1993;189:795–801.
20 Somberg KA, Lake JR, Tomlanovich SJ, et al: Transjugular intrahepatic portosystemic shunt for refractory ascites: assessment of clinical and humoral response and renal function. Hepatology 1995;21:709–716.
21 Quiroga J, Sangro B, Nunez M, et al: Transjugular intrahepatic portal-systemic shunt in the management of refractory ascites: effect on clinical, renal, humoral and hemodynamic parameters. Hepatology 1995;21:986–994.
22 Guevara M, Gines P, Bandi JC, et al: Transjugular intrahepatic portosystemic shunt in hepatorenal syndrome: effects on renal function and vasoactive systems. Hepatology 1998;28:416–422.
23 Lebrec D, Giuily N, Hadengue A, et al: Transjugular intrahepatic portosystemic shunts: comparison with paracentesis in patients with cirrhosis and refractory ascites. J Hepatol 1996;25:135–144.
24 Rossle M, Ochs A, Gulberg V, et al: A comparison of paracentesis and transjugular intrahepatic portosystemic shunting in patients with ascites. N Engl J Med 2000;342:1701–1707.
25 Gines P, Uriz J, Calahorra B, et al: Transjugular intrahepatic portosystemic shunting versus paracentesis plus albumin for refractory ascites in cirrhosis. Gastroenterology 2002;123:1839–1847.
26 Sanyal AJ, Genning C, Reddy KR, et al: The North American study for the treatment of refractory ascites. Gastroenterology 2003;124:634–641.
27 Salerno F, Merli M, Riggio O: Randomized controlled study of TIPS versus paracentesis plus albumin in cirrhosis with severe ascites. Hepatology 2004;40:629–635.
28 Albillos A, Banares R, Gonzalez M, et al: A meta-analysis of transjugular intrahepatic portosystemic shunt versus paracentesis for refractory ascites. J Hepatol 2005;43:990–996.
29 D'amico G, Luca A, Morabito A, et al: Uncovered transjugular intrahepatic portosystemic shunt for refractory ascites: a meta-analysis. Gastroenetero-logy 2005;129:1282–1293.
30 Salerno F, Camma A, Enea M, et al: Transjugular intrahepatic portosystemic shunt for refractory ascites: a meta-analysis of individual patient data. Gastroenterology 2007;133:825–834.
31 Sanyal AJ, Freedman AM, Shiffman ML, et al: Portosystemic encephalopathy after transjugular intrahepatic portosystemic shunt: results of a prospective controlled study. Hepatology 1994;20:46–55.
32 Kerlan RK Jr, LaBerge JM, Baker EL, et al: Successful reversal of hepatic encephalopathy with intentional occlusion of transjugular intrahepatic portosystemic shunts. J Vasc Interv Radiol 1995;6:917–921.
33 Kleber G, Steudel N, Behrmann C, et al: Hepatic arterial flow volume and reserve in patients with cirrhosis: use of intra-arterial Doppler and adenosine infusion. Gastroenterology 1999;116:906–914.
34 Gulberg V, Haag K, Rossle M, Gerbes AL: Hepatic arterial buffer response in patients with advanced cirrhosis. Hepatology 2002;35:630–634.
35 Malinchoc M, Kamath PS, Gordon FG, et al: A model to predict poor survival in patients undergoing transjugular intrahepatic portosystemic shunts. Hepatology 2000;31:864–871.
36 Biggins SW, Kim WR, Terrault NA, et al: Evidence-based incorporation of serum sodium concentration into MELD. Gastroenterology 2006;130: 1652–1660.
37 Guy J, Somsouk M, Shibosky S, et al: New model for end-stage liver disease improves prognostic capability after transjugular intrahepatic portosystemic shunt. Clin Gastroenterol Hepatol 2009;7:1236–1240.
38 Cazzaniga M, Salerno F, Pagnozzi G, et al: Diastolic dysfunction is associated with poor survival in patients with cirrhosis with transjugular intrahepatic portosystemic shunt. Gut 2007;56:869–875.

39 Rabie RN, Cazzaniga M, Salerno F, Wong F: The use of E/A ratio as a predictor of outcome in cirrhotic patients treated with transjugular intrahepatic portosystemic shunt. Am J Gastroenterol 2009;104: 2458–2464.
40 Thalheimer U, Leandro G, Samonakis DN, et al: TIPS for refractory ascites: a single-centre experience. J Gastroenterol. 2009;44:1089–1095.
41 Harrod-Kim P, Saad W, Waldman D: Predictors of early mortality after transjugular intrahepatic portosystemic shunt creation for the treatment of refractory ascites. J Vasc Interv Radiol 2006;17:1605–1610.
42 Gülberg V, Liss I, Bilzer M, et al: Improved quality of life in patients with refractory or recidivant ascites after insertion of transjugular intrahepatic portosystemic shunts. Digestion 2002;66:127–130.
43 Campbell MS, Brensinger CM, Sanyal AJ, et al: Quality of life in refractory ascites: transjugular intrahepatic portal-systemic shunting vs. medical therapy. Hepatology 2005;42:635–640.
44 Riggio O, Angeloni S, Salvatori FM, et al: Incidence, natural history, and risk factors of hepatic encephalopathy after transjugular intrahepatic portosystemic shunt with polytetrafluoroetylene-covered stent graft. Am J Gastroenterol 2008;103:2738–2746.
45 Angermayr B, Cejna M, Koenig F, et al: Survival in patients undergoing transjugular intrahepatic portosystemic shunt: a PTFE-covered stent graft vs. bare stents. Hepatology 2003;38:1043–1050.
46 Chalasani N, Scott Clark W, Martin LG, et al: Determinants of mortality in patients with advanced cirrhosis after transjugular intrahepatic portosystemic shunting. Gastroenterology 2000;118:138–144.
47 Ochs A, Rossle M, Hag K, et al: Transjugular intrahepatic portosystemic stent-shunt procedure for refractory ascites. N Engl J Med 1995;332:1192–1197.

Francesco Salerno, MD
IRCCS Policlinico San Donato
Via Morandi, 30
IT–20097 San Donato Milanese (Italy)
Tel./Fax +39 025 277 4462, E-Mail francesco.salerno@unimi.it

Gerbes AL (ed): Ascites, Hyponatremia and Hepatorenal Syndrome: Progress in Treatment.
Front Gastrointest Res. Basel, Karger, 2011, vol 28, pp 65–82

Spontaneous Bacterial Peritonitis – Prophylaxis and Treatment

R. Wiest[a] · G. Garcia-Tsao[b]

[a]Klinik und Poliklinik für Innere Medizin I, Universitätsklinikum Regensburg, Regensburg, Deutschland; [b]Digestive Diseases Section, Yale University School of Medicine, New Haven, Conn., and Digestive Diseases Section, VA-CT Healthcare System, West Haven, Conn., USA

Abstract

Cirrhosis predisposes to the development of severe bacterial infections, mainly spontaneous bacteremia and spontaneous bacterial peritonitis (SBP). These life-threatening infections occur in up to 50% of cirrhotic patients during hospitalization and are responsible for 20–40% of deaths in these patients. Therefore, prompt effective therapy and prophylaxis of these spontaneous infections are crucial in order to improve the prognosis of patients with cirrhosis and ascites. Patients with a history of SBP or those presenting with gastrointestinal hemorrhage require antibiotic prophylaxis. Despite substantial improvement in the identification of patients at high risk of developing the first episode of SBP, antibiotic prophylaxis in this setting is still controversial. This is mostly related to the emergence of bacterial resistance to antibiotics induced by widespread and long-term antibiotic treatment. In fact, SBP caused by bacteria resistant to currently recommended antibiotics is increasing and associated with increased risk of treatment failure and mortality. Therefore, this chapter discusses the current guidelines and available data on the prophylaxis and therapy of SBP as well as the potential drawbacks and limitations necessitating further well-designed clinical trials.

Definition and Clinical Importance

Spontaneous bacterial peritonitis (SBP) is a frequent and life-threatening complication in cirrhotic patients with ascites. The diagnosis is based on the absence of any evident intra-abdominal source of infection (e.g. pancreatitis, perforation, tuberculosis) and the presence of an inflammatory reaction to the peritoneal infection [1, 2] evidenced by a polymorphonuclear leukocyte count (PMN) in ascitic fluid greater than $250/mm^3$ (0.25×10^9/l), a cutoff that has been shown to result in the highest sensitivity. Despite improvements in culture techniques ascites culture is negative in more than 40% of patients fulfilling these criteria. However, treatment cannot be delayed until microbiological results are available and, hence, positive culture result is not an essential criterion for the definition of SBP.

The prevalence of SBP in cirrhotic outpatients is usually very low at about 5% whereas SBP develops in about 10–12% of patients admitted to the hospital. Moreover, SBP will develop in up to 30% of patients already hospitalized, making it the most frequent type of bacterial infection in cirrhosis. SBP-related mortality exceeded 90% when it was first described but has been reduced to about 20% due to early diagnosis and treatment [3].

SBP may present with local symptoms of peritonitis, systemic signs of infection, deterioration of liver or renal function, hepatic encephalopathy, shock or gastrointestinal bleeding. However, it is important to point out that up to 30% of patients with SBP are asymptomatic [4]. Therefore, it is recommended to perform a diagnostic paracentesis in all patients with cirrhosis and ascites at admission to rule out SBP. Moreover, a diagnostic paracentesis should be performed in patients with fever or other signs of infection, gastrointestinal symptoms as well as worsening liver and/or renal function, gastrointestinal bleeding and hepatic encephalopathy [1].

The 1-year survival rate after the first episode of SBP ranges between 7 and 69% underscoring the negative prognostic character of this event in the individual course of disease [4–8]. Different independent predictive factors for a poor prognosis among SBP patients have been reported including age [8, 9], Child-Pugh score [8, 10, 11], intensive care [9, 11], nosocomial genesis [11], hepatic encephalopathy [12, 13], creatinine and bilirubin [14], treatment failure and positive culture result per se [15, 16] as well as the development of bacteremia [17]. In a systematic review of the literature, the most robust independent predictors of death in SBP are the presence of acute kidney injury, the MELD score and lack of SBP resolution [Tandon and Garcia-Tsao, unpubl. obs.].

Pathogenesis and Risk Factors

Two facts point to the gut as the main source of bacteria in the development of community-acquired SBP. First, more than 70% of cases of SBP are caused by aerobic Gram-negative bacilli [18], and, second, selective gut decontamination with oral antibiotics is able to prevent most of these infections [19–21]. Intestinal bacteria reach the bloodstream and ascites through a process denominated bacterial translocation which is defined as the passage of viable bacteria from the gut to mesenteric lymph nodes and/or other extraintestinal sites [22]. Three factors have been implicated in the development of BT in liver cirrhosis: intestinal bacterial overgrowth (IBO), increased intestinal permeability and impaired immunity. It is important to stress that, although studied separately, these factors most likely act jointly, e.g. community-acquired SBP is the result of failure of the gut to contain bacteria and failure of the immune system to kill bacteria once they have escaped the gut.

IBO, predominantly with aerobic Gram-negative bacteria, has been demonstrated both in cirrhotic rats and in patients with cirrhosis, especially in severe liver disease [23–25]. An imbalance of the intestinal microflora is crucial for the process of microbial translocation since anaerobic bacteria, which represent approximately 99% of the gut flora, do not translocate readily, while aerobic Gram-negative bacilli translocate easily, even across a histologically intact intestinal epithelium [26, 27]. The majority of bacteria translocating in cirrhosis are exactly these Gram-negative bacteria, especially *Enterobacteriaceae* (mainly *E. coli*) [25, 28–32]. In addition, mucosal intestinal barrier dysfunction has been demonstrated in experimental and human advanced cirrhosis [33, 34] and is thought to be mediated at least in part by ultrastructural changes [35], oxidative stress [36] as well as alterations in the secretory barrier component, e.g. immunoglobulin A or bile acids [37]. Host defense mechanisms are defective in advanced cirrhosis including impaired innate immune response as well as changes in adaptive immunity. For instance, dysfunction of the reticuloendothelial and mononuclear system due to lack of opsonization and migratory capabilities results in reduced phagocytic and killing capacity [38, 39]. This impairment in host immune response acts synergistically with bacterial overgrowth to promote bacterial translocation and may play a crucial role in the spreading of translocated pathogenic bacteria [40]. In hospital-acquired SBP these defects in the host defense predispose to the acquisition of bacterial infections, e.g. during invasive procedures. Therefore, organisms responsible for nosocomial SBP are not exclusively enteric Gram-negative flora but predominantly nonenteric Gram-positive infections [41].

All cirrhotic patients with ascites are at risk of SBP; however, there is a wide range in incidence, depending on the presence of additional risk factors. Patients presenting with any of the following are prone to the development of SBP: (a) gastrointestinal bleeding, (b) low-protein ascitic fluid (<1.5 g/dl) or (c) a previous history of SBP. Gastrointestinal hemorrhage can trigger spontaneous bacterial infections via multiple mechanisms including increased intestinal permeability, enhanced bacterial translocation and reduced RES function [42]. Ascites protein levels correlate with local concentrations of complement factors and opsonic activity [43] and, thus, a low protein level indicates a lack of local ascites defenses. In patients with ascites protein levels >1.5 g/dl, the incidence of SBP is as low as 0–3% as compared to 14–23% in patients with an ascites protein <1.5 g/dl [5, 44]. Additional factors shown to be predictive of SBP include serum bilirubin >3.2 mg/dl and platelet count <98,000/mm [45]. Also, the risk of SBP is associated with the use of proton pump inhibitors [46] as well as increasing MELD-score [47]. Interestingly, SBP has also been shown to be increased in carriers of NOD2/CARD15 variants known to be linked with impaired intestinal mucosal barrier function [48]. In patients who have recovered from SBP, the recurrence rate is very high, ranging between 30 and 68% [6, 19] reflecting the persistence of risk factors that led to the first episode.

Prophylaxis

Since 30–50% of deaths in patients with cirrhosis are attributable to infections, prophylaxis is of crucial relevance when aiming to improve survival. Development of the first episode of SBP is an important risk factor for future episodes of SBP and is a predictor of mortality [49]. Therefore, secondary prophylaxis after the first episode of SBP is well accepted and recommended by current guidelines [1, 3]. The use of quinolones in this setting reduces the risk of recurrent SBP from 68 to 20% [19]. With the same strong consensus agreement, prophylactic antibiotic treatment is recommended in the setting of gastrointestinal bleeding in patients with cirrhosis. Meta-analyses have evidenced that this approach significantly reduces the risk of SBP and/or bacteremia with a significant improvement in survival [50, 51]. Regarding the choice of antibiotic in this setting, norfloxacin has been recommended by consensus [62]. However, in patients with advanced cirrhosis defined by two of the following criteria (severe malnutrition, hepatic encephalopathy or bilirubin >3 mg/dl) ceftriaxone i.v. has been demonstrated to be superior to oral norfloxacin after upper GI hemorrhage regarding the probability of remaining free from spontaneous bacterial infections (SBP or bacteremia) [52]. This benefit most likely reflects the extended spectrum of bacteria including Gram-positive rods as well as quinolone-resistant bacteria. Although a prospective evaluation is not available, the antibiotic treatment should be started as soon as possible, at best before endoscopy, and should last for at least 7 days [2]., although it could be discontinued if the patient is ready to be discharged from the hospital before the 7-day course is completed.

In the absence of GI hemorrhage, the use of antibiotics in the prevention of a first episode of SBP in patients with low-protein ascites (<1.5 g/dl) is still controversial despite two meta-analyses [53, 54]. Table 1 summarizes randomized-controlled trials on primary prophylaxis in high-risk cirrhotic patients. However, it needs to be emphasized that four of these trials had significant deficiencies as they included a substantial number of patients with a previous history of SBP [21, 55–57], i.e. a population with a significantly higher risk of SBP. The remaining four better-designed trials were analyzed in two recent meta-analyses achieving different conclusions [53, 54]. However, one of them has mistakenly mixed up numbers of events for primary endpoints and thus is erroneous [54, 58]. The second analysis revealed a significant reduction in incidence of SBP as well as mortality in patients treated with quinolones compared to placebo. However, this analysis also had studies that included patients with a significantly different risk of developing SBP, with the first three having a 1-year rate of ~13% [59–61] while the most recent one [27] that selected a subgroup of patients among those with low ascites protein had a 1-year rate of 30%. In the three studies with low-risk patients, antibiotics reduced SBP significantly but survival was not different. The study by Fernandez et al. [62] subselected a group of patients with low ascites protein presenting with at least one of the following additional factors: severe liver insufficiency (Child-Pugh score ≥9 with bilirubin ≥3 mg/dl), or renal insufficiency (serum creatinine ≥1.2 mg/dl, serum urea ≥25 mg/dl or serum sodium ≤130 mEq/l). In this well-defined far-advanced stage of disease norfloxacin treatment over 1 year did achieve a marked reduction in incidence of SBP (7% vs. 61%, $p < 0.001$) as well as improvement in 1-year survival (60% vs. 48%, $p < 0.05$). However, this survival benefit was most marked in the first 3 months after the start of antibiotic prophylaxis (94% vs. 62%, $p < 0.003$) and degraded thereafter. This has been suggested to be due to the increased mortality independent of spontaneous infections and/or development of resistant bacteria over time [54, 62, 63]. Thus, a rational approach may be to use primary prophylactic antibiotics only in highly selected patients with advanced liver cirrhosis fulfilling the criteria stated above and limited for short or medium terms, particularly for bridging to liver transplantation.

Future Developments for Prophylaxis

Any chronic antibiotic prophylaxis has serious drawbacks, specifically the emergence of bacterial resistance and a change in the spectrum of bacteria causing infections, namely a shift towards Gram-positive bacteria. Cirrhotic patients undergoing selective intestinal decontamination using quinolones have an increased rate of quinolone-resistant Gram-negative enteric bacteria [41] which can subsequently cause spontaneous infections, e.g. SBP [64, 65]. Intermittent or even once-a-week quinolone treatment schedules have been proposed as effective antibiotic prophylaxis in cirrhotic patients [56], but have a higher risk of developing resistant bacteria [66] and should thus be avoided. In addition, due to the widespread use of antibiotic prophylaxis, the rate of multidrug-resistant organisms isolated from cirrhotic ascites increased from 8 to 38% in an earlier (1991–1995) compared to a later (1996–2001) cohort [65]. In recent years, these numbers have increased further, with 53% quinolone resistance, 34% ESBL and 24% multidrug-resistant organism rates [67, 68]. Also, resistance to third-generation cephalosporins has been reported in up to a third of SBP cases [64, 68] with use of antibiotics in the 3 previous months being the most important independent risk factor (OR 5.98 [3.58–9.97] $p < 0.0001$) [69]. Furthermore, prior quinolone prophylaxis in cirrhotic patients has been shown to increase the risk of Gram-positive bacterial infections [41], *Clostridium difficile* infections [70] and carriage of methicillin-resistant *Staphylococcus aureus* (MRSA) [71–73], leading to the emergence of infections due to this organism [74]. Thus, any benefit achievable by prophylactic antibiotic treatment as outlined above has to be weighed against these major drawbacks and associated consequences. These include not only an increased risk of morbidity, excess length of hospital stay and increased health care costs but also an increased mortality [75] and the potential of further transmission of these resistant organisms to other patients.

Table 1. Randomized controlled trials on antibiotic primary prophylaxis of SBP

Author, year	Intervention, control/ comparator	Patient number verum/ placebo	Follow-up	Previous SBP	GI bleed	Ascites-protein content g/l	Bilirubin mg/dl	Creatinine mg/dl	Child-Pugh score class A/B/C	Exclusion criteria
Soriano, 1991 [20]	norfloxacin 400 mg/day vs. no therapy	32/31	n.a.	6%	4/61 (6.6%)	all <1.5 TP: 0.71+0.3 vs.control: 0.67+0.3	TP: 5.67+7.07 control: 4.66+5.91	TP: 1.07+0.49 control: 1.16+0.74	TP: 2/3/17 control: 1/14/16	active infection GI bleed
Rolachon, 1995 [56]	ciprofloxacin 750 mg/week vs.placebo	28/32	6 months	11%	no	all <1.5 TP: 0.94+0.3 vs.control: 1.03+0.3	TP: 2.46+1.81 control: 2.8+2.7	TP:0.89+0.19 control: 0.83+0.27	TP: 0/17/11 control: 1/18/13	HCC GI-bleed HE Crea > 1.35 mg/dl
Singh, 1995 [57]	trimetoprim-sulfameth-oxacole double-strength 1×/day (5 days/week) vs.no therapy	30/30	median 90 days (7–682)	22%	13%	no data	TP: 2.2 (no SD) control: 2.0 (no SD)	TP: 1.1 (no SD) control: 0.9	no data	no data
Novella, 1997 [60]	norfloxacin 400 mg/day vs. norfloxacin 400 mg/day	56/53	43 + 3 weeks	no	23/109 (>21%)	TP: 1.0+0.2 vs. control: 0.9+0.1	TP: 3.8+0.3 control: 4.1+0.3	TP: 1.1+0.8 control: 0.9+0.06	TP: 0/29/27 control: 0/24/29	HCC bilirubin >15 mg/dl

SBP incidence	Survival	Comment	Resistance	Allocation sequence	Allocation conceal-ment	Blinding	Outcome data complete	ITT	Approxi-mate number of cases	Compliance/ drop-out
TP: 0/32 (0%) control: 7/31 (22.5%) $p < 0.05$	TP: 30/32 (93.7%) control: 26/31 (83.9%) n.s.	1 bacterocytes in each group extraperitoneal infection reduced (1/32 [3.1%] vs. 7/31 [22.5%], $p = 0.052$)	no data	?	?	–	+	+	–	
TP: 1/28 (3.6%) control: 7/32 (22%) $p < 0.05$	TP: 24/28 (85.7%) control: 26/32 (81.2%) n.s.	no effect on extraperitoneal infections (11 % vs. 12.5%) hospitalization shorter in cipro-group (9.3+4.5 vs. 17.6 + 6.2 days, $p < 0.05$)	10/28 patients feces: no cipro-resistance within 6 months	?	?	+	+	+	+	n = 3 non-compliant n = 5 withdrawal or lost to follow-up in total 13%
TP: 1/30 (3%) control: 7/30 (23.3%) 8/30 (27%) for endpoint *$p < 0.05$	TP: 28/30 (93%) control: 24/30 (80%) n.s.	primary endpoint =SBP or spontaneous bacteremia in-exclusion criteria wide – risk factors (total protein ascites <1, bilirubin >3, creatinine >2) only stratified not selected	no data	?	?	–	?	+	–	
TP: 1/56 (1.8%) control: 9/53 (16.9%) $p < 0.01$	TP: 75% control: 62% n.s.	no effect on nosocomial SBP	90% *E. coli* (9/19) in norfloxacin-group chinolone-resistant: among those 5 with clinical infection, all sensitive to ceftriaxone	?	+	–	?	?	–	drop-out rate: >10%

Table 1. Continued

Author, year	Intervention, control/ comparator	Patient number verum/ placebo	Follow-up	Previous SBP	GI bleed	Ascites-protein content g/l	Bilirubin mg/dl	Creatinine mg/dl	Child-Pugh score class A/B/C	Exclusion criteria
Grange, 1998 [59]	norfloxacin 400 mg/ day vs. placebo	53/54	6 months	no	no	all < 1.5 TP: 0.93+0.29 control: 1.04+ 0.0.28	TP: 5.1+0.8 control: 3.8+0.6	TP: 0.8+0.2 control: 0.8+0.1	no data	active GI bleed HCC
Alvarez, 2005 [55]	norfloxacin 400 mg/day vs. trimetoprim-sulfameth-oxacole (160/800 mg) 5 days/week	32/25	3–547 days	39%	no	also patients with TP > 1.5 norfloxacin: 0.96+0.55 SMT: 1.37+0.84 p < 0.05 between groups	norfloxacin: 4.94+ 6.88 SMT: 3.53+3.77	norfloxacin: 1.76+2.07 SMT: 1.0+ 0.43 p < 0.01	norfloxacin: 1/10/21 SMT: 0/8 /17	AB within 2 weeks GI bleed within 1 week HCC/ malignancy
Fernandez, 2007 [62]	norfloxacin 400 mg/ day vs. placebo	35/33	12 months	no	3/68 (4.4%)	all <1.5 g/l TP: 0.93+0.29 control: 1.04+0.28	TP: 3.5+2.3 control: 4.4+4.6	TP: 1.2+0.4 control: 1.2+0.4	TP: 9.9+1.5 control: 10.4+1.5	HCC HIV organic kidney disease
Terg, 2008 [61]	ciprofloxacin 500 mg/day vs. placebo	50/50	12 months	no	no data	all <1.5 g/l TP: 0.84+0.01 control: 0.85+0.36	TP: 2.9+4.6 control: 2.7+3.2	TP: 0.9+0.3 control: 0.9+0.2	TP: 8.3+1.3 control: 8.5+1.5	HE HCC/ malignancy creatinine >3 mg/dl thrombo-cytes <98,000

Bilirubin mg/dl *17.1 = μmol. Creatinine mg/dl *88.4 = μmol.

SBP incidence	Survival	Comment	Resistance	Allocation sequence	Allocation concealment	Blinding	Outcome data complete	ITT	Approximate number of cases	Compliance/drop-out
SBP or bacteremia TP: 1/53 (1.9%) control: 9/54 (16.7%) $p < 0.05$	TP: 45/53 (84.9%) control: 44/54 (81.5%) n.s.	primary endpoint = rate of Gram-negative infection no information on SBP rate	10/24 norfloxacin patients chinolone-resistant bacteria in faeces (but no clinical infection)13% infectious problems in norflox acin group: Gram-positive cocci; mainly Streptococci	?	?	?	+	+	+	4/53 and 4/54 lost to follow-up drop-out-rate 7.5% 3/53 and 2/54 noncompliant 2/53 withdrawal side effects in total 14%
norfloxacin: 3/32 (9.4%) SMT: 4/25 (16%) n.s.	norfloxacin: 25/32 (78.1%) SMT: 20/25 (75%) n.s.	no placebo significant differences in risk factors between study groups	1/32 in norfloxacin-group culture-positive urinary tract infection with chinolone-resistant Enterococcus	+	+	–	?	?	–	no data
TP: 2/35 (5.7%) control: 10/33 (30.3%) $p<0.05$	TP: 25/35 (71.4%) control: 20/33 (60.6%) n.s.	frequency of other infections not affected 3 months mortality reduced in treatment group	11/13 Gram-negative infections in the norfloxacin group chinolone-resistant vs. 1/6 in placebo group	+	+	+	+	+	?	3/35 and 2/33 lost to follow-up 1 protocol violation 3/35 and 3/33 non-compliant
TP: 2/50 (4%) control: 7/50 (14%) n.s.	TP: 44/50 (80%) control: 36/50 (72%) $p<0.05$	mortality not primary endpoint	2/2 isolated *E. coli* in verum group chinolone resistant	+	+	+	+	+	+	5/50 and 4/50 lost to follow-up 1/50 cipro-stop 1/50 cipro-withdrawal

Therefore, individualization of timing and cautious selection of prophylactic measures should be the focus of future research. Moreover, studies on the duration of secondary prophylaxis are needed defining endpoints of which resolution of ascites or improvement in Child-Pugh class could be reasonable options. Moreover, the potential advantage of antibiotic cycling or combined treatment regimens lowering the risk of emerging resistant bacteria has to be evaluated prospectively. Finally, an alternative nonantibiotic method that would decrease bacterial translocation and be safe and inexpensive would be desirable. This indeed could be the case for probiotics which have been reported to correct bacterial overgrowth, stabilize mucosal barrier function, and decrease BT in experimental conditions. However, prospective randomized trials in cirrhotic patients utilizing probiotics aiming at prevention of spontaneous infections are lacking. The use of prokinetics may also be beneficial since experimental data indicate that they decrease bacterial translocation [76]. However, two small studies in cirrhotic patients did not show an effect of cisapride in decreasing the incidence of SBP [77, 78]. Notably, one of them showed that 2/10 patients on placebo developed SBP and urinary infection while infections did not occur in patients on antibiotics or cisapride [77]. Cisapride is no longer available, but the efficacy of another prokinetic, prucalopride, could be investigated in the future.

Therapy

Any cirrhotic patient with an ascitic fluid PMN count $\geq 250/mm^3$ compatible with SBP must receive empiric antibiotic therapy [1, 2]. This treatment should be started immediately and independently of results of bacterial culture of ascitic fluid samples. Before starting antibiotic treatment, blood cultures should be performed since concomitant bacteremia is observed in up to 30% of the cases and is associated with a worse prognosis [17]. Potentially nephrotoxic antibiotics (e.g. aminoglycosides) should not be used as empirical therapy. Several antibiotics can be used for the initial therapy of SBP: cephalosporins, amoxicillin-clavulanic acid or quinolones (table 2), with third-generation cephalosporins being considered the drug of choice since they usually cover 95% of the flora including the most common isolates, namely *Escherichia coli, Klebsiella pneumonia* and pneumococci. The optimal cost-effective dosage has only been investigated for cefotaxime being a minimum dose of 2 g/ 12 h i.v. for a minimum duration of 5 days [79, 80]. In a single small study, amoxicillin/ clavulanic acid, first given intravenously then orally, has similar results with respect to SBP resolution and mortality compared with cefotaxime [81]. There have been more studies using quinolones [82–84]. Ciprofloxacin, either for 7 or for 2 days i.v. followed by 5 days orally, results in a similar SBP resolution rate and hospital survival compared with cefotaxime [84]. Oral ofloxacin has given similar results as cefotaxime in uncomplicated SBP [83] (absence of renal failure, hepatic encephalopathy, gastrointestinal bleeding, ileus or shock).

The emergence of bacteria resistant to the recommended first-line antibiotic regimens has been an increasingly observed problem. In fact, increased rates of treatment failure have been observed utilizing recommended antibiotics in nosocomial SBP [68] and have been associated with a worse outcome [65, 68]. Particularly alarming are increased rates of multidrug-resistant organisms causing nosocomial SBP being likewise associated with a higher mortality rate as compared to SBP due to common bacteria [65]. In fact, the mortality is higher in patients with SBP due to multidrug-resistant organisms and in those in whom antibiotic therapy needs to be changed due to treatment failure of first-line therapy [68]. This suggests that broader-spectrum first-line antibiotics, such as carbapenems or glycopeptides, should be considered in patients with nosocomial SBP.

Major risk factors independently associated with the occurrence of (multiple) resistant bacteria are hospitalization before the development of SBP and/or prior prophylactic antibiotics [85]. Therefore, quinolones should not be used in patients who (a) are on norfloxacin prophylaxis, (b) in settings with high prevalence of quinolone-resistant organisms, or (c) in nosocomial SBP. In community-acquired SBP multidrug-resistant bacteria are isolated in less than 3% of the patients. Thus, cefotaxime or other third-generation cephalosporins, or amoxicillin-clavulanic acid can still be used as the initial therapy of SBP in these patients.

SBP resolves with adequate antibiotic therapy in approximately 90% of patients. Usually, this is associated with resolution of clinical symptoms and normalization of laboratory changes indicating infection if present at diagnosis. However, clinical evolution is not sufficiently reliable and, therefore, control of treatment success is recommended. A corresponding treatment algorithm is presented in figure 1. Resolution of SBP should be proven by demonstrating a decrease in ascitic PMN count to <250/ mm^3 or at least below 25% of PMN value before antibiotic treatment [2]. Moreover, sterile culture of ascitic fluid should be evidenced if positive at diagnosis.

Future Developments for Therapy

In nosocomial SBP, appropriate well-designed clinical trials are needed to define selection criteria for patients in need of first-line treatment with carbapenems and glycopeptides. These studies should address the potential drawback of such an aggressive approach, namely the induction of even more complex resistance profiles including carbapenem- and vancomycin-resistant bacteria. Finally, the pharmacokinetic properties of the antibiotics selected should be adequate to treat peritoneal infection (e.g. antibiotic concentration in ascitic fluid >MIC90 of causative micro-organisms). Pharmacokinetic data on carbapenems and vancomycin in cirrhotic patients with ascites (and SBP) are lacking.

Regarding patients with bacterascites (positive culture but PMN <250), it is currently recommended to treat these patients only in case of signs of systemic inflammation

Table 2. Clinical trials on antibiotic treatment of SBP

Author, year	Intervention, control/comparator	Number of patients	SBP resolution	In-hospital mortality
Felisart, 1985 [86]	tobramycin (1.75 mg/kg 8 h i.v.) plus ampicillin (2 g/4 h i.v.) vs. cefotaxime (2 g/4 h i.v.)	36/37	18/32 (56%) vs. 28/33 (85%) $p < 0.02$	14/32 (39%) 10/33 (27%) n.s.
Rimola, 1995 [79]	cefotaxime (2 g/6 h i.v.) vs. cefotaxime (2 g/12 h i.v.)	71/72	51/66 (77%) vs. 55/70 (79%) n.s.	22/71 (31%) vs. 15/72 (21%) n.s.
Navasa, 1996 [83]	ofloxacin (400 mg/12 h p.o.) vs. cefotaxime (2 g/6 h i.v.)	64/59	54/64 (84%) vs. 50/59 (85%) n.s.	12/64 (19%) 11/59 (19%) n.s.
Ricart, 2000 [81]	amoxicillin/ clavulanic acid (1/0.2 g/8 h i.v.) followed by 0.5/0.125 g/8 h p.o.) vs. cefotaxime 1 g/6 h i.v.)	24/24	21/24 (87.5%) vs. 20/24 (83.8%) n.s.	3/24 (12.5%) vs. 5/24 (20.8%) n.s.
Tuncer, 2003 [87]	ciprofloxacin (500 mg/12 h) vs. cefotaxime (2 g/8 h i.v.) vs. ceftriaxone (2 g/24 h i.v.) for 5 days	15/17/17	12/15 (80%) vs. 13/17 (76.4%) vs. 14/17 (82.3%) n.s.	2/15 (13.3%) vs. 2/17 (11.7%) vs. 3/17 (17.6%) n.s.
Terg, 2000 [84]	ciprofloxacin (200 mg/12 h for 7 days) vs. ciprofloxacin (200 mg/12 h i.v. for 2 days followed by 500 mg/12 h p.o. for 5 days	40/40	30/40 (76%) vs. 31/40 (78%)	77% vs.77% n.s.
Angeli, 2006 [82]	ciprofloxacin (200 mg/12 h i.v.) followed by 500 mg/12 h p.o. (total 8 days) vs. cetazidim (2 g/12 h i.v.)	61/55	49/61 (80%) vs. 46/55 (84%) n.s.	5/61 (8.2%) vs. 7/55 (13%) n.s.

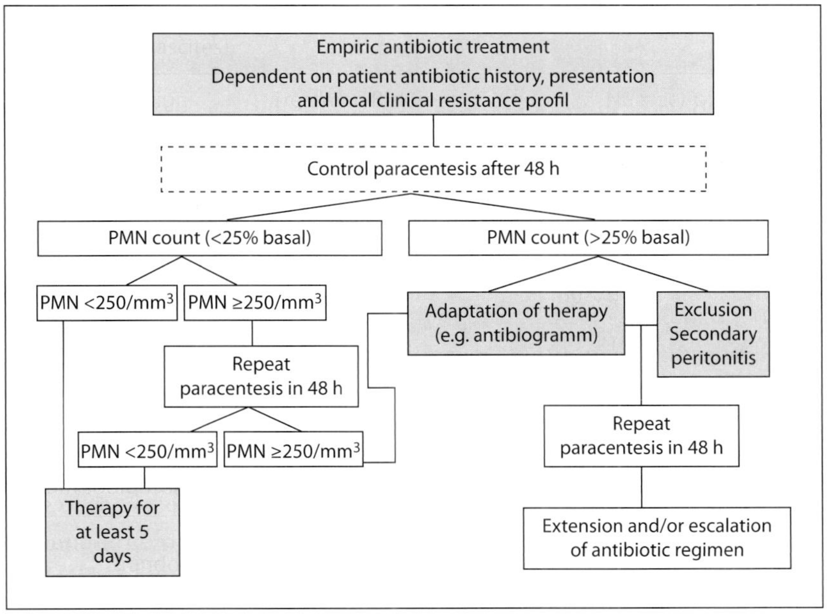

Fig. 1. Therapeutic algorithm for control of treatment failure.

or infection [1]. Otherwise, the patient should undergo a second paracentesis at the time culture results come back positive. This recommendation is based on a single-center experience showing that only the presence of signs or symptoms of infection appears to separate patients with bacterascites that progresses to SBP and those that resolve ascitic fluid colonization spontaneously [88]. However, further studies need to clarify the significance and mechanisms of bacterascites. Deficiencies in chemotaxis due to either genetic polymorphisms or acquired co-factors such as inhibition of sympathoadrenergic signaling have been shown to affect the neutrophilic response upon peritoneal bacterial stimulation in experimental cirrhosis [89]. In this context, in a retrospective study the use of a nonselective beta-blocker has recently been reported to lower the probability of community-acquired SBP in advanced cirrhosis [90] and a recent meta-analysis concluded that this protective effect is independent of the hemodynamic response achieved [91]. However, prospective randomized trials are lacking and are needed to establish the use of beta-blockers for the prevention and/or treatment of SBP.

Key Messages

- Definition: SBP is defined by PMN count in ascitic fluid ≥250/mm^3. Its development has been related to bacterial overgrowth, intestinal barrier failure and defects in host defense.
- Prophylaxis: Patients with gastrointestinal bleeding and severe liver disease should receive ceftriaxone, while patients with less severe liver disease and presentation may be given oral quinolone to prevent the development of SBP. Patients with low-protein ascites and no prior history of SBP may be started on primary antibiotic prophylaxis with quinolones in highly selected cases. After successful treatment and resolution of SBP, secondary prophylaxis has to be performed.
- Treatment: Empiric antibiotics should be started immediately following the diagnosis of SBP. First-line antibiotic treatment is third-generation cephalosporines. Alternatives include amoxicillin/clavulanic acid and quinolones. However, quinolones should not be used in patients who (a) are on prophylaxis using these drugs; (b) in areas with high prevalence of quinolone resistance, or (c) in nosocomial SBP. Potentially nephrotoxic antibiotics should not be used in cirrhotic patients.
- In nosocomial SBP, increased rates of bacterial resistance and multiple and/or complex resistance profiles have to be considered in treatment algorithms.
- Follow-Up: Treatment failure should be suspected and thus antibiotic therapy should be adapted when (a) clinical presentation worsens, or (b) follow-up paracentesis after 48 h of start of treatment fails to demonstrate a decrease of ascitic PMN counts to at least <25% of basal value before treatment.
- Future Studies: These should particularly focus on individualization and duration as well as optimization of prophylactic and therapeutic measures without increasing bacterial resistance.

References

1 Gines P, Angeli P, Lenz K, Moller S, Moore K, Moreau R: EASL clinical practice guidelines on the management of ascites, spontaneous bacterial peritonitis and hepatorenal syndrome in cirrhosis. J Hepatol 2010;in press.

2 Rimola A, Garcia-Tsao G, Navasa M, Piddock LJ, Planas R, Bernard B, Inadomi JM: Diagnosis, treatment and prophylaxis of spontaneous bacterial peritonitis: a consensus document. International Ascites Club. J Hepatol 2000;32:142–153.

3 Runyon BA: Management of adult patients with ascites due to cirrhosis: an update. Hepatology 2009;49:2087–2107.

4 Evans LT, Kim WR, Poterucha JJ and Kamath PS: Spontaneous bacterial peritonitis in asymptomatic outpatients with cirrhotic ascites. Hepatology 2003;37:897–901.

5 Andreu M, Sola R, Sitges-Serra A, Alia S, Gallen M, Vila MC, Coll S, Oliver MI: Risk factors for spontaneous bacterial peritonitis in cirrhotic patients with ascites. Gastroenterology 1993;104:1133–1138.

6 Tito L, Rimola A, Gines P, Llach J, Arroyo V, Rodes J: Recurrence of spontaneous bacterial peritonitis in cirrhosis: frequency and predictive factors. Hepatology 1988;8:27–31.

7 Terg R, Levi D, Lopez P, Rafaelli C, Rojter S, Abecasis R, Villamil F, Aziz H, Podesta A: Analysis of clinical course and prognosis of culture-positive spontaneous bacterial peritonitis and neutrocytic ascites. Evidence of the same disease. Dig Dis Sci 1992;37:1499–1504.

8 Silvain C, Besson I, Ingrand P, Mannant PR, Fort E, Beauchant M: Prognosis and long-term recurrence of spontaneous bacterial peritonitis in cirrhosis. J Hepatol 1993;19:188–189.

9 Thuluvath PJ, Morss S, Thompson R: Spontaneous bacterial peritonitis: in-hospital mortality, predictors of survival, and health care costs from 1988 to 1998. Am J Gastroenterol 2001;96:1232–1236.

10 Altman C, Grange JD, Amiot X, Pelletier G, Lacaine F, Bodin F, Etienne JP: Survival after a first episode of spontaneous bacterial peritonitis: prognosis of potential candidates for orthotopic liver transplantation. J Gastroenterol Hepatol 1995;10:47–50.
11 Toledo C, Salmeron JM, Rimola A, Navasa M, Arroyo V, Llach J, Gines A, Gines P, Rodes J: Spontaneous bacterial peritonitis in cirrhosis: predictive factors of infection resolution and survival in patients treated with cefotaxime. Hepatology 1993;17:251–257.
12 Weinstein MP, Iannini PB, Stratton CW, Eickhoff TC: Spontaneous bacterial peritonitis: a review of 28 cases with emphasis on improved survival and factors influencing prognosis. Am J Med 1978;64: 592–598.
13 Almdal TP, Skinhoj P: Spontaneous bacterial peritonitis in cirrhosis. Incidence, diagnosis, and prognosis. Scand J Gastroenterol 1987;22:295–300.
14 Terg R, Gadano A, Cartier M, Casciato P, Lucero R, Munoz A, Romero G, Levi D, Terg G, Miguez C, Abecasis R: Serum creatinine and bilirubin predict renal failure and mortality in patients with spontaneous bacterial peritonitis: a retrospective study. Liver Int 2009;29:415–419.
15 Franca AV, De Souza JB, Silva CM, Soares EC: Long-term prognosis of cirrhosis after spontaneous bacterial peritonitis treated with ceftriaxone. J Clin Gastroenterol 2001;33:295–298.
16 Kamani L, Mumtaz K, Ahmed US, Ali AW, Jafri W: Outcomes in culture positive and culture negative ascitic fluid infection in patients with viral cirrhosis: cohort study. BMC Gastroenterol 2008;8:59.
17 Cho JH, Park KH, Kim SH, Bang JH, Park WB, Kim HB, Oh MD, Lee HS, Choe KW: Bacteremia is a prognostic factor for poor outcome in spontaneous bacterial peritonitis. Scand J Infect Dis 2007;39:697–702.
18 Garcia-Tsao G, Wiest R: Gut microflora in the pathogenesis of the complications of cirrhosis. Best Pract Res Clin Gastroenterol 2004;18:353–372.
19 Gines P, Rimola A, Planas R, Vargas V, Marco F, Almela M, Forne M, Miranda ML, Llach J, Salmeron JM: Norfloxacin prevents spontaneous bacterial peritonitis recurrence in cirrhosis: results of a double-blind, placebo- controlled trial. Hepatology 1990;12:716–724.
20 Llovet JM, Bartoli R, Planas R, Vinado B, Perez J, Cabre E, Arnal J, Ojanguren I, Ausina V, Gassull MA: Selective intestinal decontamination with norfloxacin reduces bacterial translocation in ascitic cirrhotic rats exposed to hemorrhagic shock. Hepatology 1996;23:781–787.
21 Soriano G, Guarner C, Teixido M, Such J, Barrios J, Enriquez J, Vilardell F: Selective intestinal decontamination prevents spontaneous bacterial peritonitis. Gastroenterology 1991;100:477–481.
22 Deitch EA: Bacterial translocation of the gut flora. J Trauma 1990;30:S184–S189.
23 Casafont F: Small bowel bacterial overgrowth in patients with alcoholic cirrhosis. Dig Dis Sci 1995; 40:1252–1256.
24 Chesta J: Small intestinal bacterial overgrowth in patients with hepatic cirrhosis. Rev Med Chil 1991; 119:626–632.
25 Guarner C, Runyon BA, Young S, Heck M, Sheikh MY: Intestinal bacterial overgrowth and bacterial translocation in cirrhotic rats with ascites. J Hepatol 1997;26:1372–1378.
26 Steffen EK, Berg RD: Relationship between cecal population levels of indigenous bacteria and translocation to the mesenteric lymph nodes. Infect Immun 1983;39:1252–1259.
27 Wells CL: Colonization and translocation of intestinal bacterial flora. Transplant Proc 1996;28:2653–2656.
28 Garcia-Tsao G: Cirrhotic ascites: pathogenesis and management. Gastroenterologist 1995;3:41–54.
29 Garcia-Tsao G, Albillos A, Barden GE, West AB: Bacterial translocation in acute and chronic portal hypertension. Hepatology 1993;17:1081–1085.
30 Garcia-Tsao G, Lee FY, Barden GE, Cartun R, West AB: Bacterial translocation to mesenteric lymph nodes is increased in cirrhotic rats with ascites. Gastroenterology 1995;108:1835–1841.
31 Llovet JM, Bartoli R, Planas R, Cabre E, Jimenez M, Urban A, Ojanguren I, Arnal J, Gassull MA: Bacterial translocation in cirrhotic rats: its role in the development of spontaneous bacterial peritonitis. Gut 1994;35:1648–1652.
32 Llovet JM, Bartoli R, March F, Planas R, Vinado B, Cabre E, Arnal J, Coll P, Ausina V, Gassull MA. Translocated intestinal bacteria cause spontaneous bacterial peritonitis in cirrhotic rats: molecular epidemiologic evidence. J Hepatol 1998;307–313.
33 Campillo B, Pernet P, Bories PN, Richardet JP, Devanlay M, Aussel C: Intestinal permeability in liver cirrhosis: relationship with severe septic complications. Eur J Gastroenterol Hepatol 1999;11:755–759.
34 Natarajan SK, Ramamoorthy P, Thomas S, Basivireddy J, Kang G, Ramachandran A, Pulimood AB, Balasubramanian KA: Intestinal mucosal alterations in rats with carbon tetrachloride-induced cirrhosis: changes in glycosylation and luminal bacteria. Hepatology 2006;43:837–846.

35 Such J, Guardiola JV, de Juan J, Casellas JA, Pascual S, Aparicio JR, Sola-Vera J, Perez-Mateo M: Ultrastructural characteristics of distal duodenum mucosa in patients with cirrhosis. Eur J Gastroenterol Hepatol 2002;14:371–376.
36 Ramachandran A, Prabhu R, Thomas S, Reddy JB, Pulimood A, Balasubramanian KA: Intestinal mucosal alterations in experimental cirrhosis in the rat: role of oxygen free radicals. Hepatology 2002;35:622–629.
37 Wiest R, Garcia-Tsao G: Bacterial translocation (BT) in cirrhosis. Hepatology 2005;41:422–433.
38 Hassner A, Kletter Y, Jedvab M, Aronson M, Shibolet S: Impaired monocyte function in liver cirrhosis. Lancet 1979;i:329–330.
39 Rajkovic IA, Williams R: Abnormalities of neutrophil phagocytosis, intracellular killing and metabolic activity in alcoholic cirrhosis and hepatitis. Hepatology 1986;6:252–262.
40 Berg RD, Wommack E, Deitch EA: Immunosuppression and intestinal bacterial overgrowth synergistically promote bacterial translocation. Arch Surg 1988;123:1359–1364.
41 Fernandez J, Navasa M, Gomez J, Colmenero J, Vila J, Arroyo V, Rodes J: Bacterial infections in cirrhosis: epidemiological changes with invasive procedures and norfloxacin prophylaxis. Hepatology 2002;35:140–148.
42 Goulis J, Patch D, Burroughs AK: Bacterial infection in the pathogenesis of variceal bleeding. Lancet 1999;353:139–142.
43 Runyon BA, Morrissey RL, Hoefs JC, Wyle FA: Opsonic activity of human ascitic fluid: a potentially important protective mechanism against spontaneous bacterial peritonitis. Hepatology 1985;5:634–637.
44 Llach J, Rimola A, Navasa M, Gines P, Salmeron JM, Gines A, Arroyo V, Rodes J: Incidence and predictive factors of first episode of spontaneous bacterial peritonitis in cirrhosis with ascites: relevance of ascitic fluid protein concentration. Hepatology 1992;16:724–727.
45 Guarner C, Sola R, Soriano G, Andreu M, Novella MT, Vila MC, Sabat M, Coll S, Ortiz J, Gomez C, Balanzo J: Risk of a first community-acquired spontaneous bacterial peritonitis in cirrhotics with low ascitic fluid protein levels. Gastroenterology 1999;117:414–419.
46 Bajaj JS, Zadvornova Y, Heuman DM, Hafeezullah M, Hoffmann RG, Sanyal AJ, Saelan K: Association of proton pump inhibitor therapy with spontaneous bacterial peritonitis in cirrhotic patients with ascites. Am J Gastroenterol 2009;104:1130–1134.
47 Obstein KL, Campbell MS, Reddy KR, Yang YX: Association between model for end-stage liver disease and spontaneous bacterial peritonitis. Am J Gastroenterol 2007;102:2732–2736.
48 Appenrodt B, Grunhage F, Gentemann MG, Thyssen L, Sauerbruch T, Lammert F: Nucleotide-binding oligomerization domain containing 2 (NOD2) variants are genetic risk factors for death and spontaneous bacterial peritonitis in liver cirrhosis. Hepatology 2010;51:1327–1333.
49 Andreu M, Sola R, Sitges-Serra A, Alia C, Gallen M, Vila MC, Coll S, Oliver MI: Risk factors for spontaneous bacterial peritonitis in cirrhotic patients with ascites. Gastroenterology 1993;104:1133–1138.
50 Bernard B, Grange JD, Khac EN, Amiot X, Opolon P, Poynard T: Antibiotic prophylaxis for the prevention of bacterial infections in cirrhotic patients with gastrointestinal bleeding: a meta-analysis. Hepatology 1999;29:1655–1661.
51 Soares-Weiser K, Brezis M, Leibovici L: Antibiotics for spontaneous bacterial peritonitis in cirrhotics. Cochrane Database Syst Rev 2001;CD002232.
52 Fernandez J, Ruiz dA, Gomez C, Durandez R, Serradilla R, Guarner C, Planas R, Arroyo V, Navasa M: Norfloxacin vs ceftriaxone in the prophylaxis of infections in patients with advanced cirrhosis and hemorrhage. Gastroenterology 2006;131:1049–1056.
53 Loomba R, Wesley R, Bain A, Csako G, Pucino F: Role of fluoroquinolones in the primary prophylaxis of spontaneous bacterial peritonitis: meta-analysis. Clin Gastroenterol Hepatol 2009;7:487–493.
54 Saab S, Hernandez JC, Chi AC, Tong MJ: Oral antibiotic prophylaxis reduces spontaneous bacterial peritonitis occurrence and improves short-term survival in cirrhosis: a meta-analysis. Am J Gastroenterol 2009;104:993–1001.
55 Alvarez RF, Mattos AA, Correa EB, Cotrim HP, Nascimento TV: Trimethoprim-sulfamethoxazole versus norfloxacin in the prophylaxis of spontaneous bacterial peritonitis in cirrhosis. Arq Gastroenterol 2005;42:256–262.
56 Rolachon A, Cordier L, Bacq Y, Nousbaum JB, Franza A, Paris JC, Fratte S, Bohn B, Kitmacher P, Stahl JP: Ciprofloxacin and long-term prevention of spontaneous bacterial peritonitis: results of a prospective controlled trial. Hepatology 1995;22:1171–1174.
57 Singh N, Gayowski T, Yu VL, Wagener MM: Trimethoprim-sulfamethoxazole for the prevention of spontaneous bacterial peritonitis in cirrhosis: a randomized trial. Ann Intern Med 1995;122:595–598.
58 Krag A, Wiest R, Gluud LL: Fluoroquinolones in the primary prophylaxis of spontaneous bacterial peritonitis. Am J Gastroenterol 2010;105:1444–1445.

59 Grange JD, Roulot D, Pelletier G, Pariente EA, Denis J, Ink O, Blanc P, Richardet JP, Vinel JP, Delisle F, Fischer D, Flahault A, Amiot X: Norfloxacin primary prophylaxis of bacterial infections in cirrhotic patients with ascites: a double-blind randomized trial. J Hepatol 1998;29:430–436.
60 Novella M, Sola R, Soriano G, Andreu M, Gana J, Ortiz J, Coll S, Sabat M, Vila MC, Guarner C, Vilardell F: Continuous versus inpatient prophylaxis of the first episode of spontaneous bacterial peritonitis with norfloxacin. Hepatology 1997;25:532–536.
61 Terg R, Fassio E, Guevara M, Cartier M, Longo C, Lucero R, Landeira C, Romero G, Dominguez N, Munoz A, Levi D, Miguez C, Abecasis R: Ciprofloxacin in primary prophylaxis of spontaneous bacterial peritonitis: a randomized, placebo-controlled study. J Hepatol 2008;48:774–779.
62 Fernandez J, Navasa M, Planas R, Montoliu S, Monfort D, Soriano G, Vila C, Pardo A, Quintero E, Vargas V, Such J, Gines P, Arroyo V: Primary prophylaxis of spontaneous bacterial peritonitis delays hepatorenal syndrome and improves survival in cirrhosis. Gastroenterology 2007;133:818–824.
63 Runyon BA: A pill a day can improve survival in patients with advanced cirrhosis. Gastroenterology 2007;133:1029–1031.
64 Park YH, Lee HC, Song HG, Jung S, Ryu SH, Shin JW, Chung YH, Lee YS, Suh DJ: Recent increase in antibiotic-resistant microorganisms in patients with spontaneous bacterial peritonitis adversely affects the clinical outcome in Korea. J Gastroenterol Hepatol 2003;18:927–933.
65 Singh N, Wagener MM, Gayowski T: Changing epidemiology and predictors of mortality in patients with spontaneous bacterial peritonitis at a liver transplant unit. Clin Microbiol Infect 2003;9:531–537.
66 Terg R, Llano K, Cobas SM, Brotto C, Barrios A, Levi D, Wasen W, Bartellini MA: Effects of oral ciprofloxacin on aerobic Gram-negative fecal flora in patients with cirrhosis: results of short- and long-term administration, with daily and weekly dosages. J Hepatol 1998;29:437–442.
67 Borzio M, Salerno F, Pedicino C, et al: Prevalence of bacterial resistance in cirrhotic patients with bacterial infection: A preliminary report. Hepatology 2009;50(suppl): 447A (abstract).
68 Umgelter A, Reindl W, Miedaner M, Schmid RM, Huber W: Failure of current antibiotic first-line regimens and mortality in hospitalized patients with spontaneous bacterial peritonitis. Infection 2009; 37:2–8.
69 Castellote J, Ariza J, Girbau A, Rodriguez L, Vazquez X, Salord S, Baliellas C, Xiol X: Risk factors to cefotaxime-resistant spontanous bacterial peritonitis. J Hepatol 2010;52
70 Bajaj JS, Ananthakrishnan AN, Hafeezullah M, Zadvornova Y, Dye A, McGinley EL, Saeian K, Heuman D, Sanyal AJ, Hoffmann RG: *Clostridium difficile* is associated with poor outcomes in patients with cirrhosis: a national and tertiary center perspective. Am J Gastroenterol 2010;105:106–113.
71 Dupeyron C, Mangeney N, Sedrati L, Campillo B, Fouet P, Leluan G: Rapid emergence of quinolone resistance in cirrhotic patients treated with norfloxacin to prevent spontaneous bacterial peritonitis. Antimicrob Agents Chemother 1994;38:340–344.
72 Dupeyron C, Campillo SB, Mangeney N, Richardet JP, Leluan G: Carriage of *Staphylococcus aureus* and of Gram-negative bacilli resistant to third-generation cephalosporins in cirrhotic patients: a prospective assessment of hospital-acquired infections. Infect Control Hosp Epidemiol 2001;22:427–432.
73 Scarpellini E, Valenza V, Gabrielli M, Lauritano EC, Perotti G, Merra G, Dal Lago A, Ojetti V, Ainora ME, Santoro M, Ghirlanda G, Gasbarrini A: Intestinal permeability in cirrhotic patients with and without spontaneous bacterial peritonitis: is the ring closed? Am J Gastroenterol 2010;105:323–327.
74 Campillo B, Dupeyron C, Richardet JP: Epidemiology of hospital-acquired infections in cirrhotic patients: effect of carriage of methicillin-resistant *Staphylococcus aureus* and influence of previous antibiotic therapy and norfloxacin prophylaxis. Epidemiol Infect 2001;127:443–450.
75 Cosgrove SE, Sakoulas G, Perencevich EN, Schwaber MJ, Karchmer AW, Carmeli Y: Comparison of mortality associated with methicillin-resistant and methicillin-susceptible *Staphylococcus aureus* bacteremia: a meta-analysis. Clin Infect Dis 2003;36:53–59.
76 Zhang SC, Wang W, Ren WY, He BM, Zhou K, Zhu WN: Effect of cisapride on intestinal bacterial and endotoxin translocation in cirrhosis. World J Gastroenterol 2003;9:534–538.
77 Madrid AM, Hurtado C, Venegas M, Cumsille F, Defilippi C: Long-Term treatment with cisapride and antibiotics in liver cirrhosis: effect on small intestinal motility, bacterial overgrowth, and liver function. Am J Gastroenterol 2001;96:1251–1255.
78 Pardo A, Bartoli R, Lorenzo-Zuniga V, Planas R, Vinado B, Riba J, Cabre E, Santos J, Luque T, Ausina V, Gassull MA: Effect of cisapride on intestinal bacterial overgrowth and bacterial translocation in cirrhosis. Hepatology 2000;31:858–863.

79 Rimola A, Salmeron JM, Clemente G, Rodrigo L, Obrador A, Miranda ML, Guarner C, Planas R, Sola R, Vargas V: Two different dosages of cefotaxime in the treatment of spontaneous bacterial peritonitis in cirrhosis: results of a prospective, randomized, multicenter study. Hepatology 1995;21:674–679.
80 Runyon BA, McHutchison JG, Antillon MR, Akriviadis EA, Montano AA: Short-course versus long-course antibiotic treatment of spontaneous bacterial peritonitis: a randomized controlled study of 100 patients. Gastroenterology 1991;100:1737–1742.
81 Ricart E, Soriano G, Novella MT, Ortiz J, Sabat M, Kolle L, Sola-Vera J, Minana J, Dedeu JM, Gomez C, Barrio JL, Guarner C: Amoxicillin-clavulanic acid versus cefotaxime in the therapy of bacterial infections in cirrhotic patients. J Hepatol 2000;32:596–602.
82 Angeli P, Guarda S, Fasolato S, Miola E, Craighero R, Piccolo F, Antona C, Brollo L, Franchin M, Cillo U, Merkel C, Gatta A: Switch therapy with ciprofloxacin vs. intravenous ceftazidime in the treatment of spontaneous bacterial peritonitis in patients with cirrhosis: similar efficacy at lower cost. Aliment Pharmacol Ther 2006;23:75–84.
83 Navasa M, Follo A, Llovet JM, Clemente G, Vargas V, Rimola A, Marco F, Guarner C, Forne M, Planas R, Banares R, Castells L, Jimenez De Anta MT, Arroyo V, Rodes J: Randomized, comparative study of oral ofloxacin versus intravenous cefotaxime in spontaneous bacterial peritonitis. Gastroenterology 1996;111:1011–1017.
84 Terg R, Cobas S, Fassio E, Landeira G, Rios B, Vasen W, Abecasis R, Rios H, Guevara M: Oral ciprofloxacin after a short course of intravenous ciprofloxacin in the treatment of spontaneous bacterial peritonitis: results of a multicenter, randomized study. J Hepatol 2000;33:564–569.
85 Song KH, Jeon JH, Park WB, Park SW, Kim HB, Oh MD, Lee HS, Kim NJ, Choe KW: Clinical outcomes of spontaneous bacterial peritonitis due to extended-spectrum beta-lactamase-producing *Escherichia coli* and *Klebsiella* species: a retrospective matched case-control study. BMC Infect Dis 2009;9:41.
86 Felisart J, Rimola A, Arroyo V, Perez-Ayuso RM, Quintero E, Gines P, Rodes J: Cefotaxime is more effective than is ampicillin-tobramycin in cirrhotics with severe infections. Hepatology 1985;5:457–462.
87 Tuncer I, Topcu N, Durmus A, Turkdogan MK: Oral ciprofloxacin versus intravenous cefotaxime and ceftriaxone in the treatment of spontaneous bacterial peritonitis. Hepatogastroenterology 2003; 50:1426–1430.
88 Runyon BA: Monomicrobial nonneutrocytic bacterascites: a variant of spontaneous bacterial peritonitis. Hepatology 1990;12:710–715.
89 Wiest R, Worlicek M, Knebel K, Moleda L, Linde H. Schölmerich J, Straub RH: Splanchnic sympathectomy prevents translocation and spreading of E. coli in experimental cirrhosis. Gut 2010;59:1127–1134.
90 Gonzalez-Suarez B, Guarner C, Villanueva C, Minana J, Soriano G, Gallego A, Sainz S, Torras X, Cusso X, Balanzo J: Pharmacologic treatment of portal hypertension in the prevention of community-acquired spontaneous bacterial peritonitis. Eur J Gastroenterol Hepatol 2006;18:49–55.
91 Senzolo M, Cholongitas E, Burra P, Leandro G, Thalheimer U, Patch D, Burroughs AK: Beta-blockers protect against spontaneous bacterial peritonitis in cirrhotic patients: a meta-analysis. Liver Int 2009;29:1189–1193.

Reiner Wiest
Klinik und Poliklinik für Innere Medizin I, Universitätsklinikum Regensburg
Franz-Josef-Strauss-Allee 11
DE–93053 Regensburg (Germany)
Tel. +49 941 944 7010, Fax +49 941 944 7073, E-Mail Reiner.Wiest@klinik.uni-regensburg.de

Gerbes AL (ed): Ascites, Hyponatremia and Hepatorenal Syndrome: Progress in Treatment.
Front Gastrointest Res. Basel, Karger, 2011, vol 28, pp 83–90

Clinical Implications of Hyponatremia in Cirrhosis

Douglas M. Heuman

Virginia Commonwealth University, GI Section (111-N) Hunter Holmes McGuire Department of Veterans Affairs Medical Center, Richmond, Va., USA

Abstract

Hyponatremia in cirrhosis is caused by a generalized circulatory disorder, features of which include vasodilation, portal hypertension, reduced systemic vascular resistance, increased cardiac output and systemic hypotension. Hypotension activates baroreceptor neurons in the heart and great vessels, causing the hypothalamus to override its normal osmotic controls and release antidiuretic hormone. The resulting renal water retention, mediated via vasopressin V2 receptors in the collecting ducts, leads to systemic hypo-osmolality and hyponatremia. Low serum sodium is a predictor of mortality in cirrhosis, as well as in other disorders associated with circulatory failure such as congestive heart failure or pneumonia. Low serum sodium often accompanies other manifestations of advanced cirrhosis, including refractory ascites, hepatorenal syndrome and hepatic encephalopathy. Hyponatremia worsens with diuretic therapy in cirrhosis and may render patients diuretic-intolerant. Low sodium predicts cirrhotic mortality independently of MELD score, and inclusion of sodium in MELD-based survival models improves their predictive accuracy. Hyponatremia, even when severe, is well tolerated if it develops slowly, though there is some evidence that hyponatremia per se may aggravate cognitive impairment and hepatic encephalopathy. Patients with hyponatremia at the time of liver transplantation have higher post-transplant morbidity and mortality, and are particularly at risk to develop osmotic demyelination. Cirrhotic hyponatremia may improve with water restriction, diuretic withdrawal, albumin infusion, pressor therapy or administration of aquaretic vaptan agents, but it is not known whether these treatments improve outcomes. Pretransplant correction of serum sodium may be indicated to prevent post-transplant osmotic demyelination.

Hyponatremia in Cirrhosis: Pathophysiology

Ascites, hyponatremia and hepatorenal syndrome are now recognized to be components of a generalized circulatory disorder of cirrhosis [1]. This circulatory disorder is characterized by vasodilation, with reduced systemic vascular resistance, increased cardiac output, and hypotension. The vasodilatory signals responsible for the hyperdynamic circulation remain incompletely understood. Candidate mediators include bacterial endotoxins, cytokines such as TNF-α and IL-6, endogenous cannabinoids, and nitric oxide, among others. Sinusoidal and portal hypertension play a role in release of these mediators, and portosystemic shunting may contribute to their systemic accumulation. In response to vasodilatation, a variety of compensatory mechanisms are activated, including the sympathetic nervous system and the renin-angiotensin-aldosterone axis. These changes partially correct the circulatory disorder, but at a cost of avid renal sodium retention. In the setting of hypoalbuminemia with low plasma oncotic pressure, as well as sinusoidal portal hypertension, this sodium retention results in transudation of fluid from the vascular space, leading to accumulation of ascites and edema.

Above a critical threshold, progressive vasodilation with hypotension activates baroreceptor neurons in the central circulation that communicate with the hypothalamus. This causes the hypothalamus to override its normal osmotic control pathway and release antidiuretic hormone (vasopressin). At the level of the kidney, vasopressin acts on V2 receptors in the collecting ducts, causing aquaporins to translocate from the cytosol to the apical plasma membrane [2]. The previously impermeable collecting duct now becomes permeable to water, which diffuses into the renal medulla driven by the osmotic gradient there. The resulting water retention produces systemic hypo-osmolality, of which hyponatremia is the most prominent manifestation. The mechanism teleologically represents an 'emergency override' by which the body sacrifices osmolar homeostasis to maintain volume when confronted with impending circulatory collapse.

Prognostic Significance of Sodium in Cirrhosis and Liver Transplantation

The presence of hyponatremia is often a sign of impending circulatory failure, with strong prognostic implications. Low serum sodium is a predictor of mortality in many disorders associated with circulatory failure, ranging from congestive heart failure [3] to acute pneumonia [4]. Low serum sodium also predicts overall mortality in general hospital [5] and intensive care settings [6].

The importance of hyponatremia as a prognostic indicator in cirrhosis has long been recognized [7]. In the 1960s, Summerskill and colleagues [8] noted the association of hyponatremia with renal insufficiency in cirrhosis. Sherlock et al. [9] observed that hyponatremia worsens with diuretic therapy in cirrhosis and may render patients diuretic-intolerant. A multicenter point prevalence survey in Europe and the USA [10] found that low serum sodium was present in nearly half of cirrhotic patients, and was associated with increased incidence of spontaneous bacterial peritonitis, hepatic encephalopathy, and hepatorenal syndrome.

Recognition of the prognostic significance of sodium in liver disease has assumed new importance in recent years. Because of the growing gap between demand for liver transplantation and supply of deceased donor organs, governments in the USA, Europe and elsewhere have mandated allocation of scarce donor livers on a 'sickest first' basis. This approach requires a reliable model of short term prognosis for cirrhotic patients awaiting transplantation. The Model for End-Stage Liver Disease (MELD) was adopted for this purpose in the USA in 2002 [11, 12]. MELD provided a reasonably good indicator of 90-day pretransplant survival in a number of cirrhotic populations, with concordance statistics in the order of 0.8.

Creatinine is a component of MELD, and it was initially thought that increases in serum creatinine would effectively capture the risk associated with the circulatory derangement of cirrhosis. However, we reported in 2004 [13] that low serum sodium and uncontrolled ascites were predictive of 6-month pretransplant mortality in cirrhotic veterans, independently of MELD score. The added predictive value of sodium and ascites in this study was most apparent in patients with MELD ≤20; in the absence of low sodium or ascites, 180-day mortality for patients with MELD ≤20 was less than 6%, whereas if both were present or if sodium was <130 mEq/l, mortality was 40–50%. This finding suggested that while MELD may adequately identify those cirrhotic patients who are dying with hepatorenal syndrome, uncontrolled ascites and low sodium are additional important markers of advanced circulatory failure that can identify cirrhotic patients who are at risk for terminal decompensation leading to hepatorenal syndrome. Our data were also consistent with the earlier finding of Fernandez-Esparrach et al. [14], who showed in patients hospitalized with cirrhotic ascites that a failure to increase urinary volume in response to a free water challenge (indicating failure of the hypothalamus to suppress vasopressin secretion in response to hypo-osmolality) was a key predictor of mortality independent of serum creatinine.

The independent prognostic significance of low sodium and MELD in pretransplant cirrhotics was subsequently confirmed by a number of groups worldwide. A variety of prognostic models incorporating sodium and MELD have been proposed. The most sophisticated is that of Kim et al. [15], based upon analysis of mortality data from the USA national liver transplant waiting list. These authors found that mortality increased incrementally with decline in sodium from 140 to 125 mEq/l, and that the prognostic significance of sodium was greatest at low values of MELD. In the United Kingdom, a model termed UKELD that incorporates sodium along with creatinine, bilirubin and INR was adopted in 2008 to determine eligibility for liver transplantation [16].

In the USA, despite a near consensus regarding the independent prognostic value of sodium and MELD in end-stage liver disease, the liver transplant community has not embraced efforts to incorporate sodium into the survival model for organ allocation. One concern is the labile nature of hyponatremia. A number of treatments can improve serum sodium at least transiently. As a consequence, especially in the hospitalized cirrhotic patient, composite MELD-sodium prognostic scores may improve in response to short-term treatments that have little effect on the severity or prognosis of the underlying disease. In cirrhotic subjects referred for transplantation, we found that the lowest serum sodium in the preceding 90 days was a better predictor of pretransplant mortality than the current serum sodium [17]. Among cirrhotics with currently normal sodium, those who had experienced low serum sodium in the previous 90 days had substantially higher mortality risk, and risk increased with severity of prior hyponatremia. Thus, treatment to correct hyponatremia may mask the underlying risk and attenuate or nullify the prognostic value of sodium.

A second concern is the possibility that low serum sodium at transplantation can be associated with poorer transplant outcomes, and preferential organ allocation to cirrhotics with hyponatremia may therefore reduce overall benefit. Londono et al. [18] from Barcelona reported that cirrhotic patients whose serum sodium was <130 mEq/l at the time of liver transplantation had significantly higher rates of early post-transplant complications, including infections, neurological complications and renal insufficiency, as well as poorer 3-month post-transplant survival. Similar findings were reported from the United Kingdom by Dawwas et al. [19]. Yun et al. [20] reviewed outcomes of 2,321 liver transplants performed between 1990 and 2000 at a number of USA sites and found an association of pretransplant hyponatremia with prolonged post-transplant ICU and hospital stay, though early survival was not affected. Hackworth et al. [21] reported that cirrhotics whose hyponatremia had been corrected prior to transplantation nonetheless experienced higher rates of post-transplant complications than those who had not experienced hyponatremia, suggesting that hyponatremia in part may be a surrogate marker for other elements of disease severity that determine transplant risk.

A dreaded complication associated with cirrhotic hyponatremia in the transplant setting is osmotic demyelination (formerly known as central pontine myelinolysis), a type of brain injury caused by rapid increases in osmolality [22]. During the course of liver transplantation and subsequent intensive care, hyponatremic patients undergoing liver transplantation often receive massive volumes of isotonic fluids, leading to rapid normalization of serum sodium. A few of these individuals will develop osmotic demyelination [20], sometimes leading to death, coma, or permanent severe neurological deficits. Many programs are reluctant to transplant patients with severe hyponatremia. An organ allocation formula that offers priority to patients with hyponatremia would need to be constructed in such a way as to avoid penalizing clinicians and patients for taking steps to correct hyponatremia preoperatively. To date, no consensus exists on such a formula.

Hyponatremia in Cirrhosis: Treatment Options

Treatments to correct cirrhotic hyponatremia can be divided into two general groups: those that specifically seek to reduce excess free water and correct hyposmolality, and those that suppress vasopressin secretion by addressing the underlying hemodynamic derangement.

The mainstay of free water removal traditionally has been water restriction. Humans have obligatory daily water losses from skin, the respiratory tract, feces and urine in the order of 1,000–1,500 ml. If the obligatory losses exceed water intake, osmolality increases. The major limitation of water restriction as a treatment strategy is intolerable thirst, leading to noncompliance. A newer approach to free water removal is administration of vaptan diuretics, antagonists of the renal vasopressin V2 receptor. Vaptans produce rapid dilution of urine with excretion of free water, leading to an increase in serum sodium and osmolality that is sustained with continued treatment. The orally active agent tolvapatan, a selective V2 antagonist, was approved in the USA in 2009 for treatment of hyponatremia in a number of disorders, including cirrhosis. Vaptans are discussed in detail in the next chapter.

Treatments that improve sodium by correcting the underlying hemodynamics include albumin, pressors, antibiotics, and transjugular intrahepatic portosystemic shunts. These are discussed in more detail elsewhere in this volume in the context of treatment of ascites and hepatorenal syndrome. In general, aside from shunts, their efficacy is transitory, though recent studies of Tandon et al. [23] suggest that midodrine and octreotide given chronically to improve peripheral resistance and raise blood pressure in patients with cirrhotic ascites may improve hyponatremia along with renal function and diuretic response, and reduce the need for therapeutic paracentesis.

Should We Treat Cirrhotic Hyponatremia?

Hyponatremia in cirrhosis generally develops slowly, and is well tolerated. Rapid onset of hyponatremia, for example in marathon runners, can lead to fatal brain edema, but this is not seen with gradual onset of hyponatremia, since cells in the brain and elsewhere adapt to the hypo-osmolar environment over days to weeks by reducing the content of osmotically active solute [24]. Whether correction of chronic cirrhotic hyponatremia per se yields significant benefits is controversial. There is some evidence that stable chronic hyponatremia may be associated with reversible neurocognitive deficits. Chronic hyponatremia induced in rats by vasopressin administration was found to be associated with memory impairment that corrected following reversal of hyponatremia with tolvaptan [25]. In a mixed population of patients with mild chronic hyponatremia, Renneboog et al. [26] found abnormalities of attention and gait with increased risk of falls. Hyponatremic cirrhotics have reduced brain concentration of solutes such as myoinositol, and are at increased risk to develop overt hepatic encephalopathy [27]. In a preliminary report, improvement of cirrhotic hyponatremia with satavaptan therapy was found to improve complex information processing ability, as measured by the trail-making test B [28].

Aside from the potential cognitive benefits, there is little evidence that simple correction of hyponatremia, without improvement in the underlying circulatory disorder, can improve major outcomes such as survival in cirrhosis. Until recently, treatments available for outpatient management of cirrhotic hyponatremia were only transiently effective. Newer agents such as vaptan diuretics can produce sustained improvement in hyponatremia, but the role of these agents in advanced liver disease remains to be established. If transplant is imminent, a case can be made for use of vaptans or other aggressive measures to improve sodium preoperatively in a controlled manner over days to weeks, in hopes of reducing likelihood of post-transplant osmotic demyelination and other complications, even though the benefits of this approach have not yet been supported by clinical trials. However, simple correction of serum sodium is unlikely to alter substantially the natural history of cirrhosis, and use of water restriction and/or vaptans in advanced cirrhosis, especially as a measure to overcome diuretic resistance, could further aggravate circulatory failure. A prospective, randomized, placebo controlled clinical trial of satavaptan for cirrhotic hyponatremia was stopped in 2009 after excess mortality was noted in the satavaptan-treated group [29]. Optimism is further tempered by experience in patients with hyponatremia caused by heart failure. In the EVEREST trial [30], a 2-year prospective study of over 1,000 heart failure patients with hyponatremia randomized to treatment with tolvaptan versus placebo, chronic treatment with tolvaptan improved serum sodium but failed to improve survival. Similar prospective studies are needed in cirrhotics with hyponatremia before firm recommendations can be made regarding the risks and benefits of correcting hyponatremia in patients with end stage liver disease.

Key Messages

- Hyponatremia in cirrhosis is one manifestation of a systemic hemodynamic derangement, characterized by low peripheral vascular resistance, increased cardiac output, hypotension, and avid renal retention of sodium and water.
- Hyponatremia in a cirrhotic patient indicates poor prognosis, independently of MELD score.
- Cirrhotics who are hyponatremic prior to liver transplantation are at higher risk of early post-transplant complications, including osmotic demyelination.
- Hyponatremia may contribute to cognitive impairment in patients with hepatic encephalopathy.
- Cirrhotic hyponatremia often improves with water restriction, aquaretic therapy, or other treatments, but correction of hyponatremia has not been shown to improve survival.

References

1 Gines P, Schrier RW: Renal failure in cirrhosis. N Engl J Med 2009;361:1279–1290.

2 Schrier RW: Vasopressin and aquaporin 2 in clinical disorders of water homeostasis. Semin Nephrol 2008;28:289–296.

3 Tribouilloy C, Buiciuc O, Rusinaru D, Malaquin D, Levy F, Peltier M: Long-term outcome after a first episode of heart failure: a prospective 7-year study. Int J Cardiol 2010;140:309–314.

4 Nair V, Niederman MS, Masani N, Fishbane S: Hyponatremia in community-acquired pneumonia. Am J Nephrol 2007;27:184–190.

5 Whelan B, Bennett K, O'Riordan D, Silke B: Serum sodium as a risk factor for in-hospital mortality in acute unselected general medical patients. Q J Med 2009;102:175–182.

6 Stelfox HT, Ahmed SB, Khandwala F, Zygun D, Shahpori R, Laupland K: The epidemiology of intensive care unit-acquired hyponatraemia and hypernatraemia in medical-surgical intensive care units. Crit Care 2008;12:R162.

7 Arroyo V, Rodes J, Gutierrez-Lizarraga MA, Revert L: Prognostic value of spontaneous hyponatremia in cirrhosis with ascites. Am J Dig Dis 1976;21:249–256.

8 Baldus WP, Feichter RN, Summerskill WH: The kidney in cirrhosis. I. Clinical and biochemical features of azotemia in hepatic failure. Ann Intern Med 1964;60:353–365.

9 Sherlock S, Senewiratne B, Scott A, Walker JG: Complications of diuretic therapy in hepatic cirrhosis. Lancet 1966;i:1049–1052.

10 Angeli P, Wong F, Watson H, Gines P: Hyponatremia in cirrhosis: results of a patient population survey. Hepatology 2006;44:1535–1542.

11 Kamath PS, Wiesner RH, Malinchoc M, et al: A model to predict survival in patients with end-stage liver disease. Hepatology 2001;33:464–470.

12 Freeman RB Jr, Wiesner RH, Harper A, et al: The new liver allocation system: moving toward evidence-based transplantation policy. Liver Transpl 2002;8:851–858.

13 Heuman DM, Abou-Assi SG, Habib A, et al: Persistent ascites and low serum sodium identify patients with cirrhosis and low MELD scores who are at high risk for early death. Hepatology 2004;40:802–810.

14 Fernandez-Esparrach G, Sanchez-Fueyo A, Gines P, et al: A prognostic model for predicting survival in cirrhosis with ascites. J Hepatol 2001;34:46–52.

15 Kim WR, Biggins SW, Kremers WK, et al: Hyponatremia and mortality among patients on the liver-transplant waiting list. N Engl J Med 2008;359:1018–1026.

16 Neuberger J, Gimson A, Davies M, et al: Selection of patients for liver transplantation and allocation of donated livers in the UK. Gut 2008;57:252–257.

17 Heuman DM, Yilmaz N, Stravitz RT, Gilles HS, Fisher RA: MELD-Na90:an improved index for predicting pre-liver transplant mortality in cirrhotic patients. (abstract). Am J Transplant 2008;8:S219–S220.

18 Londono MC, Guevara M, Rimola A, et al: Hyponatremia impairs early posttransplantation outcome in patients with cirrhosis undergoing liver transplantation. Gastroenterology 2006;130:1135–1143.

19 Dawwas MF, Lewsey JD, Neuberger JM, Gimson AE: The impact of serum sodium concentration on mortality after liver transplantation: a cohort multicenter study. Liver Transpl 2007;13:1115–1124.

20 Yun BC, Kim WR, Benson JT, et al: Impact of pretransplant hyponatremia on outcome following liver transplantation. Hepatology 2009;49:1610–1615.

21 Hackworth WA, Heuman DM, Sanyal AJ, et al: Effect of hyponatraemia on outcomes following orthotopic liver transplantation. Liver Int 2009;29:1071–1077.

22 Laureno R, Karp BI: Myelinolysis after correction of hyponatremia. Ann Intern Med 1997;126:57–62.

23 Tandon P, Tsuyuki RT, Mitchell L, et al: The effect of 1 month of therapy with midodrine, octreotide-LAR and albumin in refractory ascites: a pilot study. Liver Int 2009;29:169–174.

24 Verbalis JG: Adaptation to acute and chronic hyponatremia: implications for symptomatology, diagnosis, and therapy. Semin Nephrol 1998;18:3–19.

25 Miyazaki T, Ohmoto K, Hirose T, Fujiki H: Chronic hyponatremia impairs memory in rats: effects of vasopressin antagonist tolvaptan. J Endocrinol 2010;206:105–111.

26 Renneboog B, Musch W, Vandemergel X, Manto MU, Decaux G: Mild chronic hyponatremia is associated with falls, unsteadiness, and attention deficits. Am J Med 2006;119:71–78.

27 Guevara M, Baccaro ME, Torre A, et al: Hyponatremia is a risk factor of hepatic encephalopathy in patients with cirrhosis: a prospective study with time-dependent analysis. Am J Gastroenterol 2009;104:1382–1389.

28 Cordoba J, Guevara M, Watson HR, Le Guennec S, Gines P: Improvement of hyponatremia in cirrhosis increases speed of complex information processing (abstract). Hepatology 2009;50(4S):451A–452A.
29 Wong F, Gines P, Nevens F, et al: Double-blind, placebo-controlled study of satavaptan in the management of recurrent ascites: the SPARE-1 study (abstract). Hepatology 2010;50(4S):448A.
30 Konstam MA, Gheorghiade M, Burnett JC Jr, et al: Effects of oral tolvaptan in patients hospitalized for worsening heart failure: the EVEREST Outcome Trial. JAMA 2007;297:1319–1331.

Douglas M. Heuman, MD
Virginia Commonwealth University, GI Section (111-N) Hunter Holmes McGuire
Department of Veterans Affairs Medical Center
1201 Broad Rock Blvd., Richmond VA 23249 (USA)
Tel. +1 804 675 5802, Fax +1 804 675 5816, E-Mail dmheuman@vcu.edu

Gerbes AL (ed): Ascites, Hyponatremia and Hepatorenal Syndrome: Progress in Treatment.
Front Gastrointest Res. Basel, Karger, 2011, vol 28, pp 91–101

Vaptans for Ascites – Chances and Risks

Florence Wong

Department of Medicine, Toronto General Hospital, University of Toronto, Toronto, Ont., Canada

Abstract

Ascites is a common complication of cirrhosis. The presence of ascites is associated with significant morbidity and mortality. Traditional treatments of ascites with diuretics and repeat large-volume paracenteses have their limitations. Definitive treatments of ascites such as the insertion of a transjugular intrahepatic portosystemic shunt or liver transplantation are available to suitably selected patients. The development of vasopressin V_2 receptor antagonists or vaptans as a treatment for hyponatremia associated with ascites has proven to be a welcoming addition to the management of these patients. Six vaptans have been assessed and all have been shown to be effective in correcting hyponatremia. Tolvaptan, conivaptan and moxivaptan are approved worldwide for clinical use for the correction of hyponatremia from any etiology. Satavaptan and tolvaptan have also been shown to improve the quality of life of patients once hyponatremia is corrected. The sodium-correcting effect of the vaptans can only be maintained while patients are taking it. Satavaptan, tolvaptan and M0002 may also have an ascites-reducing effect. Satavaptan has been studied for 52 weeks in several phase III trials and renal impairment and hyperkalemia seem to be two consistent side effects. All of the other vaptans have only been studied for less than 30 days. Therefore, the full risks or benefits related to the other vaptans are unknown. Until the long-term results of the other vaptans are known, it is prudent to start with a low dose and titrate upwards to find the appropriate dose for the desired effect.

The Clinical Problem

Ascites is a common complication of liver cirrhosis, occurring in 60% of cirrhotic patients within 10 years of diagnosis of compensated cirrhosis [1]. Ascites affects 5–7% of cirrhotic patients at any one time. The development of ascites in the natural history of cirrhosis heralds a worsening of the prognosis to 50% survival at 2 years [1], and this deteriorates to 30–50% at 1 year when the ascites becomes refractory to medical therapy [2, 3]. Ascites also worsens the quality of life of cirrhotic patients, and predisposes them to complications such as abdominal hernias, restrictive ventilatory dysfunction, malnutrition, spontaneous bacterial peritonitis and hepatorenal syndrome, some of which are life threatening. Traditionally, the management of ascites consists of dietary sodium restriction and the judicious use of diuretics [4]. With progression of liver cirrhosis, increasingly higher doses of diuretics are required in order to control the accumulation of ascites. Eventually, either diuretic-induced complications such as electrolyte abnormalities or renal dysfunction occur, or the patient no longer has a diuretic response despite very high doses of diuretics such as 160 mg of furosemide and 400 mg of spironolactone daily [4]. These patients with refractory ascites will require second-line treatments of their ascites, especially if the ascites is large enough to interfere with patient comfort and daily activities. These include large-volume paracentesis (LVP), the insertion of a transjugular intrahepatic portosystemic stent shunt (TIPS) in the suitable patients, or liver transplantation [4].

Therapeutic Limitations in the Management of Refractory Ascites

Repeat LVPs have been shown to have low complication rates [5, 6]. Although LVPs can provide a rapid relief of the symptoms related to abdominal distension, they do not correct the underlying pathophysiology of ascites formation, namely renal sodium retention. Therefore, re-accumulation of ascites invariably occurs. Although repeat LVPs are manageable, they involve significant medical manpower and inconvenience to the patients. The insertion of a TIPS shunt corrects portal hypertension, which is one of the pathogenetic factors for ascites formation, but the diversion of blood from the splanchnic to the systemic circulation through the TIPS is associated with its unique set of complications [7], especially for older patients or those with moderate underlying liver dysfunction or cardiopulmonary abnormalities [8]. Therefore, TIPS insertion is only suitable for carefully selected patients, representing approximately 40–50% of all patients with ascites. Liver transplantation corrects portal hypertension, liver dysfunction and the hemodynamic abnormalities of advanced cirrhosis. However, with the shortage of donor organs, only a small percentage of patients will receive timely liver transplantation.

Recent Novel Therapeutic Agents for the Management of Ascites

One of the pathogenetic pathways that is involved in renal sodium retention and ascites formation in cirrhosis is the development of systemic and splanchnic arterial vasodilatation, leading to relatively effective arterial underfilling that activates various renal sodium-retaining mechanisms [9]. Therefore, therapeutic agents that can potentially reduce the relative effective arterial underfilling have been tried as novel treatments for ascites in cirrhosis. These include various systemic vasoconstrictors in order to reduce the extent of arterial vasodilatation, and plasma expanders such as albumin to fill the arterial circulation.

Selective nonpeptide vasopressin V_2 receptor antagonists, or 'vaptans' as they are known, belong to a newer class of drugs that is emerging as a plausible treatment for cirrhotic ascites. These are aquaretic agents that have been developed for the treatment of hyponatremia. The development of hyponatremia in cirrhosis is common, especially in patients with advanced cirrhosis and refractory ascites. This is related to the excess secretion of arginine vasopressin (AVP) from nonosmotic stimulation. There is also resetting of the osmoreceptors in cirrhosis, so that the secretion of AVP is only suppressed at a lower serum osmolality when compared to healthy individuals [10]. The development of hyponatremia in patients with cirrhosis and ascites precludes continued use of diuretic therapy. By correcting hyponatremia, the vaptans may allow the continued use of diuretics and therefore help in the management of ascites in cirrhosis. More recently, there are emerging data that the vaptans may also be effective in the management of ascites in patients with cirrhosis but without hyponatremia [11].

The Vaptans

Vasopressin V_2 receptors are located on the basolateral surface of the principal cells of the collecting duct of the nephron, which is impermeable to water in the absence of vasopressin. Vasopressin, by binding to the V_2 receptor, stimulates a series of reactions, which ultimately leads to the insertion of aquaporin 2 on the luminal side of the collecting duct. Aquaporins 2 are water channels. Their insertion allows water to be reabsorbed from the luminal side to the basolateral side of the collecting duct (fig. 1a), and the urine is concentrated. The vaptans compete with vasopressin for attachment onto the V_2 receptors, but they lack the ability to stimulate the insertion of aquaporin 2 into the collecting duct. Therefore, the use of vaptans can effectively inhibit the reabsorption of water in the collecting duct (fig. 1b), reducing the serum water content, thereby correcting hyponatremia.

More recently, the vaptans have also been assessed as an agent for the treatment of ascites independent of the presence of hyponatremia [11–13]. Intuitively, it seems unlikely that an aquaretic agent could effect a reduction in ascites accumulation. However, the loss of a significant volume of water induced by the aquaretic agent could lead to a reduction in the intravascular volume. This could be compensated for by an increase in oral fluid intake and/or activation of various physiological mechanisms to replenish the effective intravascular volume. One of the possible mechanisms for replenishing the intravascular volume can be achieved through an increased movement of water from the interstitial and/or intracellular compartment to the vascular compartment. Another mechanism could be an increased reabsorption of ascitic fluid, leading to a reduction in ascites accumulation (fig. 2). Given the fact that reabsorption of ascitic fluid is relatively fixed, maximally at approximately 400 ml/day [14], the rate of ascites reduction will be gradual and

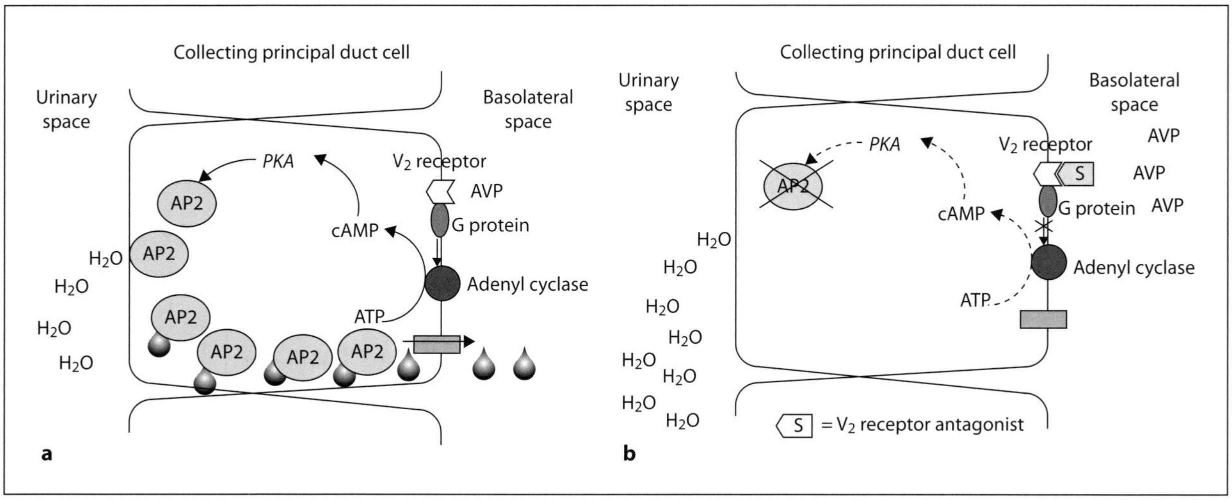

Fig. 1. **a** Mechanism of action of vasopressin in mediating water reabsorption at the principal cell of the renal collecting duct. **b** Blocking of the vasopressin V2 receptor by a vaptan.

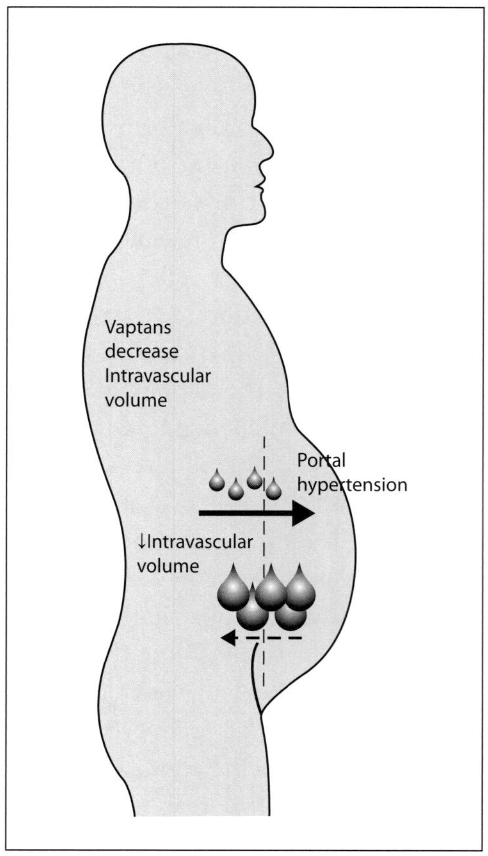

Fig. 2. The presence of portal hypertension in cirrhosis favours the transfer of fluid from the intravascular space to the peritoneal cavity. Vaptans, by decreasing the intravascular volume, favours the reabsorption of fluid from the peritoneal cavity back to intravascular compartment.

Table 1. Vaptans that have been assessed for the management of hyponatremia and/or ascites in cirrhosis

Vaptan	Compound	Receptor type	Route of administration	Current status
Conivaptan	YM-087	V_1/V_2	intravenous	approved in the United States for the treatment of hyponatremia in hospitalized patients
Tolvaptan	OPC-41061	V_2	oral	approved in the United States for the treatment of hyponatremia of all etiologies
Moxivaptan	OPC-31260	V_2	oral	approved in Japan for the treatment of hyponatremia associated with the syndrome of inappropriate anti diuretic hormone secretion
Satavaptan	SR-121463	V_2	oral	several phase III studies for the indication of treatment of ascites; development has been permanently discontinued
Lixivaptan	VPA-985	V_2	oral	phase II studies in cirrhosis for the indication of hyponatremia; further development currently postponed
M0002	RWJ-354617	V_2	oral	small phase II study in cirrhosis for the treatment of ascites; further development currently postponed

this appears to be what was observed in a medium-term study using one of the aquaretic agents, satavaptan [12].

To date, 6 vaptans have been assessed for the management of hyponatremia of all causes and/or ascites in cirrhosis (table 1). All are selective V_2 receptor antagonists, with the exception of conivaptan, which is a combined V_1/V_2 receptor antagonist. Currently, only conivaptan and tolvaptan are approved in the United States for the treatment of hyponatremia in euvolemic and hypervolemic states. Mozavaptan is approved in Japan only for the treatment of hyponatremia associated with the syndrome of inappropriate antidiuretic hormone secretion. The development of the other vaptans has either been postponed (M0002, lixivaptan) or permanently discontinued (satavaptan).

Vaptans in the Management of Hyponatremia in Cirrhosis

In the first randomized, double-blind, placebo-controlled trial assessing the efficacy of a vaptan for the management of hyponatremia, lixivaptan in ascending doses of 25, 125 or 250 mg versus placebo twice daily was given without concomitant diuretics for 7 days to 44 patients, 33 of whom of were cirrhotic patients with ascites [15]. There was a dose-dependent increase in serum sodium in the lixivaptan groups, so that by day 4 of the study, the serum sodium in the 250 mg b.i.d. group had risen from a baseline of 125 ± 1 to 135 ± 1 mmol/l, and this remained at 134 ± 2 mmol/l by the end of the 7-day study. The rise in serum sodium concentration in all the lixivaptan groups was significantly higher than that in the placebo group, whose serum sodium remained unchanged at 125 ± 2 mmol/l by the end of the study [15]. In another study involving 60 cirrhotic patients with ascites, the administration of either 50 or 100 mg of lixivaptan twice daily without diuretics also resulted in a dose-dependent increase in serum sodium, so that by the end of the study, the serum sodium had increased by 6 ± 2 mmol/l. This compared significantly higher than the placebo group, whose low serum sodium concentrations virtually remained unchanged by the end of the study [16]. Normalization of serum sodium concentration was achieved in 27 and 50% of patients in the 100- and 200-mg/day groups, respectively, but in none of the patients in the placebo group ($p < 0.05$ and $p < 0.001$, respectively) [16].

Satavaptan at 5-, 12.5- or 25-mg doses versus placebo, together with 100 mg of spironolactone per day, was first tested in 110 cirrhotic patients with ascites and serum sodium ≤130 mmol/l in a 14-day study [17]. Despite the concomitant administration of a diuretic, an improvement in serum sodium was observed in the satavaptan groups almost immediately and this increase was maintained throughout the 14-day study. Overall, the serum sodium in the satavaptan groups increased by a mean value of at least 4 mmol/l, versus a mean increase in serum sodium of 1 mmol/l in the placebo group ($p < 0.01$) [17]. The same patients were then offered re-treatment and 73 agreed [18], and, together with an additional 66 patients, participated in a 52-week study assessing the longer-term effects of 5–50 mg satvaptan daily on serum sodium concentration, with flexible doses of diuretics in order to mimic real-life clinical practice [19]. The mean sodium concentration rose from 129 mmol/l at re-randomization to either normal or near normal levels throughout the study in the satavaptan groups, whereas the mean serum sodium concentration remained at <130 mmol/l for most of the time throughout the study in the placebo group [19]. Normal sodium concentrations could only be maintained while taking satavaptan. After completion of the study, hyponatremia with serum sodium of <130 mmol/l rapidly recurred.

Tolvaptan, another orally active vaptan, was assessed for its efficacy in the treatment of hyponatremia in 2 prospective randomized controlled trials (SALT-1 and SALT-2 studies), which included a total of 444 patients with serum sodium <135 mmol/l [20]. Tolvaptan was administered at an initial dose of 15 mg daily, and this was increased to 30 mg daily and, if necessary, to 60 mg daily if the serum sodium did not reach 136 mmol/l and the change in serum sodium had been <5 mmol/l on the previous day. Thirty-eight of the SALT-2 study patients randomized to tolvaptan and 36 patients randomized to placebo had underlying cirrhosis. Considering all the study patients as a whole, there was a significant increase in serum sodium on both day 4 and day 30 of the study [20]. The cirrhotic patients in SALT-2 had a rise in serum sodium of 1.94–3.48 mmol/l on day 4 and 2.45–3.09 mmol/l on day 30. Normalization of sodium levels (>135 mmol/l) occurred in 29–30 and 17–22% of cirrhotic subjects at days 4 and 30, respectively [21]. It is not clear whether the patients were given concomitant diuretics during the study. It appears not to be so, as patients were placed on fluid restriction to help improve their serum sodium concentration. Like satavaptan, hyponatremia recurred once the study was complete and tolvaptan was stopped.

Vaptans in the Management of Ascites in Cirrhosis

It was observed in some of the above studies that, apart from improving the serum sodium concentrations, the vaptans were also able to reducing the extent of ascites in cirrhotic patients [17]. It is therefore feasible that by maintaining serum sodium, the use of vaptans had permitted diuretics to be continued, thereby improving the control of ascites. The question that follows is whether the vaptans had any effects on the control of ascites independent of diuretic therapy. In a 14-day study involving 148 patients with cirrhosis and ascites but without hyponatremia, the addition of satavaptan at the doses of 5, 12.5 or 25 mg versus placebo to 100 mg of spironolactone daily, let to a significant greater weight reduction ($p < 0.05$) in all the satavaptan groups compared to the placebo group [11], suggesting that satavaptan was able to effect a reduction in ascites irrespective of diuretics. The mean volume of ascites reduction was in the range of 2.08–2.46 liters for the 2-week study period. Interestingly, there was no dose-dependent effect on ascites reduction, suggesting that the amount of ascites reabsorption from the peritoneal cavity is relatively fixed, as demonstrated by indicator studies [14]. When satavaptan was specifically studied for its effects on preventing the recurrence of ascites after a large-volume paracentesis over a 12-week period in patients with or without hyponatremia, the same doses of satavaptan were able to significantly reduce the frequency of paracentesis when compared to placebo in the presence of 100 mg of spironolactone daily [12]. However, a longer-term study in a larger cohort of cirrhotic patients with ascites over a 52-week period on the prevention of ascites recurrence was only able to show a trend towards a better control of ascites in terms of the time to the first paracentesis and the frequency of large-volume paracentesis [22]. Further randomized controlled trials using satavaptan in patients with either diuretic-responsive ascites [23] or diuretic-resistant ascites [24] also only showed a trend towards better rather than superiority of satavaptan over placebo in terms of ascites control.

Similar to satavaptan, short-term studies with either M0002 [25] or tolvaptan [13] also showed efficacy of the vaptans in improving ascites. However, the study with M0002 only involved 15 patients for a total of vaptan administration of 2 weeks, while that using tolvaptan included 18 patients for a total of 9 study days. Therefore, while the results are encouraging, it is not clear whether longer-term studies involving a larger cohort of patients with either M0002 or tolvaptan will confirm their efficacy in reducing ascites in cirrhosis.

Vaptans – the Chances

The arrival of the vaptans more than a decade ago certainly brought a lot of enthusiasm amongst the physicians caring for patients with cirrhosis, ascites and hyponatremia. The vaptans have demonstrated their efficacy in correcting hyponatremia, thereby allowing diuretics to be continued in the management of ascites. The correction of hyponatremia has resulted in an improved health-related quality of life, whether it was assessed by a 36-item (SF-36) [26] or a 12-item short form (SF-12) [20] general health survey. The vaptans as a group has also shown some promise as an agent in the management of ascites independent of hyponatremia [12, 13, 22–25]. This is the first time in several decades that a novel class of agents is being developed for the population of cirrhotic patients with ascites. As such, the vaptans are providing a real chance for improving the overall well-being of the cirrhotic patients.

Vaptans – the Risks

The potential benefits of the vaptans have to be weighed against the risks involved in their use. The vaptans are aquaretics, and excessive correction of hyponatremia can result in osmotic demyelination and neurological sequelae [27]. Thirst is the most common side effect in almost all the trials involving the vaptans, and thirst will provide some protection against excess dehydration provided the patient is allowed free access to water. Despite this, the risk of dehydration will always be present. Indeed, renal impairment is reported much more commonly with vaptans than with placebo in most of the randomized control trials, especially with satavaptan [12,

19, 22–24]. There is also the risk of hyperkalemia with satavaptan [12, 19, 22–24]. This may be related to the fact that vasopressin normally regulates Na-K-ATPase and Na-KCl cotransporter activity [28], which is crucial for sodium reabsorption and potassium excretion in the distal nephron. Satavaptan, by blocking vasopressin binding to the V_2 receptor, effectively decreases Na-K-ATPase expression, thereby reducing renal tubular potassium secretion. It appears that hyperkalemia has only been reported with satavaptan, and not with the other vaptans. The reason for this is unknown. All these risks can be minimized by starting with lower doses of the vaptan and titrate slowly towards the most effective dose. The fact that the development of satavaptan has been discontinued permanently is disappointing. Increased mortality in the patients randomized to satavaptan in the phase III studies has been reported, although no single cause of the increased mortality can be identified [pers. commun.].

The Future

Currently, 3 vaptans have been approved for use in the management of hyponatremia from whatever cause worldwide. Therefore, the vaptans will be administered to patients with cirrhosis when the indication arises. Although satavaptan is the only vaptan that has long-term data on its efficacy and risks in a significant number of cirrhotic patients with ascites, and there are risks associated with its use in cirrhosis, it is difficult to assign the same risks to the other vaptans when there have not been long-term studies with the other vaptans. Therefore, we will need to await further longer-term trials to assess the risk-benefit ratio of chronic vaptan use. In particular, we need to assess whether correcting hyponatremia will alter the overall morbidity and mortality of these patients with advanced cirrhosis.

Key Messages

- The vaptans are aquaretic agents. They increase the renal excretion of free water by blocking the action of vasopressin at the renal collecting tubule.
- The vaptans are very effective in correcting hyponatremia from any etiology even in the presence of diuretics.
- The vaptans have shown a trend towards reducing ascites in cirrhotic patients, and therefore may be used as an adjunct therapy to diuretics in the management of ascites.
- The vaptans can potentially cause dehydration and too rapid correction of hyponatremia with neurological sequelae, and possibly renal impairment.
- Hyperkalemia appears to be a common side effect of satavaptan.
- It is prudent to start a vaptan with a low dose and titrate upwards to find the appropriate dose for the desired effect.

References

1 D'Amico G, Garcia-Tsao G, Pagliaro L: Natural history and prognostic indicators of survival in cirrhosis: a systematic review of 118 studies. J Hepatol 2006;44:217–231.

2 Planas R, Montoliu S, Balleste B, Rivera M, et al: Natural history of patients hospitalized for management of cirrhotic ascites. Clin Gastroenterol Hepatol 2006;4:1385–1394.

3 Moreau R, Delegue P, Pessione F, Hillaire S, Durand F, Lebrec D, Valla DC: Clinical characteristics and outcome of patients with cirrhosis and refractory ascites. Liver Int 2004;24:457–464.

4 Moore KP, Wong F, Gines P, Ochs A, et al: The management of ascites: report on the consensus conference of the International Ascites Club. Hepatology 2003;38:258–266.

5 Gines P, Arroyo V, Quintero E, Planas R, et al: Comparison of paracentesis and diuretics in the treatment of cirrhotics with tense ascites: results of a randomized study. Gastroenterology 1987;93:234–241.

6 Salerno F, Badalamenti S, Incerti P, Tempini S, et al: Repeated paracentesis and i.v. albumin infusion to treat 'tense' ascites in cirrhotic patients: a safe alternative therapy. J Hepatol 1987;5:102–108.

7 Wong F: The use of TIPS in chronic liver disease. Ann Hepatol 2006;5:5–15.

8 Salerno F, Cammà C, Enea M, Rössle M, Wong F: Transjugular intrahepatic portosystemic shunt for refractory ascites, a meta-analysis of individual patient data Gastroenterology 2007;113:825–834.

9 Schrier RW, Arroyo V, Bernardi M, Epstein M, Henriksen JH, Rodes J: Peripheral arterial vasodilation hypothesis: a proposal for the initiation of renal sodium and water retention in cirrhosis. Hepatology 1988;8:1151–1157.

10 Gines P, Berl T, Bernardi M, Bichet DG, et al: Hyponatremia in cirrhosis: from pathogenesis to treatment. Hepatology 1998;28:851–864.

11 Gines P, Wong F, Watson HR, Dudley F, Zarski JP, Bruha R. Terg R: Effects of combination of satavaptan, a selective vasopressin V_2 receptor antagonist, and diuretics in patients with cirrhosis without hyponatremia: a randomized, double-blind, placebo-controlled study. Aliment Pharmacol Ther 2010;8:834–845.

12 Wong F, Gines P, Watson H, Horsmans Y, Angeli P, Gow P, Minini P, et al: Effects of a selective vasopressin V_2 receptor antagonist, satavaptan, on recurrence of ascites after large volume paracentesis in patients with cirrhosis. J Hepatol 2010;53:283–290.

13 Okita K, Sakaida I, Okada M, Kaneko M, et al: A multicenter, open-label, dose-ranging study to exploratively evaluate the efficacy, safety, and dose-response of tolvaptan in patients with decompensated liver cirrhosis. J Gastroenterol 2010;45:979–987.

14 Shear L, Ching S, Gabuzda GJ: Compartmentalization of ascites and edema in patients with hepatic cirrhosis. N Engl J Med 1970;282:1391–1396.

15 Wong F, Blei A, Blendis LM, Robertson G, Thuluvath PJ, North American VPA-985 Study Group: The effects of VPA-985, a vasopressin receptor antagonist, on water metabolism in patients with hyponatremia: a multi-center randomized placebo controlled trial. Hepatology 2003;37:182–191.

16 Gerbes AL, Gülberg V, Ginès P, Decaux G, Gross P, Gandjini H, Djian J, VPA Study Group: Therapy of hyponatremia in cirrhosis with a vasopressin receptor antagonist: a randomized double-blind multicenter trial. Gastroenterology 2003;124:933–939.

17 Ginès P, Wong F, Watson H, Milutinovic S, Ruiz del Arbol L, Olteanu D: Effects of Satavaptan, a selective vasopressin V_2 receptor antagonist, on ascites and serum sodium concentration in patients with cirrhosis and hyponatremia. Hepatology 2008;48:204–213.

18 Gines P, Wong F, Watson H, EXPOCAT Study Investigators: Long-term improvement of serum sodium by the V_2 receptor antagonist satavaptan in patients with cirrhosis and hyponatremia (abstract). J Hepatol 2007;46(suppl 1):S41.

19 Gines P, Wong F, Martin M, Lecorps G, Watson HR: Effects of satavaptan on hyponatremia, management of ascites and morbidity in liver cirrhosis in a long-term placebo controlled study (abstract). Hepatology 2008;48(suppl):413A.

20 Schrier RW, Gross P, Gheorghiade M, Berl T, Verbalis JG, Czerwiec FS, Orlandi C, SALT Investigators: Tolvaptan, a selective oral vasopressin V_2-receptor antagonist, for hyponatremia. N Engl J Med 2006;355:2099–2112.

21 Afdhal N, Cardenas A, Gines P, Gross P, et al: Randomized placebo-controlled trial of tolvaptan, a novel V_2 receptor antagonist in hyponatremia, results of the SALT-2 trial with emphasis on efficacy and safety in cirrhosis (abstract). Hepatology 2005;42(suppl 1):756A.

22 Wong F, Bernardi M, Horsmans Y, Cabrijan Z, Watson HR, Ginès P, exSPA Investigators: Effects of satavaptan, an oral vasopressin V_2 receptor antagonist, on management of ascites and morbidity in liver cirrhosis in a long-term, placebo-controlled study (abstract). J Hepatol 2009;50(suppl 1):S42.

23 Wong F, Ginès P, Nevens F, van Vlierberghe H, et al: Double-blind, placebo-controlled study of satavaptan in the management of recurrent ascites: the SPARe-1 study (abstract). Hepatology 2009;50 (suppl):448A.
24 Gerbes A, Wong F, Horsmans Y, Alper E, Watson HR, Badalamenti S, Ginès P: Satavaptan efficacy and safety in recurrent ascites without concomitant diuretics: the SPARe-2 study (abstract). J Hepatology 2010;52(suppl 1):S334.
25 Nevens F, Moreno C, Cools M, Thielemans L, Kerstens R, Meulemans A: Effects of M0002, a novel V_2 antagonist on sodium levels and weight gain affected by water accumulation in cirrhotic patients with ascites. J Hepatol 2009;50(suppl 1):S76.
26 Gines P, Wong F, Smadja-Lew E, Diamand F: Hyponatremia: a major determinant of impaired health related quality of life in cirrhosis with ascites (abstract). Hepatology 2007;46(suppl):567A.
27 Decaux G, Soupart A: Treatment of symptomatic hyponatremia. Am J Med Sci 2003;326:25–30.
28 Bertuccio CA, Ibarra FR, Toledo JE, Arrizurieta EE, Martin RS: Endogenous vasopressin regulates Na-K-ATPase and Na(+)-K(+)-Cl(–) cotransporter rbsc-1 in rat outer medulla. Am J Physiol Renal Physiol 2002;282:F265–F270.

Florence Wong, MB BS, MD, FRACP, FRCPC
9th floor, North Wing, Room 983
Toronto Hospital, 200 Elizabeth Street
Toronto M5G 2C4, ON (Canada)
Tel. +1 416 340 3834, Fax +1 416 340 5019, E-Mail florence.wong@utoronto.ca

Gerbes AL (ed): Ascites, Hyponatremia and Hepatorenal Syndrome: Progress in Treatment.
Front Gastrointest Res. Basel, Karger, 2011, vol 28, pp 102–111

Cardiorenal Syndrome – A New Entity?

Søren Møller[a] · Aleksander Krag[b]

Departments of [a]Clinical Physiology and Nuclear Medicine, and [b]Medical Gastroenterology, Hvidovre Hospital, Faculty of Health Sciences, University of Copenhagen, Hvidovre, Denmark

Abstract

A considerable number of patients with advanced cirrhosis develop an initial hyperdynamic circulation and renal failure, which carry a poor prognosis. The hepatorenal syndrome denotes a progressive functional renal failure, owing to pronounced renal vasoconstriction, central hypovolemia, and low arterial perfusion pressure. Cirrhotic cardiomyopathy has been described as a condition with impaired contractile responsiveness to stress and altered diastolic relaxation. There are now several observations that indicate a relation between impaired renal function and decreased cardiac systolic function in advanced cirrhosis, in particular in patients with spontaneous bacterial peritonitis or refractory ascites. This has lent support to the hypothesis of a cardiorenal syndrome in cirrhosis. A cardiorenal syndrome refers to a condition where dysfunction of one of the organs affects the other, and implies that a cardiac systolic dysfunction in cirrhosis affects kidney function and survival in patients with advanced cirrhosis and renal failure. Thus, renal failure as well as cardiac dysfunction should be targets for new treatments that ameliorate abnormal systemic vascular resistance, effective blood volume, arterial blood pressure, and cardiac systolic function. Future research should confirm the hypothesis of a cardiorenal syndrome in cirrhosis and the potential principles of treatment.

Cirrhosis with portal hypertension leads to development of portosystemic collaterals and related complications in a variety of organ systems. These include esophageal varices, ascites, bacterial infections, encephalopathy, renal failure, and hyponatremia [1]. Preceding this, many patients develop a circulatory dysfunction with a hyperdynamic circulation simultaneously characterized by low arterial pressure [2]. The presence of these complications mainly determines the course and prognosis of the disease. For example, mild ascites is associated with poor survival, with a 50% mortality rate within 3 years [3]. In about 25% of the patients, spontaneous bacterial peritonitis (SBP) further worsens the prognosis [4]. With disease progression, a substantial number of patients with ascites develop hepatorenal syndrome (HRS), which still carries a very poor prognosis [1, 5]. Hitherto, little attention has been paid to the role of cardiac dysfunction in the pathogenesis of HRS. However, recent research has

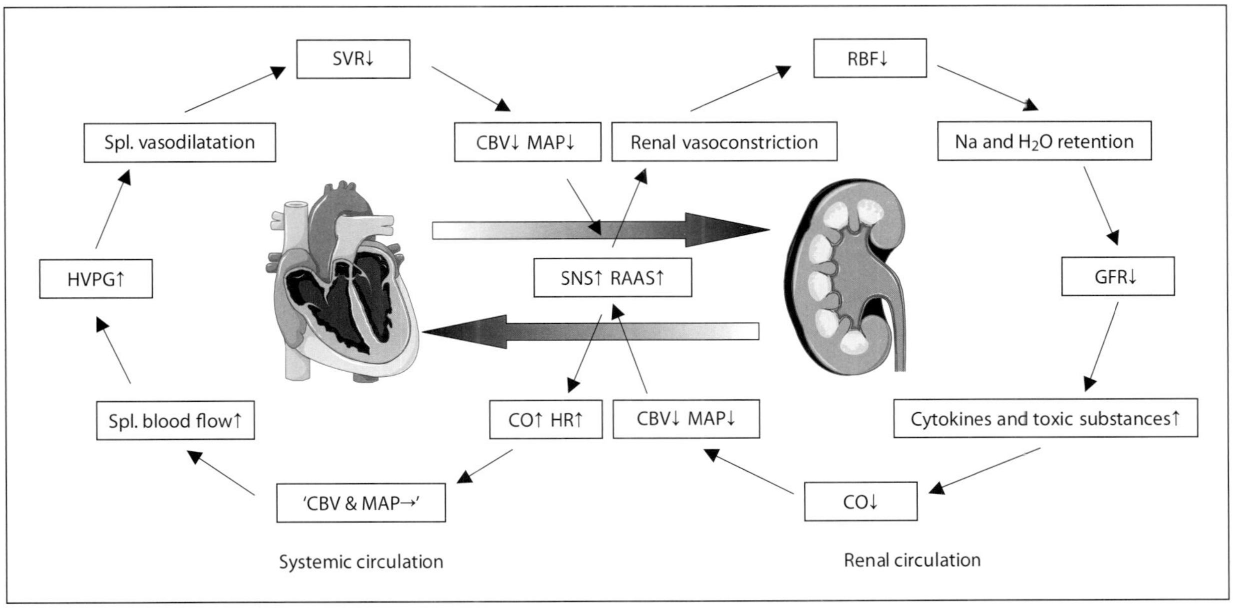

Fig. 1. Proposal for a relation between arteriolar splanchnic vasodilatation and development of a compensatory hyperdynamic circulation, partly because of central hypovolemia. As part of a vicious circle, renal vasoconstriction and impaired renal function may contribute to suppression of cardiac function at a later stage, further deteriorating renal function as a cardiorenal syndrome. The cardiorenal syndrome in cirrhosis denotes that dysfunction of an individual organ may affect the function of another. Direct or indirect cardiac effects on renal function (horizontal arrows) include low arterial blood pressure and cardiac output and increased activity of the sympathetic nervous and renin-angiotensin-aldosterone systems. Renal effects on the heart include anemia and sodium and water retention.

focused on the failing heart as a contributing factor to renal failure in cirrhosis [2]. This chapter discusses the basics of a potential cardiorenal syndrome in cirrhosis.

Hepatic Decompensation and Hemodynamic Derangements in Cirrhosis

The 'forward theory of ascites formation' combines arterial and splanchnic and central underfilling with a forward increase in splanchnic capillary pressure and filtration with increased lymph formation [1, 2]. Central hypovolemia and low arterial blood pressure are strong stimuli for the baroreceptor-induced activation of potent vasoconstricting systems, such as the sympathetic nervous system (SNS), the renin-angiotensin-aldosterone system (RAAS), and nonosmotic release of vasopressin [1, 2] (fig. 1). The pathophysiological consequence is formation of ascites in the face of increased cardiac output and low arterial blood pressure (table 1). In this sense, cardiac output can be regarded as a mediator of the effective blood volume, and

Table 1. Hemodynamic changes at rest in advanced cirrhosis

Heart	
	Heart rate ↑
	Cardiac output (→)↑(↓)
	Left atrial volume ↑
	Left ventricular volume → (↑)
	Right atrial volume → ↑ ↓
	Right atrial pressure → ↑
	Right ventricular end-diastolic pressure →
	Pulmonary artery pressure → ↑
	Pulmonary capillary wedge pressure →
	Left atrial pressure →
	Left ventricular end diastolic pressure →
Systemic circulation	
	Plasma volume ↑
	Total blood volume ↑
	Non-central blood volume ↑
	Central and arterial blood volume →↓
	Arterial blood pressure →↓
	Systemic vascular resistance ↓
Kidneys	
	Renal blood flow ↓
	Glomerular filtration rate ↓
	Sodium and water retention ↑
	Renal venous pressure ↑

↑→ ↓ = Increased, unchanged, and decreased values compared to controls.
Arrows in parentheses describe less typical changes.

underfilling of the arterial circulation occurs in later stages of the disease as a result of a further reduction in systemic vascular resistance [6]. However, at a much later stage of the disease, underfilling of the arterial circulation may also occur secondary to a reduction in the increased cardiac output, as described in patients with renal failure and SBP [7].

Renal Failure in Cirrhosis – The Clinical Problem

Renal function is disturbed even in the early phases of cirrhosis. About 75% of patients with cirrhosis develop ascites and 45% of these become infected with SBP and a further 35% of the latter develop renal failure [8]. Altogether, about 20% of cirrhotic patients with refractory ascites progress to a HRS, which is defined as a functional renal failure in patients with chronic liver disease without significant morphological changes in renal histology and with largely normal tubular function [9]. Two types of HRS have been defined depending on the rapidity and extent of the renal failure [9]. Type 1 is an acute form with a rapid decrease in renal function and renal failure as an independent predictive factor; type 2 is a chronic form with a more stable renal dysfunction [9]. The prognosis of patients with full-blown HRS is poor, ranging from days to weeks, and liver transplantation is the only radical treatment [1, 9].

SBP per se may precipitate the development of HRS, partly through release of toxic substances and cytokines, such as TNF-α, and others. Since the mortality of patients with HRS is extremely high, there is considerable interest in acquiring more insight into the pathophysiology and new potentials for treatment.

Cardiac Dysfunction

Independent observations have confirmed the presence of a latent cardiac dysfunction in cirrhosis that affects cardiac contractility as well as the electromechanical function [10]. This syndrome is termed cirrhotic cardiomyopathy, and particularly systolic dysfunction can be revealed by pharmacological or physical strain (table 2) [2]. Diastolic dysfunction reflects delayed left ventricular filling and is partly attributed to ventricular hypertrophy and altered collagen structure. Atrial natriuretic peptide (ANP) levels are increased in some patients with cirrhosis and portal hypertension [11]. In addition, the Q-T interval is prolonged in about half of the cirrhotic patients and may be normalized with β-blockers [2, 10]. Systolic dysfunction can be divided into chronotropic and inotropic incompetence. Chronotropic incompetence is a prognostic indicator of primary heart disease and mortality in other patients as well as in those with sepsis [12, 13]. Similarly, chronotropic incompetence is seen in patients with advanced cirrhosis [14, 15]. Systolic dysfunction as part of a cirrhotic cardiomyopathy has recently been implicated in renal failure in advanced disease,

Table 2. Proposal for diagnostic and supportive criteria for cirrhotic cardiomyopathy agreed upon at a working party held at the 2005 World Congress of Gastroenterology in Montreal

A working definition of cirrhotic cardiomyopathy
Cardiac dysfunction in patients with cirrhosis characterized by impaired contractile responsiveness to stress and/or altered diastolic relaxation with electrophysiological abnormalities in the absence of other known cardiac disease
Diagnostic criteria
Systolic dysfunction
Blunted increase in cardiac output with exercise, volume challenge or pharmacological stimuli
Resting left ventricular ejection fraction < 55%
Diastolic dysfunction
E/A ratio <1.0 (age-corrected)
Prolonged deceleration time (>200 ms)
Prolonged isovolumetric relaxation time (>80 ms)
Supportive criteria
Electrophysiological abnormalities
Abnormal chronotropic response
Electromechanical uncoupling/dyssynchrony
Prolonged Q-Tc interval
Enlarged left atrium
Increased myocardial mass
Increased BNP and pro-BNP
Increased troponin I

BNP = Brain natriuretic peptide.

and there are indications that this cardiorenal axis in cirrhosis may affect the function of various organs, including the kidneys.

Cardiorenal Axis in Cirrhosis

In some cirrhotic patients, increased portal pressure is accompanied by a moderate increase in renal venous pressure that may affect renal function. In cardiac failure, increased cardiac preload is associated with increased renal venous pressure. An elevated central venous pressure has been shown to decrease the glomerular filtration rate (GFR) and cause sodium and water retention; an increase in renal venous pressure can also stimulate the RAAS [16]. Cardiac failure per se can therefore contribute to renal dysfunction by increasing the renal venous pressure and not solely because of systolic dysfunction [17]. In cardiac failure too, central hypovolaemia induces high-pressure, baroreceptor-stimulated SNS and RAAS activity. Pronounced arterial vasoconstriction in the kidneys leads to decreased renal blood flow, glomerular filtration, and sodium and water excretion. In patients with hepatic nephropathy and circulatory insufficiency, it is a major clinical challenge to distinguish between HRS, hypovolemia-induced renal failure, parenchymal renal disease, and drug-induced renal failure [1]. Cardiac dysfunction may play a role in the two first instances.

Cardiorenal Syndrome

There are several indications of reduced systolic performance in cirrhosis and in particular of a renal suppressive effect on the heart when kidney function deteriorates [5]. Thus, Ruiz-Del-Arbol et al. [14] showed that cirrhotic patients with renal failure had a lower cardiac output than those without. Moreover, those patients with infections had an even lower cardiac output, which remained low even after resolution of the infection. The authors therefore concluded that cardiac output seems to decrease in SBP as a consequence of combined 'septic' and cirrhotic cardiomyopathy [14]. Later on, the same group carried out a longitudinal study in which 40% of the patients developed HRS [7]. Patients with HRS had lower arterial blood pressure as well as lower cardiac output and significant activation of the SNS and RAAS. In this study, the increased plasma renin activity and low cardiac output turned out to be strong prognostic determinants [7]. Thus, maintenance of cardiac contractility, as well as peripheral vasodilatation, seems to be of importance in the development of renal dysfunction and HRS. Anemia, often seen in cirrhotic patients for various reasons, has been discussed as a factor in the development of the hyperdynamic syndrome [18]. When adjusted for the reduced red blood cell count, cardiac output is normal [19]. In addition, inflammation and increased cytokine production can suppress erythrocytosis [16]. In both cirrhotic patients and patients with heart failure, anemia is associated with a significantly increased mortality and it is possible that normalizing blood hemoglobin per se would improve cardiac and renal function [16] (fig. 1).

Recently, Krag et al. [15] studied 24 patients with advanced cirrhosis. In patients with a low cardiac index, the GFR was significantly lower than in those with a higher cardiac index. The low cardiac index group also demonstrated lower renal blood flow and higher levels of plasma creatinine. Moreover, the number of patients who developed HRS type 1 within 3 months was significantly higher in the group with suppressed cardiac function. This study was among the first to describe the association between cardiac dysfunction and renal failure and survival in cirrhosis [15] (fig. 2).

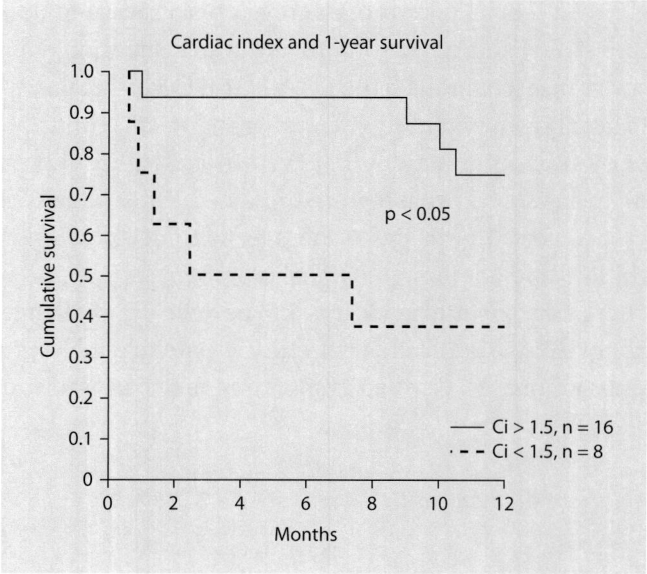

Fig. 2. Kaplan-Meier survival curves showing significantly poorer survival in patients with renal impairment and lower cardiac index (<1.5 liters • min^{-1} • m^2). From Krag et al. [15].

This cardiorenal relation in decompensated cirrhosis may very well be the result of an acute-on-chronic circulatory stress. It would therefore be tempting to suggest a relation between an acute cardiac dysfunction and the development of a type 1 HRS. This could accordingly be termed type 1 cardiorenal syndrome and would primarily be expected to be associated with acute events such as infections and alcoholic hepatitis [14, 20]. A more chronic cardiac dysfunction related to type 2 HRS could be termed type 2 cardiorenal syndrome and this would be expected to be more related to chronic activation of the vasoactive systems [7, 15, 21]. Cardiac performance can be suppressed by diverse mechanisms of depressing factors such as NO, TNF-α, endocannabinoids, carbon monoxide, and others [10, 21]. Thus, there is a profound but reversible, myocardial depression in patients with septic shock, particularly in those who are unable to increase their cardiac output [22, 23]. In patients with ascites, bacterial translocation of bacterial products from the gut into the circulation may initiate a systemic inflammatory response with generation of cytokines and other substances having potential harmful effects on renal and cardiac function [4]. This further suppresses cardiac performance, systolic function, arterial blood pressure, and renal perfusion, starting a vicious circle that among other effects leads to central hypovolemia, further deteriorating renal function (fig. 1). With the reduced GFR, the clearance of toxic substances by the liver is further reduced. Antibiotic treatment seems to ameliorate the marked immune and hemodynamic abnormalities in some patients [24].

The relationship between the failing heart and the kidney may not be unique for patients with liver disease and can be regarded as a more universal concept [25] (fig. 1). Thus, a cardiorenal relation has been described in patients with primary heart failure. This is generally defined as a pathophysiological disorder of the heart and kidneys, whereby acute or chronic dysfunction of one organ may induce acute or chronic dysfunction of the other. Various clinical subtypes have been defined. Cardiorenal syndromes types 1 and 2 appear to share most pathophysiological similarities to HRS types 1 and 2, respectively [26]. These are characterized by acute and chronic abnormalities in cardiac function causing progressive chronic kidney disease. In these patients even a slight decrease in the estimated GFR significantly increases mortality and is an independent negative prognostic factor in both diastolic and systolic ventricular dysfunction [27]. Moreover, neurohumoral abnormalities are present with excessive production of vasoconstrictive mediators such as noradrenaline, angiotensin, and endothelin.

Conclusions and Future Developments

Several observations suggest a link between the heart and the liver in hepatic nephropathy and results of independent studies have reported a lower cardiac output in cirrhotic patients with advanced renal failure.

Cirrhotic cardiomyopathy comprises systolic as well as diastolic dysfunction. After transjugular intrahepatic portosystemic shunt insertion, renal failure develops only in patients with diastolic dysfunction [28]. In addition, patients with combined systolic dysfunction and renal failure seem to have a much poorer survival.

In cirrhosis, two types of cardiorenal syndrome can be suggested: an acute type 1 related to acute events such as infections, and a chronic type 2 related to retarded events such as chronic inflammation.

Treatment of a combined cardiorenal syndrome in cirrhosis is highly speculative and complex, since potential drugs can oppose their effects in the two organs. Hence, there are drugs that should be avoided or administered cautiously and drugs with potential beneficial effects that should be tested experimentally. For instance, administration of terlipressin improves the GFR and renal blood flow in patients with refractory ascites through activation of V1 receptors that most likely induce an increase in arterial blood pressure. On the other hand, terlipressin may suppress cardiac function with a further decrease in cardiac output as the result. This response, i.e. an increased systemic vascular resistance and thereby an increase in left ventricular afterload, has also been observed with other potent vasoconstrictors, for example angiotensin II. β-Blockers may also have adverse effects with reduced cardiac output and potential to further disturb renal function directly or indirectly through a blood pressure-lowering effect.

Adenosine 1 receptor antagonists could represent a potential therapeutic approach, as adenosine concentrations are elevated in heart failure and cirrhosis. Antagonism of adenosine 1 receptors thus has the potential to improve renal function [29].

A mutual therapeutic approach to the treatment of a potential cardiorenal syndrome in cirrhosis is complex (fig. 1). However, it should be emphasized that adequate renal perfusion pressure is essential. The arterial blood pressure depends on the product of systemic vascular resistance and cardiac output. In patients with refractory ascites and HRS, the combination of terlipressin and human serum albumin has successfully improved the survival rates. These results are most likely based on the effects of terlipressin on systemic vascular resistance and of albumin on cardiac output [30]. The effects of this therapeutic approach emphasize the importance of the combination of an increasing systemic vascular resistance and improved renal volume flow to maintain renal perfusion pressure. More studies of a clearly defined cardiorenal syndrome in cirrhosis and studies of potential, new therapies that effectively combine an improvement in cardiac contractility and vascular resistance belong to the future.

Key Messages

- Cirrhotic cardiomyopathy denotes a condition of impaired contractile responsiveness to stress, altered diastolic relaxation, and the presence of electrophysiological abnormalities.
- Hepatorenal syndrome denotes functional renal failure in patients with advanced cirrhosis.
- Cardiorenal syndrome indicates a condition where dysfunction of one organ affects the other. There is evidence that a primary systolic dysfunction in cirrhosis affects the kidney function and survival of patients with advanced cirrhosis and renal failure.

References

1 Gines P, Schrier RW: Renal failure in cirrhosis. N Engl J Med 2009;361:1279–1290.
2 Møller S, Henriksen JH: Cardiovascular complications of cirrhosis. Gut 2008;57:268–278.
3 Fernandez-Esparrach G, Sanchez-Fueyo A, Gines P, Uriz J, Quinto L, Ventura PJ, Cardenas A, Guevara M, Sort P, Jimenez W, Bataller R, Arroyo V, Rodes J: A prognostic model for predicting survival in cirrhosis with ascites. J Hepatol 2001;34:46–52.
4 Wiest R, Garcia-Tsao G: Bacterial translocation (BT) in cirrhosis. Hepatology 2005;41:422–433.
5 Arroyo V, Terra C, Gines P: Advances in the pathogenesis and treatment of type-1 and type-2 hepatorenal syndrome. J Hepatol 2007;46:935–946.
6 Schrier RW: Decreased effective blood volume in edematous disorders: what does this mean? J Am Soc Nephrol 2007;18:2028–2031.
7 Ruiz-Del-Arbol L, Monescillo A, Arocena C, Valer P, Gines P, Moreira V, Maria MJ, Jimenez W, Arroyo V: Circulatory function and hepatorenal syndrome in cirrhosis. Hepatology 2005;42:439–447.
8 Fasolato S, Angeli P, Dallagnese L, Maresio G, Zola E, Mazza E, Salinas F, Dona S, Fagiuoli S, Sticca A, Zanus G, Cillo U, Frasson I, Destro C, Gatta A: Renal failure and bacterial infections in patients with cirrhosis: epidemiology and clinical features. Hepatology 2007;45:223–229.
9 Salerno F, Gerbes A, Gines P, Wong F, Arroyo V: Diagnosis, prevention and treatment of the hepatorenal syndrome in cirrhosis: a consensus workshop of the international ascites club. Gut 2007;56:1310–1318.
10 Alqahtani SA, Fouad TR, Lee SS: Cirrhotic cardiomyopathy. Semin Liver Dis 2008;28:59–69.
11 Gerbes AL, Wernze H, Arendt RM, Riedel A, Sauerbruch T, Paumgartner G: Atrial natriuretic factor and renin-aldosterone in volume regulation of patients with cirrhosis. Hepatology 1989;9:417–422.
12 Lauer MS, Okin PM, Larson MG, Evans JC, Levy D: Impaired heart rate response to graded exercise: prognostic implications of chronotropic incompetence in the Framingham Heart Study. Circulation 1996;93:1520–1526.

13 Kumar A, Schupp E, Bunnell E, Ali A, Milcarek B, Parrillo JE: Cardiovascular response to dobutamine stress predicts outcome in severe sepsis and septic shock. Crit Care 2008;12:R35.
14 Ruiz-Del-Arbol L, Urman J, Fernandez J, Gonzalez M, Navasa M, Monescillo A, Albillos A, Jimenez W, Arroyo V: Systemic, renal, and hepatic hemodynamic derangement in cirrhotic patients with spontaneous bacterial peritonitis. Hepatology 2003;38: 1210–1218.
15 Krag A, Bendtsen F, Henriksen JH, Møller S: Low cardiac output predicts development of hepatorenal syndrome and survival in patients with cirrhosis and ascites. Gut 2010;59:105–110.
16 Sarraf M, Masoumi A, Schrier RW: Cardiorenal syndrome in acute decompensated heart failure. Clin J Am Soc Nephrol 2009;4:2013–2026.
17 Firth JD, Raine AEG, Ledingham JGG: Raised venous pressure: a direct cause of renal sodium retention in oedema. Lancet 1988;i:1033–1038.
18 Cirera I, Elizalde JI, Pique JM, Feu F, Casadevall M, Goldin E, Teres J, Bosch J, Rodes J: Anemia worsens hyperdynamic circulation of patients with cirrhosis and portal hypertension. Dig Dis Sci 1997;42:1697–1702.
19 Henriksen JH, Bendtsen F, Møller S: Normal red cell cardiac output in the hyperkinetic syndrome of alcoholic cirrhosis. J Hepatol 2001;34:782–783.
20 Tristani FE, Cohn JN: Systemic and renal hemodynamics in oliguric hepatic failure: effect of volume expansion. J Clin Invest 1967;46:1894–1906.
21 Ros J, Claria J, Jimenez W, Boschmarce M, Angeli P, Arroyo V, Rivera F, Rodes J: Role of nitric oxide and prostacyclin in the control of renal perfusion in experimental cirrhosis. Hepatology 1995;22:915–920.
22 Parker MM, Shelhamer JH, Bacharach SL, Green MV, Natanson C, Frederick TM, Damske BA, Parrillo JE: Profound but reversible myocardial depression in patients with septic shock. Ann Intern Med 1984;100:483–490.
23 Parrillo JE, Burch C, Shelhamer JH, Parker MM, Natanson C, Schuette W: A circulating myocardial depressant substance in humans with septic shock: septic shock patients with a reduced ejection fraction have a circulating factor that depresses in vitro myocardial cell performance. J Clin Invest 1985;76:1539–1553.
24 Albillos A, de la HA, Gonzalez M, Moya JL, Calleja JL, Monserrat J, Ruiz-Del-Arbol L, Alvarez-Mon M: Increased lipopolysaccharide binding protein in cirrhotic patients with marked immune and hemodynamic derangement. Hepatology 2003;37:208–217.
25 Neubauer S: The failing heart – an engine out of fuel. N Engl J Med 2007;356:1140–1151.
26 Ronco C, Haapio M, House AA, Anavekar N, Bellomo R: Cardiorenal syndrome. J Am Coll Cardiol 2008;52:1527–1539.
27 McAlister FA, Ezekowitz J, Tonelli M, Armstrong PW: Renal insufficiency and heart failure: prognostic and therapeutic implications from a prospective cohort study. Circulation 2004;109:1004–1009.
28 Rabie RN, Cazzaniga M, Salerno F, Wong F: The use of E/A ratio as a predictor of outcome in cirrhotic patients treated with transjugular intrahepatic portosystemic shunt. Am J Gastroenterol 2009.
29 Stanley AJ, Forrest EH, Dabos K, Bouchier IAD, Hayes PC: Natriuretic effect of an adenosine-1 receptor antagonist in cirrhotic patients with ascites. Gastroenterology 1998;115:406–411.
30 Brinch K, Møller S, Bendtsen F, Becker U, Henriksen JH: Plasma volume expansion by albumin in cirrhosis: relation to blood volume distribution, arterial compliance and severity of disease. J Hepatol 2003;39:24–31.

Søren Møller, MD, DMSc
Department of Clinical Physiology and Nuclear Medicine
239, Hvidovre Hospital, Faculty of Health Sciences, University of Copenhagen
DK–2650 Hvidovre (Denmark)
Tel. +45 3632 3568, Fax +45 3632 3750, E-Mail soeren.moeller@hvh.regionh.dk

Gerbes AL (ed): Ascites, Hyponatremia and Hepatorenal Syndrome: Progress in Treatment.
Front Gastrointest Res. Basel, Karger, 2011, vol 28, pp 112–121

Renal Failure in Cirrhosis

Thierry Gustot[a,b] · Richard Moreau[b–d]

[a]Department of Gastroenterology and Hepato-Pancreatology, Erasme Hospital, Université Libre de Bruxelles, Brussels, Belgium; [b]INSERM U773, Centre de Recherche Biomédicale Bichat Beaujon CRB3, Clichy/Paris, [c]Liver Unit, Hôpital Beaujon, Clichy, and [d]Université Denis Diderot-Paris 7, Paris, France

Abstract

In patients with cirrhosis, acute kidney injury (AKI) is mainly due to prerenal factors (including type 1 hepatorenal syndrome; HRS) and ischemic acute tubular necrosis (ATN). Patients with cirrhosis may also develop chronic kidney disease (CKD) due to type 2 HRS, IgA nephropathy, hepatitis C virus-related membranoproliferative glomerulonephritis, hepatitis B-related membranous glomerulopathy, diabetic nephropathy, nondiabetic glomerulosclerosis and ischemic nephropathy. Some patients have 'acute-on-chronic' kidney injury. In patients with cirrhosis and CKD waiting for liver transplantation, renal biopsy may be indicated because histopathological analysis of renal-biopsy specimens provides diagnostic and prognostic information. In these patients, the transjugular route can be safely used. Treatments of AKI should target the cause of renal hypoperfusion (e.g. fluid replacement to treat intravascular volume depletion; vasoconstrictor therapy for type 1 HRS). There is no specific treatment for ATN; renal-replacement therapy may be used. Treatments of CKD depend on the cause: there is no established therapy for type 2 HRS or IgA nephropathy; patients with chronic hepatitis C and membranoproliferative glomerulonephritis may benefit from antiviral therapy. Combined liver and kidney transplantation (CLKT) may be used in some patients with cirrhosis and CKD. The decision is based on the value of glomerular filtration rate (GFR) (ideally one should use measured and not estimated GFR) and the results of renal biopsy.

Renal failure is common in patients with advanced cirrhosis [1, 2]. It is a syndrome which associates a decline in glomerular filtration rate, alteration of extracellular fluid volume, electrolyte and acid-base homeostasis, and retention of nitrogenous waste from protein catabolism [1, 2]. The model of end-stage liver disease (MELD) score which takes into account serum creatinine, serum bilirubin and the international normalized ratio of prothrombin time, is accurate in assessing the short-term probability of death in patients with cirrhosis [3]. Use of the MELD score has increased the number of patients with renal failure who receive a liver transplant and has reduced mortality among patients awaiting liver transplantation [2, 3]. In addition, pretransplant renal failure is a predisposing factor for post-transplant renal failure and poor outcome [4]. Together these findings indicate that the management of pretransplant renal failure is of major importance. On the clinical scene, renal failure may be related to an acute process, referred to as acute kidney injury (AKI), or a chronic process, referred to as chronic kidney disease (CKD) or the combination of an acute process superimposed to chronic kidney changes.

Acute Kidney Injury

Definition

Until now, the diagnosis of AKI is based on changes in serum creatinine levels. In cirrhotic patients without renal impairment at admission, a diagnosis of AKI is based on an increases in serum creatinine level by more than 50% of the baseline value and exceeding 1.5 mg/dl (133 μmol/l) [1]. In patients with preexisting renal impairment, AKI is diagnosed when serum creatinine increases by more than 50% above the baseline value [1]. It should be noted that the Acute Kidney Injury Network (AKIN) defined AKI as an abrupt (≤48 h) reduction in kidney function manifested by either an absolute increase in serum creatinine level of more than 0.3 mg/dl (26.5 μmol/l), an increase by more than 50% (by a factor of 1.5 from baseline) or a reduction in documented urinary output (<0.5 ml/kg body weight/h for >6 h) [5]. Once AKI is established, a staging system then defines its severity [5]. The AKIN definition was not specifically designed for patients with cirrhosis and should therefore be validated by large observational studies in these patients. However, one should have in mind that compared to healthy subjects, patients with cirrhosis have lower serum creatinine due to decreased production and reduced muscle mass [6]. Therefore, normal serum creatinine values do not exclude low GFR. Creatinine-based equations (Cockcroft, MDRD and CDK-EPI) are also inappropriate. Theoretically, the clearance of endogenous agents (inulin or iohexol, for example) is the only reliable way to assess precisely GFR in cirrhotic patients [6]. Unfortunately, direct measurement of GFR is costly and impractical for routine use.

Causes

Causes are divided as being due to prerenal, intrarenal or postrenal factors [1]. Prerenal factors range from marked renal hypoperfusion in patients with hypotension or hemorrhage to more subtle renal hypoperfusion such as that seen in patients with cirrhosis and type 1 hepatorenal syndrome (HRS). Postrenal AKI occurs because of obstruction of the urinary outflow tract. Intrarenal causes of AKI can be divided into diseases of the vasculature, tubulointerstitium, and glomerulus [1].

Table 1. Expected causes of AKI in patients with cirrhosis (modified from Moreau and Lebrec [1])

Underlying problem	Possible causes
Prerenal	
Intravascular volume depletion	hemorrhage, vomiting, diarrhea, bacterial sepsis, diuretic therapy
Decreased effective perfusion volume to kidneys	hepatorenal syndrome, heart failure, nephrotic syndrome
Impaired renal blood flow from exogenous agents	inhibitors of angiotensin II biological activity, NSAIDs, COX-2 inhibitors, contrast medium
Intrarenal	
Acute tubular necrosis	ischemia; toxins, including drugs (e.g. aminoglycosides), NSAIDs, COX-2 inhibitors,contrast medium; sepsis
Glomerular disease	postinfectious glomerulonephritis
Interstitial disease	pyelonephritis

For unexpected causes, see Moreau and Lebrec [1].

The expected causes of AKI in cirrhosis are shown in table 1. The most common causes are 'prerenal factors' and ischemic acute tubular necrosis [1, 7, 8]. In other words, renal hypoperfusion can explain most cases of cirrhosis-associated AKI [1]. Moreover, one should bear in mind that prerenal AKI is a pre-ischemic state which is reversible if renal perfusion is restored by the appropriate treatment. However, prerenal AKI may progress very rapidly to ischemic ATN in patients with shock [1, 8]. In the absence of shock, the progression of prerenal AKI to ATN may result from the absence of appropriate treatment [1]. Pathological analysis of renal-biopsy specimens obtained in patients with cirrhosis without shock has shown that lesions (e.g. endarteritis or arteriolosclerosis) of afferent glomerular arterioles are common and significantly associated with the existence ischemic ATN [9]. Patients with lesions of afferent arterioles have impaired GFR autoregulation resulting in abnormal susceptibility to ischemic ATN (the so-called 'normotensive ischemic ATN'); in these patients, ATN may develop in response to subtle decreases in arterial pressure [10].

Diagnosis

Information may be obtained from urinalysis. For example, pigmented granular casts are typical of ischemic and toxic acute renal failure and red cell casts of glomerulonephritis. Patients with renal azotemia due to acute or subacute glomerulonephritis have significant proteinuria (around 3 g/day) [1]. In contrast, proteinuria is absent or moderate in other causes of acute renal failure [1]. However, there are limitations to urinalysis: (1) expert personnel for the analyses of the urinary sediment are not available everywhere, and (2) it has recently been shown that some patients with cirrhosis have parenchymal kidney disease (shown by pathological analysis of renal-biopsy specimens) while they have neither proteinuria nor microscopic hematuria [9].

It has been suggested that urine indices (urine osmolality, urinary sodium concentration and fractional excretion of sodium) may help distinguish prerenal failure (including type 1 HRS) from tubular necrosis [1, 2]. The tubular ability to reabsorb sodium and to concentrate urine is preserved in prerenal azotemia and impaired in tubular necrosis [1, 2]. Patients with prerenal failure have low urinary sodium concentrations (below 20 mmol/l) and elevated urine osmolality (higher than 500 mosm/kg). Patients with tubular necrosis have high urinary sodium concentrations (above 40 mmol/l) and urine osmolality below 350 mosm/kg. However, the urinary sodium concentration may be low early in the course of certain processes that lead to tubular necrosis such as sepsis, exposure to radiocontrast agents or obstruction [1, 2]. In addition, some cases of HRS with elevated urinary sodium concentrations have been reported [1]. Therefore, it may be difficult to differentiate type 1 HRS from ATN or other causes of AKI. The International Ascites Club has suggested that five major criteria must be present to confirm the diagnosis of HRS [11]. However, a recent clinicopathological study has shown that patients with the clinical diagnosis of HRS may have intrarenal lesions [9]. These findings suggest that kidney biopsy (via the transjugular route, see below) may be useful for the diagnosis of AKI in patients with cirrhosis. However, transjugular kidney biopsy is not feasible everywhere. Clearly, biomarkers for renal lesions need to be identified.

Chronic Kidney Disease

Definition

CKD is defined by guidelines from the Kidney Disease Outcomes Quality Initiatives (KDOQI) Workgroup [12] as the presence for at least 3 months of either kidney damage (manifested by the presence of pathological abnormalities or other markers of kidney damage, including abnormalities in the composition of the blood or urine or abnormalities in imaging tests) or reduced kidney function (estimated GFR <60 ml/min/1.73 m^2 body surface area; BSA) [6]. However, as discussed above, estimation of GRF in cirrhosis using creatinine-based equations is with a source of inaccuracies [6] and GFR should rather be assessed using clearance of exogenous agents. In addition, a proportion of cirrhotic patients with CKD have type 2 HRS, i.e. functional renal disease related to refractory ascites.

Causes

Causes include type 2 HRS, IgA nephropathy, HCV-related membranoproliferative glomerulonephritis, HBV-related membranous glomerulopathy, diabetic nephropathy, nondiabetic glomerulosclerosis and ischemic nephropathy [6, 9].

Diagnosis

Diagnosis is based on clinical and biological evaluation [1]. An important point is that the absence of significant proteinuria does not exclude significant glomerular changes in cirrhosis [9]. Renal biopsy may be useful before the occurrence of end-stage renal disease. Theoretically, percutaneous kidney biopsy represents the ideal route since, most often, it allows obtain adequate tissue samples. However, patients with advanced cirrhosis have contra-indications to percutaneous biopsy due to coagulation disorders. Transjugular renal biopsy has been developed to overcome these limitations. In a large series of cirrhotic patients, the transjugular route was found efficient: the average number of glomeruli for optical microscopy was >10 and there were no major complications [9]. Indications of kidney biopsy depend on the GFR [6]: there is no indication for GFR <15 ml/min/1.73 m^2 BSA or GFR >60 ml/min/1.73 m^2 BSA. Biopsy is mandatory for GFR between 15 and 30 ml/min/1.73 m^2 BSA. Biopsy is required in patients with GFR between 30 and 60 ml/min/1.73 m^2 BSA if there is suspicion of parenchymal kidney disease as indicated by proteinuria >500 mg/day, microscopic hematuria (>50 red blood cells per high power field) and/or a recognized cause of chronic kidney disease (diabetes, past history of hypertension, HBV and HCV infection).

'Acute-on-Chronic' Kidney Injury

Results of renal biopsy in patients with cirrhosis and impaired renal function have shown that 40% of patients have complex renal lesions, including chronic tubulointerstitial injury (interstitial fibrosis and/or tubular atrophy), acute tubulointerstitial lesions (ATN, osmotic nephrosis, interstitial inflammation) and arteriolar lesions (endarteritis, hyalinosis, arteriolosclerosis) [9]. Therefore, a significant proportion of cirrhotic patients with an acute deterioration in renal function mimicking acute kidney diseases may have acute kidney changes superimposed to chronic changes. Unless no prospective study has been conducted in this context, patients with acute-on-chronic kidney injury may have lower chances of recovery compared to patients with AKI.

Management of Acute Kidney Injury

In most cases, patients should be managed in an intensive care unit.

Prerenal Causes

Treatment is directed at the cause of renal hypoperfusion [1].

Intravascular Volume Depletion
In patients with gastrointestinal hemorrhage, transfusions of packed red blood cells maintain the hematocrit between 25 and 30% and plasma expanders maintain hemodynamic stability [1]. In patients with intestinal or renal fluid losses, crystalloids (and sometimes colloids) are administered and diuretic therapy is stopped [1].

Severe Sepsis
The treatment is based on early broad-spectrum antibiotic therapy, correction of volume depletion, and vasopressor therapy (for patients in whom circulatory failure 'resists' to fluid replacement therapy) [1]. Treatments such as early goal-directed therapy or activated protein C administration have been shown to be effective in noncirrhotic patients with severe sepsis but have not yet been evaluated in cirrhotic patients with severe sepsis [13].

Type 1 HRS
Randomized clinical trials have shown that treatment with a combination of the vasopressin analogue terlipressin and intravenous albumin improved renal function in patients with type 1 HRS [14–16]. In patients with type 1 HRS, terlipressin is associated with a significant improvement of renal function [14–16]. However, the survival benefit is modest. In most responders, discontinuation of terlipressin is rapidly followed by a rapid decline in urine output and an increase in creatinine. Sustained administration of terlipressin for a few weeks as a bridge to liver transplantation has been reported occasionally [14].

Other treatments are under evaluation [reviewed in 1, 14], including vasoconstrictor therapy with noradrenaline (combined with albumin) or midodrine (combined with octreotide and albumin), and artificial liver support devices. Albumin dialysis using the MARS® system was also associated with a significant improvement in survival compared with conventional treatment. However, as with terlipressin, survival benefit was modest. Albumin dialysis should only be considered as a bridge to transplantation.

Other Causes
There are no specific measures for treatment of AKI induced by contrast medium, NSAIDs or COX-2 inhibitors [1]. In any case, these latter drugs should be withdrawn.

Intrarenal Causes

Acute Tubular Necrosis
Management is based on general care (see below) and renal-replacement therapy (when necessary) [1]. To date, there is no specific treatment capable of accelerating tubular compensation in patients with ATN [1].

Acute Glomerulonephritis
Patients with postinfectious glomerulonephritis should receive appropriate antibiotic therapy [1].

Acute Interstitial Nephritis
Patients with pyelonephritis should receive the appropriate antibiotic therapy [1].

General Care

The goals of general care are to avoid further kidney injury in patients with prerenal or intrarenal AKI. Nonselective β-blockers should not be used in patients with refractory ascites because they increase mortality in these patients [17].

Prevention of AKI

Spontaneous bacterial peritonitis (SBP) and other bacterial infections are known to precipitate type 1 HRS [1]. The administration of a combination of cefotaxime (a third-generation cephalosporin) plus intravenous albumin to patients with SBP has been shown to significantly decrease the incidence of HRS and mortality [18].

Subclinical, 'noninfectious' systemic inflammation is common in patients with advanced cirrhosis. Two randomized clinical trials have shown that the 'anti-inflammatory' pentoxifylline prevented the development of renal failure in patients with severe acute alcoholic hepatitis [19] and in patients with Child-Pugh C cirrhosis [20].

Primary SBP prophylaxis using the oral quinolone antibiotic norfloxacin is beneficial in selected patients with cirrhosis, i.e. patients with low protein ascites (<15 g/l) and advanced liver failure or impaired renal function. In these patients, norfloxacin administration was found to reduce the 1-year probability of developing spontaneous bacterial peritonitis and HRS and to improve the 3-month and the 1-year probability of survival compared to a placebo [21].

Intravenous saline is recommended to prevent contrast medium-induced acute kidney injury in noncirrhotic patients who are at risk of developing this complication, i.e. mainly patients with chronic renal failure and/or diabetes [22]. Saline infusion should also be used to prevent contrast medium-induced nephropathy in cirrhotic patients with chronic increases in serum creatinine levels and/or diabetes.

Management of Chronic Kidney Disease

Type 2 HRS

Patients with type 2 HRS have refractory ascites. The management should focus on treatment of refractory ascites. To date, there is no established treatment for type 2 HRS per se. Vasoconstrictor therapy plus intravenous albumin and transjugular intrahepatic portosystemic shunting should be evaluated in this indication [14].

Other Causes

There is no established treatment for IgA nephropathy. Patients with HCV-related membranoproliferative glomerulonephritis and cryoglobulinemia may benefit from antiviral therapy [1].

Selection of Candidates for Combined Liver and Kidney Transplantation

Patients with serum creatinine >2 mg/dl (176 μmol/l) do better with combined liver and kidney transplantation (CLKT) than with liver transplantation alone [23]. In the setting of AKI, CLKT should be considered in patients who have been on dialysis for more than 8 weeks because, in this situation, recovery is highly unlikely [24]. Otherwise, only patients with CKD should be considered for CLKT. Candidates to CLKT are patients with GFR below 30 ml/min and no evidence for an additional factor related to liver disease which could improve with liver transplantation. Borderline patients should have a biopsy. CLKT should be preferred to liver transplantation alone when pathology demonstrates more than 30% glomerulosclerosis and/or more than 30% interstitial fibrosis [24]. CLKT should also be considered if pathology shows prominent vascular changes [9] since they might be at higher risk of developing end-stage renal disease with calcineurin inhibitors.

Conclusions

In cirrhosis, AKI is mainly due to renal hypoperfusion which results in prerenal AKI (including type 1 HRS) and in some cases ATN. CKD has different causes: type 2 HRS, IgA nephropathy or membranoproliferative glomerulonephritis. Some patients have 'acute-on-chronic' kidney injury. In some patients with cirrhosis and CKD, renal biopsy may be useful because morphological analysis of renal-biopsy specimens provides diagnostic and prognostic information. In these patients, the transjugular route can be safely used. Treatments for AKI should target the cause of renal hypoperfusion Treatments for CKD depend on the cause: there is no established therapy for type 2 HRS or IgA nephropathy; patients with chronic hepatitis C and membranoproliferative glomerulonephritis may benefit from antiviral therapy. CLKT may be used in some patients with cirrhosis and CKD. The decision is based on the value of GFR (ideally one should use measured GFR and not estimated GFR) and the results of renal biopsy.

Key Messages

- In cirrhosis, AKI is mainly due to prerenal factors (including type 1 HRS) and ischemic ATN.
- CKD may be due to type 2 HRS, IgA nephropathy or membranoproliferative glomerulonephritis. Some patients have 'acute-on-chronic' kidney injury.
- In patients with cirrhosis and CKD waiting for liver transplantation, renal biopsy may be indicated because histopathological analysis of renal-biopsy specimens provides diagnostic and prognostic information. In these patients, the transjugular route can be safely used.
- Treatments for AKI should target the cause of renal hypoperfusion (e.g. fluid replacement to treat intravascular volume depletion; vasoconstrictor therapy for type 1 HRS). There is no specific treatment for ATN; renal-replacement therapy may be used.
- Treatments for CKD depend on the cause: there is no established therapy for type 2 HRS or IgA nephropathy; patients with chronic hepatitis C and membranoproliferative glomerulonephritis may benefit from antiviral therapy.
- CLKT may be used in some patients with cirrhosis and CKD. The decision is based on the GFR value (ideally one should use measured and not estimated GFR) and the results of renal biopsy.

References

1 Moreau R, Lebrec D: Acute renal failure in patients with cirrhosis: perspectives in the age of MELD. Hepatology 2003;37:233–243.

2 Ginès P, Schrier RW: Renal failure in cirrhosis. N Engl J Med 2009;361:1279–1290.

3 Kamath PS, Kim WR: The model for end-stage liver disease (MELD). Hepatology 2007;45:797–805.

4 Ojo AO, Held PJ, Port FK, et al: Chronic renal failure after transplantation of a nonrenal organ. N Engl J Med 2003;349:931–940.

5 Mehta RL, Kellum JA, Shah SV, et al: Acute Kidney Injury Network: report of an initiative to improve outcomes in acute kidney injury. Crit Care 2007;11: R31.

6 Francoz C, Glotz D, Moreau R, et al: The evaluation of renal function and disease in patients with cirrhosis. J Hepatol 2010;52:605–613.

7 Thabut D, Massard J, Gangloff A, et al: Model for end-stage liver disease score and systemic inflammatory response are major prognostic factors in patients with cirrhosis and acute functional renal failure. Hepatology 2007;46:1872–1882.

8 Garcia-Tsao G, Parikh CR, Viola A: Acute kidney injury in cirrhosis. Hepatology 2008;48:2064–2077.

9 Trawalé JM, Paradis V, Rautou PE, et al: The spectrum of renal lesions in patients with cirrhosis: a clinicopathologic study. Liver Int 2010;30:725–732.

10 Abuelo JG: Normotensive ischemic acute renal failure. N Engl J Med 2007;357:797–805.

11 Salerno F, Gerbes A, Ginès P, et al: Diagnosis, prevention and treatment of hepatorenal syndrome in cirrhosis. Gut 2007;56:1310–1318.
12 K/DOQI Clinical Practice Guidelines for Chronic Kidney Disease: Evaluation, classification, and stratification. Am J Kidney Dis 2002;39(suppl 2): S1–S246.
13 Gustot T, Durand F, Lebrec D, Vincent JL, Moreau R: Severe sepsis in cirrhosis. Hepatology 2009;50: 2022–2033.
14 Moreau R, Lebrec D: The use of vasoconstrictors in patients with cirrhosis: type 1 HRS and beyond. Hepatology 2006;43:385–394.
15 Sanyal AJ, Boyer T, Garcia-Tsao G, et al: A randomized prospective double blind placebo controlled trial of terlipressin for type 1 hepatorenal syndrome. Gastroenterology 2008;134:1360–1368.
16 Martín-Llahí M, Pépin MN, Guevara M, et al: Terlipressin and albumin versus albumin in patients with cirrhosis and hepatorenal syndrome: a randomized study. Gastroenterology 2008;134:1352–1359.
17 Serste T, Melot C, Francoz C, et al: Deleterious effects of beta-blockers on survival in patients with cirrhosis and refractory ascites. Hepatology 2010;in press.
18 Sort P, Navasa M, Arroyo V, et al: Effect of intravenous albumin on renal impairment and mortality in patients with cirrhosis and spontaneous bacterial peritonitis. N Engl J Med 1999;341:403–409.
19 Akriviadis E, Botla R, Briggs W, et al: Pentoxifylline improves short-term survival in severe acute alcoholic hepatitis: a double-blind, placebo-controlled trial. Gastroenterology 2000;119:1637–1648.
20 Lebrec D, Thabut D, Oberti F, Perarnau JM, Condat B, Barraud H, Saliba F, Carbonell N, Renard P, Ramond MJ, Moreau R, Poynard T: Pentoxifylline does not decrease short-term mortality but does reduce complications in patients with advanced cirrhosis. Gastroenterology 2010;138:1755–1762.
21 Fernández J, Navasa M, Planas R, et al: Primary prophylaxis of spontaneous bacterial peritonitis delays hepatorenal syndrome and improves survival in cirrhosis. Gastroenterology 2007;133:818–824.
22 Barrett BJ, Parfrey PS: Preventing nephropathy induced by contrast medium. N Engl J Med 2006; 354:379–386.
23 Jeyarajah DR, Gonwa TA, McBride M, et al: Hepatorenal syndrome: combined liver kidney transplants versus isolated liver transplant. Transplantation 1997;64:1760–1765.
24 Eason JD, Gonwa TA, Davis CL, Sung RS, Gerber D, Bloom RD: Proceedings of consensus conference on simultaneous liver-kidney transplantation (SLK). Am J Transplant 2008;8:2243–2251.

Richard Moreau, MD
INSERM U773 and Liver Unit
Pavillon Abrami, Hôpital Beaujon
FR–92118 Clichy (France)
Tel. +33 1 57 27 75 10, Fax +33 1 47 30 17 11, E-Mail richard.moreau@inserm.fr

Gerbes AL (ed): Ascites, Hyponatremia and Hepatorenal Syndrome: Progress in Treatment.
Front Gastrointest Res. Basel, Karger, 2011, vol 28, pp 122–129

Novel Definition of Hepatorenal Syndrome: Clinical Consequences

Javier Fernandez · Vicente Arroyo

Liver Unit, Institute of Digestive and Metabolic Diseases, Hospital Clinic, University of Barcelona, Barcelona, Spain

Abstract

Renal failure is common in cirrhosis, especially in patients with ascites. It is typically secondary to one or more intercurrent events, which further compromise renal perfusion on a background of a relative reduction in renal perfusion and may have a negative impact on survival. An accurate and prompt diagnosis and treatment of renal complications in cirrhosis is therefore essential to improve the management of these patients. However, several factors decrease the diagnostic accuracy of serum creatinine in patients with cirrhosis. The International Ascites Club has set out clear diagnostic criteria for both type 1 and type 2 hepatorenal syndrome, the most characteristic forms of renal failure in cirrhosis. However, no specific guidelines have been delineated for the diagnosis of other forms of acute or chronic renal failure. Recently, nephrology and critical care medicine societies have proposed definitions and staging systems for acute kidney injury (AKI) and chronic kidney disease, terms and definitions that could help to better define renal impairment in cirrhosis. Although hepatorenal syndrome is the most recognized form of AKI in patients with liver disease, it only accounts for less than 10% of cases in current clinical practice, as volume unresponsive AKI or acute tubular necrosis is now much more common. The present chapter will discuss the current definitions of hepatorenal syndrome and AKI in cirrhosis, their limitations and their possible impact on clinical practice and on future research.

Hepatorenal Syndrome: Concept, Clinical Types and Diagnostic Caveats

Concept

Hepatorenal syndrome (HRS) is a frequent complication in patients with cirrhosis, ascites and advanced liver failure. Its annual incidence in patients with ascites is about 8% [1]. HRS is a functional renal failure due to renal vasoconstriction and low renal perfusion [1–4]. Kidney histology is normal or shows lesions that do not justify the decrease in the glomerular filtration rate (GFR). It is characterized by impaired renal function and marked abnormalities in the arterial circulation and activity of

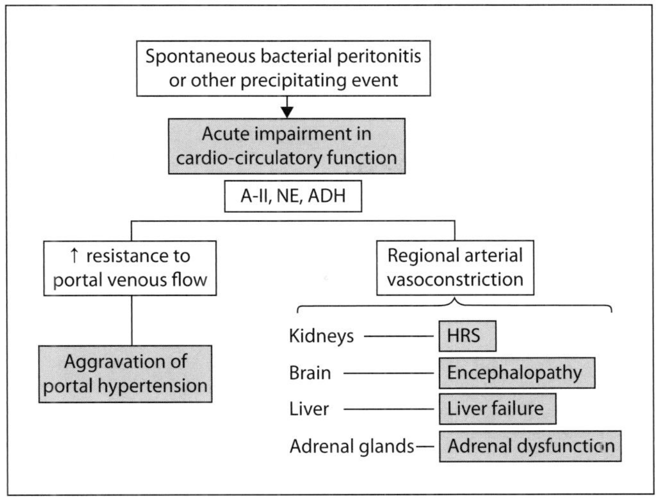

Fig. 1. Hepatorenal syndrome as part of a multiorgan failure. A-II = Angiotensin II; NE = norepinephrine; ADH = antidiuretic hormone; HRS = hepatorenal syndrome.

endogenous vasoactive systems. The traditional concept is that HRS is due to deterioration in circulatory function secondary to an intense vasodilation in the splanchnic circulation (peripheral arterial vasodilation hypothesis). During the last decade, however, several features suggest a much more complex pathogenesis. In fact, two types of HRS with different clinical course, prognostic implications and treatment response have been identified. Type 1 and type 2 HRS are, therefore, not different expressions of a common disorder but probably two syndromes with distinct pathogenesis.

Types of Hepatorenal Syndrome

Type 1 HRS is an extremely unstable condition. It frequently develops in the setting of an important clinical event that acts as a precipitating factor. There is a rapid deterioration of circulatory and renal function within days after the onset of the syndrome leading to severe arterial hypotension and acute renal failure with intense oliguria. Moreover, there is also a rapid deterioration of hepatic function, with increase in jaundice and encephalopathy [5]. Recent studies in patients with spontaneous bacterial peritonitis (SBP) indicate that type 1 HRS represents a special form of acute multiple organ failure related to the rapid deterioration in circulatory function (fig. 1). The syndrome develops in the setting of a significant decrease in arterial pressure and a marked stimulation of the renin-angiotensin and sympathetic nervous systems in the absence of changes in systemic vascular resistance, which is consistent with an increase in the arterial vasodilation obscured by the vascular effect of these vasoconstrictor systems. There is also an acute decrease in the cardiac output that contributes to the effective arterial hypovolemia [6]. In addition to renal vasoconstriction, patients with type 1 HRS associated with SBP develop vasoconstriction in the intrahepatic circulation, with a marked reduction in hepatic blood flow and an increase in portal pressure [6]. The acute deterioration of hepatic function and hepatic encephalopathy may be related to this feature. Cerebral vascular resistance is increased in patients with decompensated cirrhosis and correlates directly with the activity of the renin-angiotensin and sympathetic nervous system and renal vasoconstriction [7]. Reduction in cerebral blood flow could, therefore, play a contributory role to hepatic encephalopathy.

In contrast, type 2 HRS is the chronic form of HRS. It develops imperceptibly in patients with cirrhosis and ascites who are otherwise in stable clinical condition. These patients do not differ clinically from patients with cirrhosis and ascites without renal failure. They respond poorly to diuretics but this also occurs in a significant number of patients with serum creatinine concentration below 1.5 mg/dl. Circulatory function, although severely deteriorated, remains steady or progress slowly during months as it occurs with the renal failure. Patients have advanced cirrhosis but the degree of liver failure is also stable. Hepatic encephalopathy is infrequent. The main clinical problem is refractory ascites [5].

Caveats in the Diagnosis of HRS

The first step in the diagnosis of HRS is the demonstration of a reduced GFR, and this is not easy in advanced cirrhosis. Serum creatinine measurements in cirrhosis are affected by different factors such as loss of muscle mass, reduced dietary protein intake, sex, ethnic origin as well as by interference with the standard Jaffé colorimetric method of creatinine determination by bilirubin and other compounds which accumulate in liver failure. Similarly, urea is synthesized by the liver and may be reduced as a consequence of hepatic insufficiency. Other biomarkers of kidney function such as cystatin C are not accurate in patients with liver failure. Therefore, false negative diagnosis of HRS is relatively common [8–10]. There is consensus to establish the diagnosis of HRS when serum creatinine has risen above 1.5 mg/dl [11].

The second step is the differentiation of HRS from other types of renal failure. The traditional parameters used to differentiate functional renal failure from acute tubular necrosis (oliguria, low urine sodium concentration, urine-to-plasma osmolality ratio greater than unity, normal fresh urine sediment and no proteinuria) are not useful in decompensated cirrhosis with ascites. Acute tubular necrosis in patients with cirrhosis and ascites usually occurs with oliguria, low urine sodium concentration and urine osmolality greater than plasma osmolality [12]. On the contrary, relatively high urinary sodium concentration has been observed in patients with HRS and high serum bilirubin [13]. The first guidelines for the definition and diagnosis of HRS were published in 1996 and based the diagnosis of this complex entity on the exclusion of other disorders that can cause renal failure in cirrhosis (table 1). Clinically, HRS was further divided into two types [11].

Table 1. Past and present diagnostic criteria for HRS

a Past International Ascites Club criteria [11]

Major criteria
Chronic or acute liver disease with advanced hepatic failure and portal hypertension
Low glomerular filtration rate, as indicated by serum creatinine of >1.5 mg/dl or 24-hour creatinine clearance <40 ml/min
Absence of shock, ongoing bacterial infection, and current or recent treatment with nephrotoxic drugs Absence of gastrointestinal fluid losses (repeated vomiting or intense diarrhea) or renal fluid losses (weight loss >500 g/day for several days in patients with ascites without peripheral edema or 1,000 g/day in patients with peripheral edema)
No sustained improvement in renal function (decrease in serum creatinine to ≤1.5 mg/dl or increase in creatinine clearance to ≥40 ml/min) following diuretic withdrawal and expansion of plasma volume with 1.5 liters of isotonic saline
Proteinuria <500 mg/day and no ultrasonographic evidence of obstructive uropathy or parenchymal renal disease
Additional criteria
Urine volume <500 ml/day
Urine sodium <10 mEq/l
Urine osmolality greater than plasma osmolality
Urine red blood cells <50 per high-power field
Serum sodium concentration <130 mEq/l

b New International Ascites Club criteria [21]

Cirrhosis with ascites
Serum creatinine >133 μmol/l (1.5 mg/dl)
No improvement of serum creatinine (decrease to a level of ≤133 μmol/l) after at least two days of diuretic withdrawal and volume expansion with albumin The recommended dose of albumin is 1 g/kg body weight per day up to a maximum of 100 g/day
Absence of shock
No current or recent treatment with nephrotoxic drugs
Absence of parenchymal kidney disease as indicated by proteinuria >500 mg/ day, microhematuria (>50 red blood cells per high power field) and/or abnormal renal ultrasonography

As stated before, type 1 HRS is characterized by a severe and rapidly progressive renal failure, which has been defined as doubling of serum creatinine reaching a level >2.5 mg/dl in less than two weeks. Without treatment, type 1 HRS is the complication of cirrhosis with the poorest prognosis, with a median survival time after the onset of renal failure of only two weeks [8]. On the contrary, type 2 HRS is characterized by a moderate (serum creatinine <2.5 mg/dl) and slowly progressive renal failure. These patients are predisposed to develop type 1 HRS following SBP or other precipitating events [5]. Median survival of patients with type 2 HRS (6 months) is worse than that of patients with non-azotemic cirrhosis with ascites [5, 14].

New Definition of Hepatorenal Syndrome

Investigations performed in the last decades have markedly improved our understanding on the pathophysiology of HRS [6, 15, 16], have identified effective treatments for HRS [17–20] and have shown that it occurs frequently following bacterial infections, mainly SBP. With this background, the International Ascites Club held a second consensus conference in 2005 to update the definition and diagnostic criteria for HRS and to facilitate the diagnosis of this entity, therefore allowing the prompt institution of treatment [21]. The revised definition states that 'HRS is a potentially reversible syndrome occurring in patients with cirrhosis, ascites and liver failure. It is characterized by impaired renal failure, marked alterations in the cardiovascular function and over-activity of the endogenous vasoactive systems. Marked vasoconstriction in the kidney causes low GFR, whereas in the systemic circulation, there is decreased vascular resistance due to splanchnic and peripheral arterial vasodilatation. A similar syndrome can also occur in acute liver failure and acute alcoholic hepatitis'. In these guidelines, HRS remained as a diagnosis of exclusion but its diagnostic criteria were simplified (table 1). The following changes were made:

- Creatinine clearance was removed because it is more complicated that serum creatinine for clinical practice and it does not increase the accuracy of renal function assessment in cirrhosis.
- Renal failure in the setting of an ongoing bacterial infection, but in the absence of septic shock, was considered HRS. This new criteria enables the physicians to start the treatment of HRS without waiting for a complete infection resolution.
- Plasma volume expansion should be performed with albumin rather than saline, as saline is isotonic to serum and will be transferred to the peritoneal cavity, without having effects on the central blood volume.
- Minor diagnostic criteria of HRS were also eliminated, as they were not essential for the diagnosis.

These latest diagnostic criteria for HRS set out clearly which patients should be considered as having HRS, and therefore receive treatment promptly. However, the

Table 2. Definitions and classifications of AKI

a Acute Dialysis Quality Initiative criteria: RIFLE Classification

	RIFLE R (risk)	RIFLE I (injury)	RIFLE F (failure)	RIFLE L (loss)	RIFLE E (end-stage)
Serum creatinine or GFR criteria	↑ creatinine 1.5-fold from baseline or ↓ GFR>25%	↑ creatinine 2-fold from baseline or ↓ GFR >50%	↑ creatinine 3-fold from baseline or ↓ GFR by 75% or creatinine ≥4 mg/dl with an acute rise >0.5 mg/dl	Complete loss of kidney function >4 weeks	End-stage kidney disease (>3 months)
Urine output criteria	<0.5 ml/kg/h × 6 h	<0.5 ml/kg/h × 12 h	<0.3 ml/kg/h × 24 h or anuria × 12 h		

b Acute Kidney Injury Network criteria

Stage	Serum creatinine criteria	Urine output criteria
1	↑ creatinine of ≥0.3 mg/dl (≥26.4 μmol/l) or ↑ of 150–200% (1.5- to 2-fold) from baseline	<0.5 ml/kg/h for >6 h
2	↑ creatinine >200% but ≤300% (>2- to 3-fold) from baseline	<0.5 ml/kg/h for >12 h
3	↑ creatinine >300% (>3-fold) from baseline or creatinine of ≥4.0 mg/dl (≥354 μmol/l) with an acute ↑ of ≥0.5 mg/dl (44 μmol/l)	<0.3 ml/kg/h for 24 h or anuria for 12 h

use of the rigid cut off value of serum creatinine of 1.5 mg/dl suppose that many patients with milder degrees of renal dysfunction are not considered for treatment, thus limiting the diagnosis of HRS to a very small proportion of cirrhotic patients with renal dysfunction.

Definition of Acute Kidney Injury in Cirrhosis

The term AKI has been recently coined by several nephrology and intensive care medicine societies. It encompasses the entire spectrum of acute kidney failure thus allowing patients with small increments of serum creatinine to be regarded as having significant renal dysfunction.

In 2004, a consensus conference developed the RIFLE classification (R-renal risk, I-injury, F-failure, L-loss of kidney function, E-end-stage renal disease) for AKI, which stratified renal failure into grades of increasing severity based on changes in patient's serum creatinine or GFR and/or urine output (table 2) [22]. These RIFLE criteria have been validated in the general population and in critically ill cirrhotic patients and constitute a good predictor of hospital survival [23, 24]. After the development of the RIFLE criteria the Acute Kidney Injury Network redefined AKI as an abrupt (≤48 h) reduction in kidney function manifested by an absolute increase in serum creatinine of ≥26 μmol/l (0.3 mg/dl), equivalent to a ≥50% increase in serum creatinine (1.5-fold from baseline) or a urine output of <0.5 ml/kg/h for more than 6 h [25]. Once AKI is established, a staging system then defines the severity of the AKI (table 2). The application of these AKI criteria to patients with cirrhosis could lead to the identification of many patients with acute renal dysfunction, normal serum creatinine levels but low GFR. However, the real usefulness of the AKI criteria must be tested appropriately in the cirrhotic population before recommending these criteria for clinicians to use in clinical practice. Future studies should also characterize the cirrhotic patients with AKI in terms of demographics, incidence and prevalence and describe the natural history of AKI in cirrhosis. Until then and considering their complexity, RIFLE and AKI criteria should be mainly used in the management of critically ill cirrhotic patients.

Key Messages

- Hepatorenal syndrome is the most characteristic but not the most frequent form of acute kidney injury in cirrhosis.
- The diagnostic accuracy of serum creatinine in cirrhosis is decreased.
- The clinical impact of novel definitions of hepatorenal syndrome and acute kidney injury in cirrhosis is still unknown.

References

1 Gines A, Escorsell A, Gines P, et al: Incidence, predictive factors, and prognosis of the hepatorenal-syndrome in cirrhosis with ascites. Gastroenterology 1993;105:229–236.
2 Gines P, Rodes J: Clinical disorders of renal function in cirrhosis with ascites; in Arrovo V, Gines P, Rodes J, Schrier RW (eds): Ascites and Renal Dysfunction in Liver Disease: Pathogenesis, Diagnosis, and Treatment. Malden, Blackwell Science, 1999, pp 36–62.
3 Koppel MH, Coburn JW, Mims MM, Goldstei H, Boyle JD, Rubini ME: Transplantation of cadaveric kidneys from patients with hepatorenal syndrome: evidence for functional nature of renal failure in advanced liver disease. N Engl J Med 1969;280:1367–1370.
4 Gines P, Guevara M, Arroyo V, Rodes J: Hepatorenal syndrome. Lancet 2003;362:1819–1827.
5 Arroyo V, Fernandez J, Ginès P: Pathogenesis and treatment of hepatorenal syndrome. Semin Liver Dis 2008;28:81–95.
6 Ruiz-del-Arbol L, Urman J, Fernandez J, et al: Systemic, renal, and hepatic hemodynamic derangement in cirrhotic patients with spontaneous bacterial peritonitis. Hepatology 2003;38:1210–1218.
7 Guevara M, Bru C, Gines P, et al: Increased cerebrovascular resistance in cirrhotic patients with ascites. Hepatology 1998;28:39–44.
8 Caregaro L, Menon F, Angeli P, et al: Limitations of serum creatinine level and creatinine clearance as filtration markers in cirrhosis. Arch Intern Med 1994;154:201–205.
9 Sherman DS, Fish DN, Teitelbaum I: Assessing renal function in cirrhotic patients: problems and pitfalls. Am J Kidney Dis 2003;41:269–278.
10 Cholangitas E, Marelli L, Kerry A, Senzolo M, Goodier DW, Nair D, Thomas M, Patch D, Burroughs AK: Different methods of creatinine measurement significantly affect MELD scores. Liver Transpl 2007;13:523–529.

11 Arroyo V, Gines P, Gerbes AL: Definition and diagnostic criteria of refractory ascites and hepatorenal syndrome in cirrhosis. Hepatology 1996;23:164–176.
12 Cabrera J, Arroyo V, Ballesta AM, et al: Aminoglycoside nephrotoxicity in cirrhosis: value of urinary beta-2-microglobulin to discriminate functional renal-failure from acute tubular damage. Gastroenterology 1982;82:97–105.
13 Dudley FJ, Kanel GC, Wood LJ, Reynolds TB: Hepatorenal-syndrome without avid sodium retention. Hepatology 1986;6:248–251.
14 Rodes J, Arroyo V, Bosch J: Clinical types and drug-therapy of renal impairment in cirrhosis. Postgrad Med J 1975;51:492–497.
15 Maroto A, Gines P, Arroyo V, et al: Brachial and femoral-artery blood-flow in cirrhosis: relationship to kidney dysfunction. Hepatology 1993;17:788–793.
16 Ruiz-del-Arbol L, Monescillo A, Arocena C, et al: Circulatory function and hepatorenal syndrome in cirrhosis. Hepatology 2005;42:439–447.
17 Uriz J, Gines P, Cardenas A, et al: Terlipressin plus albumin infusion: an effective and safe therapy of hepatorenal syndrome. J Hepatol 2000;33:43–48.
18 Ortega R, Gines P, Uriz J, et al: Terlipressin therapy with and without albumin for patients with Hepatorenal syndrome: results of a prospective, nonrandomized study. Hepatology 2002;36:941–948.
19 Duvoux C, Zanditenas D, Hezode C, et al: Effects of noradrenalin and albumin in patients with type I hepatorenal syndrome: a pilot study. Hepatology 2002;36:374–380.
20 Wong F, Pantea L, Sniderman K: Midodrine, octreotide, albumin, and TIPS in selected patients with cirrhosis and type 1 hepatorenal syndrome. Hepatology 2004;40:55–64.
21 Salerno F, Gerbes A, Ginès P, Wong F, Arroyo V: Diagnosis, prevention and treatment of hepatorenal syndrome in cirrhosis. Gut 2007;56:1310–1318.
22 Bellomo R, Ronco C, Kellum JA, Mehta RL, Palevsky P, Acute Dialysis Quality Initiative workgroup: Acute renal failure: definition, outcome measures, animal models, fluid therapy and information technology needs. Second International Consensus Conference of the Acute Dialysis Quality Initiative (ADQI) Group. Crit Care 2004;R204–R212.
23 Ricci Z, Cruz D, Ronco C: The RIFLE criteria and mortality in acute kidney injury: a systematic review. Kidney Int 2008;73:538–546.
24 Cholongitas E, Calvaruso V, Senzolo M, Patch D, Shaw S, O'Beirne J, Burroughs AK: RIFLE classification as predictive factor of mortality in patients with cirrhosis admitted to intensive care unit. J Gastroenterol Hepatol 2009;24:1639–1647.
25 Mehta RL, Kellum JA, Shah SV, Molitoris BA, Ronco C, Warnock DG, Levin A: Acute Kidney Injury Network: report of an initiative to improve outcomes in acute kidney injury. Crit Care 2007;11:R31.

J. Fernandez, MD
Liver Unit, Hospital Clínic
Villarroel 170
ES–08036 Barcelona (Spain)
Tel. +34 93 227 5400, Fax +34 93 451 5522, E-Mail Jfdez@clinic.ub.es

Gerbes AL (ed): Ascites, Hyponatremia and Hepatorenal Syndrome: Progress in Treatment.
Front Gastrointest Res. Basel, Karger, 2011, vol 28, pp 130–141

Role of Infections in Hepatorenal Syndrome

R. Wiest

Klinik und Poliklinik für Innere Medizin I, Universitätsklinikum Regensburg, Regensburg, Deutschland

Abstract

Bacterial infections are among the dominant precipitators of hepatorenal syndrome (HRS) in cirrhosis. This relates to aggravation of both key events in the pathophysiolgy of HRS: splanchnic vasodilation and relative insufficiency in cardiac output maintaining compensatory adequate hyperdynamic circulation. Therefore, guidelines have been adopted excluding renal failure in presence of bacterial infections now particularly allowing and recognizing bacterial infections as potent stimuli for HRS. The following chapter will therefore try to unravel the central role of pathological bacterial translocation and bacterial infections for the development of HRS in advanced cirrhosis. Furthermore, the potential differences regarding site and type of infection as well as role of underlying liver disease will be discussed.

Epidemiology and Prognosis of Bacterial Infections and Associated Renal Failure in Cirrhosis

Bacterial infections commonly observed in patients with cirrhosis are, in descending order of frequency, spontaneous bacterial peritonitis (SBP), urinary tract infection and pneumonia [1]. In general, risk for acquisition of bacterial infections is increased in advanced cirrhosis due to deficiencies in host defence at multiple levels. For instance, bacteraemia has been reported to be 10 times more frequent in cirrhosis as compared to non-cirrhotic hospitalized patients [2]. Except for pneumonia, community-acquired spontaneous bacterial infections are predominantly Gram-negative in nature and mainly caused by endogenous enteral commensal bacteria [e.g. *E. coli*; see chapter on SBP]. In contrast, nosocomial infections are more frequently are caused by Gram-positive bacteria, mainly due to the invasive procedures necessary during treatment [1, 3, 4]. Besides increased frequency of bacterial infections, associated mortality is also vastly increased in cirrhotic patients because of their lower capacity for bacterial clearance, alterations in inflammatory responses and pre-existing hemodynamic derangement. Cases in which renal dysfunction occurs during the course of bacterial infection have a poor prognosis, and renal dysfunction is a key indicator predicting death in patients with bacterial infection [5]. In fact, the lower GFR the worse survival in patients waiting for liver transplantation [6]. Particularly fatal is the development of irreversible renal dysfunction, which ultimately is always lethal.

Risk Factors for Renal Dysfunction

Liver cirrhosis per se is associated with increased risk of renal failure for which risk factors identified include ascites [7], elevated bilirubin [8], hepatic encephalopathy [9], underlying renal insufficiency [9, 10] and use of aminoglycosides [7]. However, more than 50% of hepatorenal syndrome (HRS) are induced by precipitating events, among which bacterial infections are the leading cause, being responsible for up to 60% of the cases [11]. The main risk factors for the development of renal failure after bacterial infections are (1) the severity of infection, (2) the MELD score at the diagnosis of infection, and (3) the persistence of infection despite antibiotic treatment [12, 13]. In more detail, leukocyte count in blood, most likely reflecting severity of infection, was found to be associated with the development of renal failure in several investigations [12, 14–16]. Regarding severity of liver disease and MELD score, retrospective data reveal that in presence of SBP, patients with bilirubin >4 mg/dl and serum creatinin >1 mg/dl at diagnosis are at particularly high risk [17, 18]. Indeed, this selected group of patients presents with an up to ninefold increased risk of renal failure and more than three-fold increased mortality as compared to low-risk patients. In addition, in those high-risk patients hyponatremia (<130 mEq/l) is an independent strong predictor for the development of renal failure. Moreover, the risk of type 1 HRS following a bacterial infection is higher in patients with pre-existing type 2 HRS [14, 19]. Finally, in cases of bacterial infections other than SBP, identified risk factors have been reported to be alcoholic genesis and MELD score >20, the latter being particularly predictive for development of irreversible renal dysfunction [20].

Site of Infection and Renal Dysfunction

The association of SBP and development of renal failure in cirrhosis has been well established. In fact, approximately 10–30% [1, 14] – in some reports up to 56% – of SBP cases [18] will develop renal dysfunction, despite appropriate non-nephrotoxic antibiotic treatment. Most of these cases fulfil the most recent diagnostic criteria of type 1 HRS. In patients with bacterial infections other than SBP, despite its high prevalence, the clinical significance of renal dysfunction has long been less clear. However, renal dysfunction is observed in 26–36% of cirrhotic patients presenting with non-SBP bacterial infections [13, 20]. In fact, it has been recognized recently that renal failure in advanced cirrhosis can be precipitated by most types of bacterial infections. Particularly causative can be urinary, biliary or intestinal infections, which in some cases can trigger an acute renal failure with hallmarks of type 1 HRS [12].

Key Events for Development of Renal Dysfunction in Advanced Cirrhosis with Emphasis on Bacterial Infections and Pathological Bacterial Translocation

Hemodynamics and Cardiac Function

The two main causative features in the development of HRS are excessive splanchnic arterial vasodilation and impaired ventricular contractility translating into the inability of cardiac function to prevent the severe reduction of effective circulating volume caused by splanchnic vasodilation [21]. This excessive splanchnic vasodilation is due to increased production or activity of vasodilator factors, particularly nitric oxide, carbon monoxide and cannabinoids [22, 23], and leads to blood pooling and thus, relative central hypovolemia. This in turn stimulates baroreceptors and volume receptors activating the sympathetic nervous system, renin-angiotensin-aldosterone system (RAAS) and many other vasoconstrictors as well as nonosmotic release of an antidiuretic hormone aiming to counterbalance arterial vasodilation. These mediators act on the kidney, facilitating sodium and water retention and thus plasma volume expansion, to compensate for the stated central underfilling. With progression of cirrhosis, splanchnic vasodilation worsens and activated vasoconstrictive systems lead to renal vasoconstriction, causing a marked drop in renal plasma flow and thus fraction of CO delivered to the kidney [24], resulting in deterioration of GFR. In fact, plasma renin activity >3.5 ng/ml/h, norepinephrine >544 pg/ml, hyponatremia (<130 mEq/l) and low mean arterial pressure (≤85 mm Hg), all of which indicate that severe vasodilation and a marked hyperdynamic circulatory syndrome display significant predictive value for the development of HRS [11, 14, 17]. Therefore, due to the hyperdynamic circulatory state of advanced cirrhosis and associated neurohormonal alterations, renal blood flow is very susceptible to events associated with a further decrease in effective arterial blood volume. Additionally, the heart response becomes insufficient to maintain perfusion pressure (high-output heart failure) and further contributes to a decrease in renal blood flow and renal failure. Indeed, patients who develop HRS following SBP present with lower cardiac index at the time of bacterial infection [16]. Moreover, cirrhotic ascitic patients with cardiac index <1.5 are significantly more likely to develop HRS 1 and are more likely to die within 3 months of follow-up [25]. Taken together, it is appealing to hypothesize that a hyperdynamic circulation is essential for the maintenance of an effective central blood volume and that any decrease in cardiac output due to precipitating events such as SBP or other bacterial infections can lead to a severe effective hypovolemia, therefore precipitating HRS.

SBP vs. Other Infections as Precipitating Factor for Hepatorenal Syndrome

The reason for SBP being the most frequent bacterial infection triggering HRS is most likely related to the extent and duration of inflammatory response in the peritoneal cavity induced by an episode of SBP. Patients with SBP developing renal failure present with significantly greater plasma and ascitic fluid cytokine levels (TNF and IL-6) at the time of diagnosis as compared to patients that do not [15]. In fact, the ascitic level of IL-6 represents a strong and independent predictor for the development of HRS. In this context, local ascitic levels of cytokines and endotoxin are severalfold higher than in the systemic circulation. A strong direct correlation between plasma and ascitic fluid levels of TNF and IL-6 underlines that systemic levels are mainly splanchnic/peritoneal-derived. In more detail, patients with culture-positive SBP present with a significantly stronger pro-inflammatory response and higher PMN count in ascites than patients with culture-negative SBP [15]. Moreover, Gram-negative isolates appear to associate with particularly high ascitic pro-inflammatory cytokines and PMN counts as compared to Gram-positive cases [15]. These data point towards the importance of bacterial load, subtype of causative bacteria and chemotactic capacity of the individual patient for the inflammatory response taking place. In general, however, it is important to emphasize that patients with chronic liver disease respond to sepsis and bacterial stimuli with a vastly greater and longer-lasting release in pro-inflammatory cytokines than patients without cirrhosis [26, 27]. This 'priming' phenomenon has been mainly shown in peripheral mononuclear cells but may well be likewise present or even exaggerated in the splanchnic-peritoneal compartment. This assumed splanchnic 'boost' of pro-inflammatory cytokines easily explains why SBP in particular can trigger HRS (fig. 1). (1) The hemodynamic dysregulation already present with vasodilation being most marked in the splanchnic circulation renders these patients most susceptible for further vasodilatory stimuli in this compartment [22]. (2) Endotoxins, bacterial DNA and TNF and other pro-inflammatory cytokines are known to impair cardiac function [28–30]. In fact, severe bacterial infections produce a cytokine-mediated septic cardiomyopathy which may well contribute to 'tip the tail' leading to progressive renal failure. (3) Bacterial products can exacerbate hepatic dysfunction, worsening liver insufficiency [31]. Other types of bacterial infections besides SBP may also cause renal failure in patients with cirrhosis, yet the severity of the inflammatory response and renal impairment is not as marked as in SBP [12, 13]. This in fact easily explains why infections in the splanchnic-peritoneal compartment (SBP, biliary or gastrointestinal) are more prone to trigger HRS and indeed induce more often progressive HRS than nonsplanchnic bacterial infections [12]. In other words, the splanchnic-peritoneal compartment represents the 'Achilles heal' for the development of HRS in advanced cirrhosis.

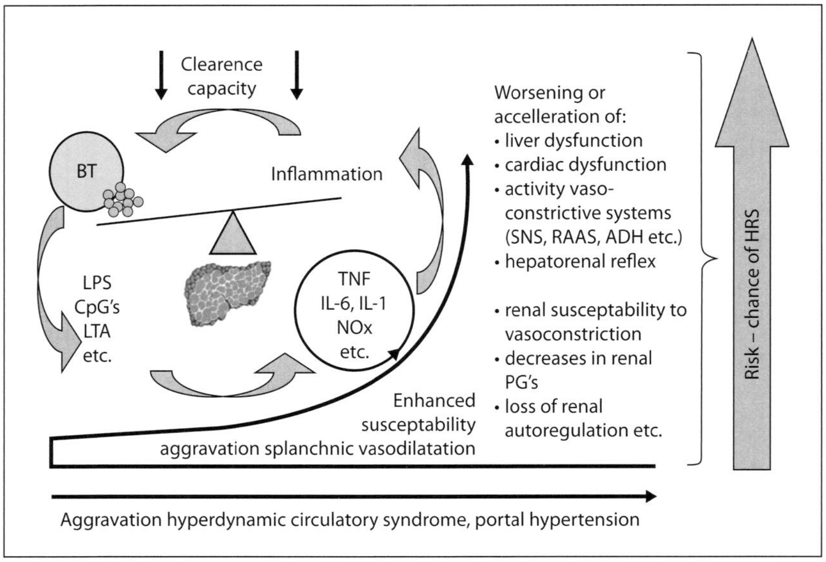

Fig. 1. Is bacterial translocation a trigger for HRS? Working hypothesis and scenario for the pathophysiological role of BT for the development of HRS in advanced cirrhosis. Pathological BT leads to influx of bacterial products into the splanchnic compartment and stimulates the release of pro-inflammatory cytokines. This inflammatory response is vastly enhanced, the clearance of bacterial products as well as pro-inflammatory cytokines reduced and thus, the stimulatory capacity most likely prolonged in cirrhosis. In addition, in the face of splanchnic arterial vasodilation susceptibility the clinical impact of any further vasodilatory stimulus is markedly increased in cirrhosis. This in sum explains the pronounced and often fatal hemodynamic derangement triggered by bacterial infections, particularly in the splanchnic compartment, such as SBP. These can include an additional potent increment in activity of vasoconstrictive systems, aggravation of HCS, portal hypertension and thus, most likely hepatorenal reflex. Associated effects also can impact on ventricular contractility and, at the level of the kidney, may include a loss of compensatory mechanisms such as perfusion autoregulation and enhanced susceptibility to any intrarenal vasoconstrictive effect as well as lack of vasodilatory prostaglandins.

Bacterial Translocation

Bacterial translocation (BT) is defined as the migration of viable microorganisms from the intestinal lumen to mesenteric lymph nodes (MLN) and other extra-intestinal organs and sites [32]. Limited BT to MLN is a physiological phenomenon that has been proposed to be essential for development and maintenance of tolerance against the intestinal flora [33]. However, any increase in rate and severity of BT may be deleterious for the patient and thus should be termed 'pathological BT'. BT has been postulated as the main mechanism in the pathogenesis of spontaneous infections in cirrhosis. Moreover, pathological BT can be considered the primary event in endotoxinemia known to be a common finding in advanced cirrhosis with increasing levels being associated with hepatic failure, encephalopathy and death [34,

35]. Experimental cirrhosis without BT exerts only low – in most cases negligible – concentrations of endotoxins in the systemic circulation whereas cirrhotic rats with BT to MLN show marked systemic endotoxinemia [36]. In fact, local mesenteric lymphatic endotoxin levels being most marked in presence of BT strongly correlate with systemic appearance of endotoxins, indicating that the source of endotoxins is the gut.

Bacterial DNA detected by a PCR-based method has recently been suggested as a surrogate marker and molecular evidence for BT in decompensated cirrhosis [37–39]. Detectable bacterial DNA in serum as well as BT to MLN in experimental cirrhosis has been shown to elicit an inflammatory response, with increased production of pro-inflammatory cytokines, such as TNF and IL-6, with concomitant NO release in the splanchnic circulation aggravating splanchnic vasodilation and accelerating the hyperdynamic circulatory syndrome [36, 40–44]. The inflammatory response to bacterial DNA has been reported to be similar in magnitude for Gram-positive and Gram-negative translocation [45, 46]. Another marker of 'pathological BT' of Gram-negative bacteria and representing long-term exposure to LPS is LPS-binding protein. Patients with increased levels of this protein present with a more than four-fold increased cumulative probability for the development of overt bacterial infection but are clinically otherwise indistinguishable [47]. Moreover, patients with increased levels of LPS-binding protein even in absence of any evidence of bacterial infection have increased serum levels of cytokines, reduced systemic vascular resistance and increased cardiac output, as compared to cirrhotic patients without evidence of BT [40, 43, 48]. It is also tempting to speculate that indeed episodes of BT are key to the stated phenomenon of 'priming' of mononuclear cells (e.g. in the splanchnic compartment) to produce an excessive inflammatory response in case of SBP. Even in the absence of SBP, MLN have been shown to release more TNF in decompensated cirrhosis (known to present with an increased rate of BT), indicating that the gut becomes a 'cytokine-releasing organ' in the presence of pathologically increased BT [34, 49]. Indeed, TNF is found in MLN of cirrhotic ascitic rats only in the presence of BT [44]. Proof of concept for this scenario comes from investigations on the clinical impact of selective gut decontamination (e.g. utilizing norfloxacin) in advanced cirrhosis. Indeed, selective gut decontamination by mainly inhibiting growth of Gram-negative commensal flora has been shown to abrogate the presence of bacterial DNA in serum and thus prevent BT [43]. This approach results in lower gut-derived cytokine release, diminished activity of vasoactive systems (RAAS, sympathetic nervous system, NO, etc.) and thus ameliorates the hyperdynamic circulation in advanced decompensated cirrhosis [44, 48, 50, 51].

However, BT-associated bacterial products and pro-inflammatory responses not only impact on splanchnic and systemic hemodynamics but also directly affect the kidney. LPS per se induces renal vasoconstriction via stimulation of endothelin, thromboxane A_2 and leukotrienes and enhances susceptibility for decreases in renal synthesis of vasodilative prostaglandins [52, 53]. Likewise, TNF causes renal vasoconstriction but also glomerular fibrin deposition leading to a reduction in GFR [54]. Finally, IL-6 with complex action on renal hemodynamic and function predicts occurrence of acute kidney injury in sepsis [55]. Therefore, it is tempting to speculate that pathological BT in cirrhosis is involved in intrarenal mechanisms contributing to the development of HRS even independent from its splanchnic and systemic hemodynamic effects. Therefore, independent of the development of any overt bacterial infection, bacterial products as well as the BT-associated pro-inflammatory cytokine response may have severe clinical consequences in advanced liver cirrhosis triggering and/or exacerbating hepatic dysfunction, aggravating hemodynamic disturbances and potentially causing HRS.

General Assessment

The evaluation of cirrhotic patients with renal failure should include not only the assessment of renal function but also evaluation of liver function and, particularly, exclusion of possible bacterial infections. In that regard, even in the absence of signs of infection, evaluation should include culture of blood, ascites and urine as well as exclusion of SBP by testing PMN count in ascitic fluid. The patient's medication has to be reviewed carefully, diuretics should be discontinued since these agents either cause or contribute to the impairment of renal function. Due to the observed increased risk of renal dysfunction any use of aminoglycosides has to be avoided. Considering the key role of central and splanchnic hemodynamics, the patient with HRS should be monitored in the ICU, at best including not only central venous line and invasive blood pressure monitoring but also evaluation of cardiac output, and systemic vascular resistance.

Therapeutic Considerations for Bacterial Infections and Their Role for Development of Hepatorenal Syndrome

The central role of circulatory dysfunction and particularly central arterial underfilling is substantiated by the observation that the risk of HRS in SBP can be markedly reduced with the i.v. administration of albumin (1.5 g/kg BW at diagnosis and 1.0 g/kg BW 48 h later) [56]. The observation of nonalbumin plasma expanders being less effective in this setting points towards other actions of albumin besides plasma volume expansion. These indeed include antioxidant properties but also binding and scavenging of metabolic waste and bacterial products [57, 58]. Most interestingly, however, this beneficial effect is basically only present in patients with bilirubin >4 mg/dl and/or increased serum creatinine at diagnosis of SBP. Therefore, most likely albumin is most effective in patients presenting with an already marked hyperdynamic circulation and pathologically increased BT. In this line, in cirrhotic patients with high risk for development of SBP, namely low-protein ascites and associated impairment in liver function, renal function or both (bilirubin above 3 mg/dl, Child-Pugh score >10, serum sodium <130 mmol/l or serum creatinine >1.2 mg/dl), long-term administration of norfloxacin not only reduces the risk of SBP but also HRS and improves survival [59]. Worthwhile mentioning is the fact that every patient developing SBP did receive preventive albumin infusions and therefore, only 1 of 10 SBP patients in the placebo group developed HRS. In other words, the lower incidence of SBP induced by long-term norfloxacin is not responsible for the observed prevention of HRS. In contrast, the most logic explanation is that (although not being assessed) norfloxacin effectively inhibited BT and thus lowered the release of pro-inflammatory cytokines and ameliorated the hyperdynamic circulation in these patients. Important to note is that norfloxacin reduced the incidence of HRS but this did not reach statistical significance. However, onset of HRS was significantly delayed, with the most marked effect being observed during the first 3 months of selective gut decontamination. This gain in time without development of HRS clearly can be of fundamental importance for those patients, particularly when waiting for liver transplantation.

Clinical Problems and Future Developments

Prophylaxis

In patients suffering SBP or other bacterial infections, risk factors for the development of HRS need to be defined in more detail. Considering the most likely central role of (1) pathological BT and associated pro-inflammatory cytokine response as well as (2) splanchnic and systemic hemodynamics this should include investigations on the following: (a) factors determining the magnitude and duration of pro-inflammatory response in individual cirrhotic patients, and (b) new tools to measure and monitor central hemodynamics such as special catheters enabling assessment of, for example, stroke volume variance, pulse pressure variation and global end-diastolic volume, all of which are known to reflect 'central volume responsiveness'.

Therapy

The lack of resolution of bacterial infection has been consistently shown to predict death in advanced cirrhosis, and thus first line therapy needs to be effective. For further details related to this point, see chapter on SBP [this vol.]. However, in some patients HRS may persist or even progress rapidly despite resolution of the infection [7, 17, 60]. For this scenario, further studies have to identify risk factors enabling stratification of patients into therapeutic algorithms preventing failure of first-line treatment.

Key Messages

- In the hospital setting, the increased risk of bacterial infections in cirrhotic patients dictates strict adherence to universal precautions and careful monitoring of catheter sites and wounds with particular emphasis in this population and in the ICU.
- Administration of non-steroidal anti-inflammatory drugs or aminoglycosides must be avoided in all patients with cirrhosis because these agents may impair renal function.
- Bacterial infections are potent precipitating events for the development of HRS, particularly when located in the splanchnic compartment. Besides this, pathological bacterial translocation per se and associated release of pro-inflammatory cytokines from the gut, most likely is one of the key triggers for development of HRS in advanced cirrhosis.
- Bacterial infection should be ruled out in all cirrhotic patients with acute renal failure or worsening of renal function. In patients with ascites, differential cell count and culture should be performed to rule out infection of ascitic fluid. Blood and urine culture should be performed even in the absence of obvious signs of infection. Chest radiograph should be carried out to exclude lung infection.
- Further studies have to identify in more detail risk factors for the development of HRS, such as individual susceptibility and capacity of pro-inflammatory response to bacterial translocation and infection. In addition, as for therapeutic optimization, predictive factors for persistence of HRS despite resolution of infection have to be delineated, and evaluation of new invasive methods for monitoring central hemodynamics is warranted.

References

1 Fernandez J, Navasa M, Gomez J, Colmenero J, Vila J, Arroyo V, Rodes J: Bacterial infections in cirrhosis: epidemiological changes with invasive procedures and norfloxacin prophylaxis. Hepatology 2002;35:140–148.

2 Thulstrup AM, Sorensen HT, Schonheyder HC, Moller JK, Tage-Jensen U: Population-based study of the risk and short-term prognosis for bacteremia in patients with liver cirrhosis. Clin Infect Dis 2000;31:1357–1361.

3 Garcia-Tsao G, Wiest R: Gut microflora in the pathogenesis of the complications of cirrhosis. Best Pract Res Clin Gastroenterol 2004;18:353–372.

4 Wiest R, Garcia-Tsao G: Bacterial translocation (BT) in cirrhosis. Hepatology 2005;41:422–433.

5 Navasa M, Rodes J: Bacterial infections in cirrhosis. Liver Int 2004;24:277–280.

6 Lim YS, Larson TS, Benson JT, Kamath PS, Kremers WK, Therneau TM, Kim WR: Serum sodium, renal function, and survival of patients with end-stage liver disease. J Hepatol 2010;52:523–528.

7 Hampel H, Bynum GD, Zamora E, El Serag HB: Risk factors for the development of renal dysfunction in hospitalized patients with cirrhosis. Am J Gastroenterol 2001;96:2206–2210.

8 Desai TK, Tsang TK: Aminoglycoside nephrotoxicity in obstructive jaundice. Am J Med 1988;85:47–50.

9 Cabrera J, Arroyo V, Ballesta AM, Rimola A, Gual J, Elena M, Rodes J: Aminoglycoside nephrotoxicity in cirrhosis: value of urinary beta 2-microglobulin to discriminate functional renal failure from acute tubular damage. Gastroenterology 1982;82:97–105.

10 Moore RD, Smith CR, Lietman PS: Predicting aminoglycoside nephrotoxicity. JAMA 1986;256:864–866.

11 Gines A, Escorsell A, Gines P, Salo J, Jimenez W, Inglada L, Navasa M, Claria J, Rimola A, Arroyo V: Incidence, predictive factors, and prognosis of the hepatorenal syndrome in cirrhosis with ascites. Gastroenterology 1993;105:229–236.

12 Fasolato S, Angeli P, Dallagnese L, Maresio G, Zola E, Mazza E, Salinas F, Dona S, Fagiuoli S, Sticca A, Zanus G, Cillo U, Frasson I, Destro C, Gatta A: Renal failure and bacterial infections in patients with cirrhosis: epidemiology and clinical features. Hepatology 2007;45:223–229.

13 Terra C, Guevara M, Torre A, Gilabert R, Fernandez J, Martin-Llahi M, Baccaro ME, Navasa M, Bru C, Arroyo V, Rodes J, Gines P: Renal failure in patients with cirrhosis and sepsis unrelated to spontaneous bacterial peritonitis: value of MELD score. Gastroenterology 2005;129:1944–1953.
14 Follo A, Llovet JM, Navasa M, Planas R, Forns X, Francitorra A, Rimola A, Gassull MA, Arroyo V, Rodes J: Renal impairment after spontaneous bacterial peritonitis in cirrhosis: incidence, clinical course, predictive factors and prognosis. Hepatology 1994;20:1495–1501.
15 Navasa M, Follo A, Jimenez W, Francitorra A, Planas R, Rimola A, Arroyo V, Rodes J: Tumor necrosis factor and interleukin-6 in spontaneous bacterial peritonitis in cirrhosis: relationship with development of renal impairment and mortality. Hepatology 1998;27:1227–1232.
16 Ruiz-Del-Arbol L, Urman J, Fernandez J, Gonzalez M, Navasa M, Monescillo A, Albillos A, Jimenez W, Arroyo V: Systemic, renal, and hepatic hemodynamic derangement in cirrhotic patients with spontaneous bacterial peritonitis. Hepatology 2003;38: 1210–1218.
17 Terg R, Gadano A, Cartier M, Casciato P, Lucero R, Munoz A, Romero G, Levi D, Terg G, Miguez C, Abecasis R: Serum creatinine and bilirubin predict renal failure and mortality in patients with spontaneous bacterial peritonitis: a retrospective study. Liver Int 2009;29:415–419.
18 Perdomo CG, Alves DM: Renal impairment after spontaneous bacterial peritonitis: incidence and prognosis. Can J Gastroenterol 2003;17:187–190.
19 Angeli P, Guarda S, Fasolato S, Miola E, Craighero R, Piccolo F, Antona C, Brollo L, Franchin M, Cillo U, Merkel C, Gatta A: Switch therapy with ciprofloxacin vs. intravenous ceftazidime in the treatment of spontaneous bacterial peritonitis in patients with cirrhosis: similar efficacy at lower cost. Aliment Pharmacol Ther 2006;23:75–84.
20 Kim JH, Lee JS, Lee SH, Bae WK, Kim NH, Kim KA, Moon YS: Renal dysfunction induced by bacterial infection other than spontaneous bacterial peritonitis in patients with cirrhosis: incidence and risk factor. Gut Liver 2009;3:292–297.
21 Angeli P, Merkel C: Pathogenesis and management of hepatorenal syndrome in patients with cirrhosis. J Hepatol 2008;48(suppl 1):S93–S103.
22 Groszmann RJ, Abraldes JG: Portal hypertension: from bedside to bench. J Clin Gastroenterol 2005;39: S125–S130.
23 Wiest R, Groszmann RJ: The paradox of nitric oxide in cirrhosis and portal hypertension: too much, not enough. Hepatology 2001;35:478–491.
24 Fernandez-Seara J, Prieto J, Quiroga J, Zozaya JM, Cobos MA, Rodriguez-Eire JL, Garcia-Plaza A, Leal J: Systemic and regional hemodynamics in patients with liver cirrhosis and ascites with and without functional renal failure. Gastroenterology 1989;97: 1304–1312.
25 Krag A, Bendtsen F, Henriksen JH, Moller S: Low cardiac output predicts development of hepatorenal syndrome and survival in patients with cirrhosis and ascites. Gut 2010;59:105–110.
26 Byl B, Roucloux I, Crusiaux A, Dupont E, Deviere J: Tumor necrosis factor alpha and interleukin 6 plasma levels in infected cirrhotic patients. Gastroenterology 1993;104:1492–1497.
27 Deviere J, Content J, Denys C, Vandenbussche P, Schandene L, Wybran J, Dupont E: Excessive in vitro bacterial lipopolysaccharide-induced production on monokines in cirrhosis. Hepatology 1990;11: 628–634.
28 Kumar A, Thota V, Dee L, Olson J, Uretz E, Parrillo JE: Tumor necrosis factor alpha and interleukin 1beta are responsible for in vitro myocardial cell depression induced by human septic shock serum. J Exp Med 1996;183:949–958.
29 Knuefermann P, Schwederski M, Velten M, Krings P, Ehrentraut H, Rudiger M, Boehm O, Fink K, Dreiner U, Grohe C, Hoeft A, Baumgarten G, Koch A, Zacharowski K, Meyer R: Bacterial DNA induces myocardial inflammation and reduces cardiomyocyte contractility: role of toll-like receptor 9. Cardiovasc Res 2008;78:26–35.
30 Ao L, Song Y, Fullerton DA, Dinarello CA, Meng X: The interaction between myocardial depressant factors in endotoxemic cardiac dysfunction: role of TNF-alpha in TLR4-mediated ICAM-1 expression. Cytokine 2007;38:124–129.
31 Han DW: Intestinal endotoxemia as a pathogenetic mechanism in liver failure. World J Gastroenterol 2002;8:961–965.
32 Berg RD, Garlington AW: Translocation of certain indigenous bacteria from the gastrointestinal tract to the mesenteric lymph nodes and other organs in a gnotobiotic mouse model. Infect Immun 1979;23: 403–411.
33 Wittig BM, Zeitz M: The gut as an organ of immunology. Int J Colorectal Dis 2003;18:181–187.
34 Bigatello LM, Broitman SA, Fattori L, DiPaoli M, Pontello M, Bevilacqua G, Nespoli A: Endotoxemia, encephalopathy, and mortality in cirrhotic patients. Am J Gastroenterol 1987;82:11–15.
35 Lumsden AB, Henderson JM, Kutner MH: Endotoxin levels measured by a chromogenic assay in portal, hepatic and peripheral venous blood in patients with cirrhosis. Hepatology 1988;8:232–236.

36 Wiest R, Tsai MH, Garcia-Tsao G, McCuskey R, Milstien S, Groszmann R: Bacterial translocation up-regulates GTP-cyclohydrolase I in mesenteric vasculature of cirrhotic rats. Hepatology 2003;38: 1508–1515.

37 Frances R, Benlloch S, Zapater P, Gonzalez JM, Lozano B, Munoz C, Pascual S, Casellas JA, Uceda F, Palazon JM, Carnicer F, Perez-Mateo M, Such J: A sequential study of serum bacterial DNA in patients with advanced cirrhosis and ascites. Hepatology 2004;39:484–491.

38 Guarner C, Gonzalez-Navajas JM, Sanchez E, Soriando G, Frances R, Chiva M, Zapater P, Benlloch S, Munoz C, Pascual S, Balanzo J, Perez-Mateo M, Such J: The detection of bacterial DNA in blood of rats with CCl4-induced cirrhosis with ascites represents episodes of bacterial translocation. Hepatology 2006;44:633–639.

39 Such J, Frances R, Munoz C, Zapater P, Casellas JA, Cifuentes A, Rodriguez-Valera F, Pascual S, Sola-Vera J, Carnicer F, Uceda F, Palazon JM, Perez-Mateo M: Detection and identification of bacterial DNA in patients with cirrhosis and culture-negative, nonneutrocytic ascites. Hepatology 2002;36:135–141.

40 Bellot P, Garcia-Pagan JC, Frances R, Abraldes J, Gonzalez-Navajas JM, Navasa M, Perez-Mateo M, Such J, Bosch J: Bacterial translocation induces proinflammatory cytokines and worsens systemic hemodynamics in cirrhotic patients with ascites. J Hepatol 2009;50(suppl 1):41.

41 Frances R, Munoz C, Zapater P, Uceda F, Gascon I, Pascual S, Perez-Mateo M, Such J: Bacterial DNA activates cell mediated immune response and nitric oxide overproduction in peritoneal macrophages from patients with cirrhosis and ascites. Gut 2004; 53:860–864.

42 Frances R, Gonzalez-Navajas JM, Zapater P, Munoz C, Cano R, Pascual S, Marquez D, Santana F, Perez-Mateo M, Such J: Bacterial DNA induces the complement system activation in serum and ascitic fluid from patients with advanced cirrhosis. J Clin Immunol 2007;27:438–444.

43 Frances R, Zapater P, Gonzalez-Navajas JM, Munoz C, Cano R, Moreu R, Pascual S, Bellot P, Perez-Mateo M, Such J: Bacterial DNA in patients with cirrhosis and noninfected ascites mimics the soluble immune response established in patients with spontaneous bacterial peritonitis. Hepatology 2008;47: 978–985.

44 Wiest R, Das S, Cadelina G, Garcia-Tsao G, Milstien S, Groszmann RJ: Bacterial translocation in cirrhotic rats stimulates eNOS-derived NO production and impairs mesenteric vascular contractility. J Clin Invest 1999;104:1223–1233.

45 Gonzalez-Navajas JM, Bellot P, Frances R, Zapater P, Munoz C, Garcia-Pagan JC, Pascual S, Perez-Mateo M, Bosch J, Such J: Presence of bacterial-DNA in cirrhosis identifies a subgroup of patients with marked inflammatory response not related to endotoxin. J Hepatol 2008;48:61–67.

46 Frances R, Gonzalez-Navajas JM, Zapater P, Munoz C, Cano R, Pascual S, Santana F, Marquez D, Perez-Mateo M, Such J: Translocation of bacterial DNA from Gram-positive microorganisms is associated with a species-specific inflammatory response in serum and ascitic fluid of patients with cirrhosis. Clin Exp Immunol 2007;150:230–237.

47 Albillos A, de la Hera A, Alvarez-Mon M: Serum lipopolysaccharide-binding protein prediction of severe bacterial infection in cirrhotic patients with ascites. Lancet 2004;363:1608–1610.

48 Albillos A, DelaHera A, Gonzalez M, Moya J, Calleja J, Monserrat J, Ruiz-Del-Arbol L, Alvarez-Mon M: Increased lipopolysaccharide binding protein in cirrhotic patients with marked immune and hemodynamic derangement. Hepatology 2003;37:208–217.

49 Genesca J, Marti R, Rojo F, Campos F, Peribanez V, Gonzalez A, Castells L, Ruiz-Marcellan C, Margarit C, Esteban R, Guardia J, Segura R: Increased tumour necrosis factor alpha production in mesenteric lymph nodes of cirrhotic patients with ascites. Gut 2003;52:1054–1059.

50 Rasaratnam B, Kaye D, Jennings G, Dudley F, Chin-Dusting J: The effect of selective intestinal decontamination on the hyperdynamic circulatory state in cirrhosis: a randomized trial. Ann Intern Med 2003;139:186–193.

51 Albillos A, de la Hera A, Reyes E, Monserrat J, Munoz L, Nieto M, Prieto I, Sanz A, Alvarez-Mon M: Tumor necrosis factor-alpha expression by activated monocytes and altered T-cell homeostasis in ascitic alcoholic cirrhosis: amelioration with norfloxacin. J Hepatol 2004;40:624–631.

52 Wang W, Zolty E, Falk S, Summer S, Stearman R, Geraci M, Schrier R: Prostacyclin in endotoxemia-induced acute kidney injury: cyclooxygenase inhibition and renal prostacyclin synthase transgenic mice. Am J Physiol Renal Physiol 2007;293:F1131–F1136.

53 Kellum JA: Endotoxin and renal blood flow. Blood Purif 1997;15:286–291.

54 Donnahoo KK, Shames BD, Harken AH, Meldrum DR: Review article: the role of tumor necrosis factor in renal ischemia-reperfusion injury. J Urol 1999; 162:196–203.

55 Yohannes S, Chawla LS: Evolving practices in the management of acute kidney injury in the ICU (intensive care unit). Clin Nephrol 2009;71:602–607.

56 Sort P, Navasa M, Arroyo V, Aldeguer X, Planas R, Ruiz-Del-Arbol L, Castells L, Vargas V, Soriano G, Guevara M, Gines P, Rodes J: Effect of intravenous albumin on renal impairment and mortality in patients with cirrhosis and spontaneous bacterial peritonitis. N Engl J Med 1999;341:403–409.
57 Fernandez J, Navasa M, Garcia-Pagan JC, Abraldes J, Jimenez W, Bosch J, Arroyo V: Effect of intravenous albumin on systemic and hepatic hemodynamics and vasoactive neurohormonal systems in patients with cirrhosis and spontaneous bacterial peritonitis. J Hepatol 2004;41:384–390.
58 Quinlan GJ, Martin GS, Evans TW: Albumin: biochemical properties and therapeutic potential. Hepatology 2005;41:1211–1219.
59 Fernandez J, Navasa M, Planas R, Montoliu S, Monfort D, Soriano G, Vila C, Pardo A, Quintero E, Vargas V, Such J, Gines P, Arroyo V: Primary prophylaxis of spontaneous bacterial peritonitis delays hepatorenal syndrome and improves survival in cirrhosis. Gastroenterology 2007;133:818–824.
60 Tandon P, Garcia-Tsao G: Bacterial infections, sepsis, and multiorgan failure in cirrhosis. Semin Liver Dis 2008;28:26–42.

Reiner Wiest
Klinik und Poliklinik für Innere Medizin I, Universitätsklinikum Regensburg
Franz-Josef-Strauss-Allee 11
DE–93053 Regensburg (Germany)
Tel. +49 941 944 7010, Fax +49 941 944 7073, E-Mail Reiner.Wiest@klinik.uni-regensburg.de

Gerbes AL (ed): Ascites, Hyponatremia and Hepatorenal Syndrome: Progress in Treatment.
Front Gastrointest Res. Basel, Karger, 2011, vol 28, pp 142–148

TIPS for HRS

Tilman Sauerbruch · Beate Appenrodt

Medical Department I, University of Bonn, Bonn, Germany

Abstract

Transjuglar intrahepatic portosystemic shunt (TIPS) improves kidney function in selected patients with liver cirrhosis and HRS types 1 and 2. The rationale for its placement is mainly the shift of the splanchnic blood pool into the central intrathoracic blood volume with de-escalation of vasoconstrictor formation which leads to a reduction of renal sodium reabsorption. There are contraindications which have to be observed. The procedure is not evidence based in the setting of HRS because controlled trials are lacking, but it may be an option to bridge for liver transplantation in some patients.

A definition of hepatorenal syndrome (HRS) is given in the chapter by Fernandez and Arroyo [this vol.]. It is a functional renal failure in patients with advanced liver insufficiency. Other causes of acute kidney impairment should be ruled out in these patients, such as renal parenchymal disease or prerenal failure due to bleeding and infections. Out of those patients with kidney dysfunction and liver cirrhosis only about one third have HRS [1–3]. HRS is linked to a high portal pressure and a systemic circulatory dysfunction characterized by low cardiac output [4, 5], low mean arterial blood pressure, renal hypoperfusion and marked activation of the renin-aldosterone-angiotensin system (RAAS) as well as increased catecholamine levels in the systemic circulation [6].

It is hypothesized that splanchnic blood pooling together with a hypovolemia of the central blood compartment is the driving pathophysiology of these phenomena. Indeed, it has been shown that the vasoconstrictor terlipressin – which redistributes abdominal blood to the central pool [7, 8] – together with albumin reverses the vicious circle and improves kidney function in about half of the patients [9–11]. However, these drugs need i.v. application and can only be given transiently.

Thus, it has been speculated that transjugular intrahepatic portosystemic shunt (TIPS) could be an alternative to repeat treatment with vasoconstrictors and infusion of albumin.

Rationale for TIPS in HRS

TIPS improves kidney function in liver cirrhosis and allows better mobilization of ascites for the following reasons:

- It has been shown that a higher hepatic venous pressure gradient, which correlates inversely with renal blood flow, is associated with a more severe renal dysfunction [6]. TIPS leads to a reduction of the portal venous pressure by around 50% and to a reduction of the sinusoidal pressure. This might improve renal perfusion by an immediate effect via nerval mediation [12], for example, via stretch receptors. Yet, it remains an open question whether such a local hepatorenal reflex really is crucial since the beneficial effect of TIPS on renal function occurs gradually and is not immediate. Nevertheless, TIPS shifts the deranged renal autoregulatory blood flow curve back to the left.
- Patients with a cardiac index <1.5 liters/min/m^2 have a reduced renal blood flow, higher serum creatinine and higher risk of developing hepatorenal syndrome than patients with values above this threshold [4]. TIPS increases the mean cardiac output [13]. At the same time central blood volume increases. However, systemic vascular resistance – which is already reduced in patients with liver cirrhosis – further declines after TIPS [13, 14]. Thus, the hyperdynamic situation of the patient with liver cirrhosis is aggravated by TIPS placement, whereas the central blood volume is increased, which has positive effects (see below).
- After establishment of an intrahepatic portosystemic shunt the activation of baroreceptors is blunted, probably due to refilling of the effective central arterial blood volume. This leads to a constant reduction of plasma renin activity and plasma aldosterone levels up to 1 month after TIPS placement. There is also a less-pronounced deactivation of norepinephrine formation [13, 15–17]. This reduced RAAS activity allows a significant reduction of (proximal) tubular reabsorption of sodium and reinstitutes sodium excretion [13, 15, 18].

Most of the above-mentioned effects counteract the development of functional impairment of the kidney in patients with liver cirrhosis. On the other hand, persistence of peripheral vasodilation and continued elevated plasma norepinephrine levels are factors in favor of sustainment of renal impairment. Furthermore, most patients with hepatorenal syndrome present with advanced liver dysfunction. In these patients, TIPS may worsen liver function towards terminal liver failure, mainly due to loss of portal venous perfusion. Last but not least, TIPS may aggravate spill over of intestinal bacteria into the systemic circulation. All these negative factors explain why only small series have been carried out on the effect of TIPS in patients with liver cirrhosis and HRS.

Table 1. Survival and kidney function after TIPS

a Survival after TIPS in patients with HRS type 1/2

Study	Survival		Study design
	HRS 1	HRS 2	
Brensing [18] (14 HRS 1, 7 HRS 2)	1-year survival with TIPS: 20%	1-year survival with TIPS: 70%	prospective, uncontrolled
Guevara [16] (7 HRS 1)	TIPS: median survival 4.7±2.0 months		prospective, uncontrolled
Wong [19] (5 HRS 1)	TIPS: mean survival 17±5 months		prospective, uncontrolled

b Kidney function after TIPS in patients with HRS type 1/2

Study	GFR	Serum creatinine	24-hour urinary sodium
Brensing [18] (14 HRS 1, 7 HRS 2)	pre-TIPS 18±15 ml/min 4 weeks after TIPS 44±28 ml/min	pre-TIPS 2.3±1.7 mg/dl 4 weeks after TIPS 1.5±1.2 mg/dl	pre-TIPS 12±16 mmol/day 4 weeks after TIPS 91±60 mmol/day
Guevara [16] (7 HRS 1)	pre-TIPS 9±4 ml/min 4 weeks after TIPS 27±7 ml/min	pre-TIPS 5.0±0.8 mg/dl 4 weeks after TIPS 1.8±0.4 mg/dl	pre-TIPS 2.4±0.4 mmol/day 4 weeks after TIPS 9.4±4.2 mmol/day
Testino [24] (18 HRS 2)	pre-TIPS 25.0±6.0 ml/min 12 weeks after TIPS 70.0±19.0 ml/min	pre-TIPS 1.9±0.5 mg/dl 12 weeks after TIPS 0.9±0.3 mg/dl	pre-TIPS 8.0±2.0 mmol/day 12 weeks after TIPS 110.0±41.0 mmol/day

Results of TIPS in Patients with HRS

All series are uncontrolled so that – strictly speaking – a putative beneficial effect of TIPS on HRS is not evidence based. From these small series (table 1), it may be derived that TIPS can be placed in selective patients without deteriorating liver function. In short, the results are as follows:

- Even in selected type 1 patients responding to TIPS, their 1-year survival was only around 20–30% for HRS type 1. Thus, every patient should be evaluated for liver transplantation (fig. 1, 2).
- Improvement of creatinine and sodium excretion occurs gradually over 1–2 months; for example, before TIPS implantation and after 4 weeks following it, 24-hour urinary sodium excretion was 12 ± 16 mmol/day and 91 ± 60 mmol/

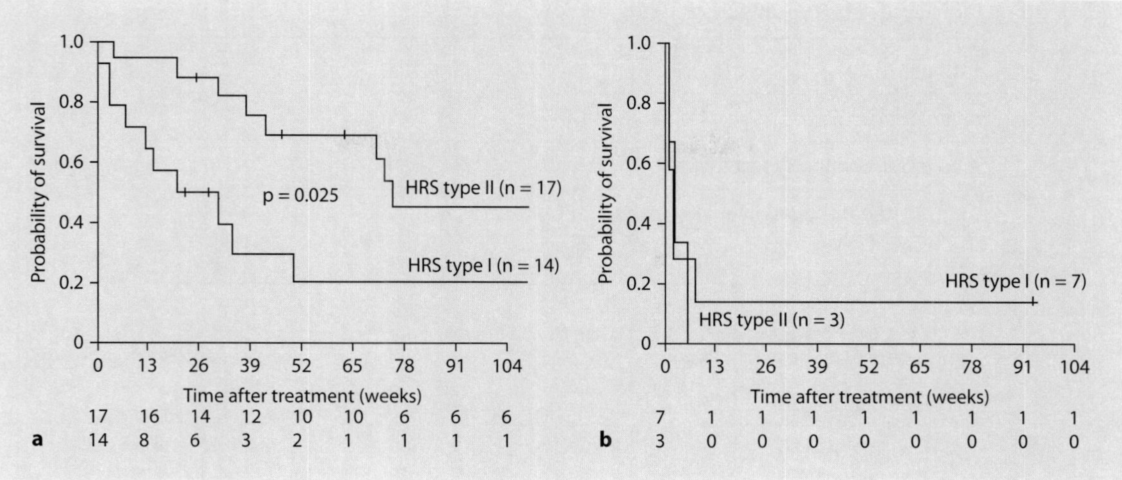

Fig. 1. Kaplan-Meier survival analysis of patients with HRS treated by TIPS (n = 31). **a** Survival analysis after TIPS. **b** Survival analysis of non-TIPS patients (n = 10). Reproduced from Brensing et al. [18].

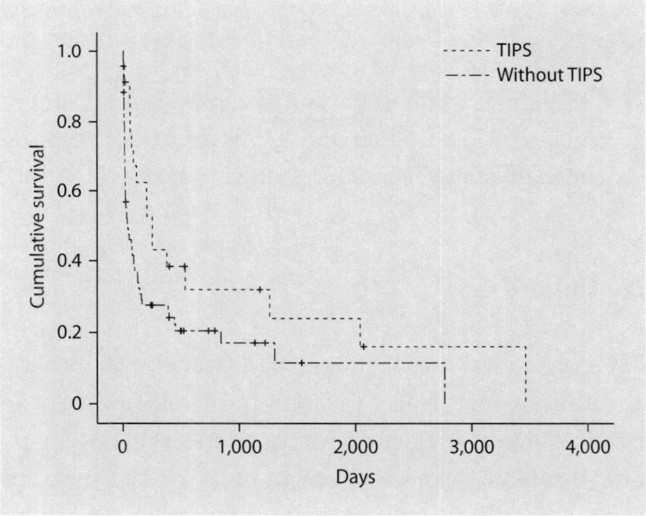

Fig. 2. Kaplan-Meier survival analysis of patients (HRS type 1) with TIPS (n = 23) and without TIPS (n = 68). Mean Child-Pugh points in group with TIPS: 10 (9; 13) and in group without TIPS: 12 (11; 13). Reproduced from Appenrodt et al. [23].

day, respectively. Glomerular filtration rate rose from 18 ± 15 ml/min to 44 ± 28 ml/min and serum creatinine decreased from 2.3 ± 1.7 to 1.5 ± 1.2 mg/dl [18].

- Patients who do not respond to TIPS have a dismal prognosis and a very short survival (3-month survival is 15%) [18].
- Response to pretreatment with vasoconstrictors and albumin could be a selection criterion for TIPS placement [19].

Table 2. Contraindications for TIPS

Absolute
Severe heart failure
Severe pulmonary hypertension
Multiple hepatic cysts, liver abscesses or multifocal HCC
Sepsis
Relative
Thrombosis of all hepatic veins
Portal vein thrombosis
Severe coagulopathy
Severe chronic hepatic encephalopathy
Bilirubin >5 mg/dl
Spontaneous bacterial peritonitis

- Diastolic dysfunction as measured by E/A ratio of ≤1 [20], a high MELD score and a very low GFR are predictive of a poor response [21, 22].
- There are some clear contraindications for TIPS in HRS (table 2).

Conclusions

TIPS reverses some but not all pathogenetic factors associated with HRS.

While it may lead to a long-term improvement of kidney function in selected patients, deterioration of liver function has to be kept in mind. Therefore, TIPS should only be placed very selectively in units where liver transplantation is available. Its role is not evidence-based since controlled trials are lacking.

Key Messages

- Some pathogenetic factors of HRS may be reversed by TIPS.
- Therefore, it can be considered in selected patients as a bridge for liver transplantation.
- Controlled trials are lacking.

References

1 Schepke M, Appenrodt B, Heller J, Zielinski J, Sauerbruch T: Prognostic factors for patients with cirrhosis and kidney dysfunction in the era of MELD: results of a prospective study. Liver Int 2006; 26:834–839.

2 Francoz C, Glotz D, Moreau R, Durand F: The evaluation of renal function and disease in patients with cirrhosis. J Hepatol 2010;52:605–613.

3 Moreau R, Lebrec D: Acute renal failure in patients with cirrhosis: perspectives in the age of MELD. Hepatology 2003;37:233–243.

4 Krag A, Bendtsen F, Henriksen JH, Møller S: Low cardiac output predicts development of hepatorenal syndrome and survival in patients with cirrhosis and ascites. Gut 2010;59:105–110.

5 Ruiz-del-Arbol L, Monescillo A, Arocena C, Valer P, Ginès P, Moreira V, Milicua JM, Jiménez W, Arroyo V: Circulatory function and hepatorenal syndrome in cirrhosis. Hepatology 2005;42:439–447.

6 Stadlbauer V, Wright GA, Banaji M, Mukhopadhya A, Mookerjee RP, Moore K, Jalan R: Relationship between activation of the sympathetic nervous system and renal blood flow autoregulation in cirrhosis. Gastroenterology 2008;134:111–119.

7 Narahara Y, Kanazawa H, Taki Y, Kimura Y, Atsukawa M, Katakura T, Kidokoro H, Harimoto H, Fukuda T, Matsushita Y, Nakatsuka K, Sakamoto C: Effects of terlipressin on systemic, hepatic and renal hemodynamics in patients with cirrhosis. J Gastroenterol Hepatol 2009;24:1791–1797.

8 Kiszka-Kanowitz M, Henriksen JH, Hansen EF, Møller S, Bendtsen F: Effect of terlipressin on blood volume distribution in patients with cirrhosis. Scand J Gastroenterol 2004;39:486–492.

9 Sanyal AJ, Boyer T, Garcia-Tsao G, Regenstein F, Rossaro L, Appenrodt B, Blei A, Gülberg V, Sigal S, Teuber P, Terlipressin Study Group: A randomized, prospective, double-blind, placebo-controlled trial of terlipressin for type 1 hepatorenal syndrome. Gastroenterology 2008;134:1360–1368.

10 Martín-Llahí M, Pépin MN, Guevara M, Díaz F, Torre A, Monescillo A, Soriano G,Terra C, Fábrega E, Arroyo V, Rodés J, Ginès P, TAHRS Investigators: Terlipressin and albumin vs. albumin in patients with cirrhosis and hepatorenal syndrome: a randomized study. Gastroenterology 2008;134:1352–1359.

11 Sagi SV, Mittal S, Kasturi KS, Sood GK: Terlipressin therapy for reversal of type 1 hepatorenal syndrome: a meta-analysis of randomized controlled trials. J Gastroenterol Hepatol 2010;25:880–885.

12 Jalan R, Forrest EH, Redhead DN, Dillon JF, Hayes PC: Reduction in renal blood flow following acute increase in the portal pressure: evidence for the existence of a hepatorenal reflex in man? Gut 1997; 40:664–670.

13 Wong F, Sniderman K, Liu P, Allidina Y, Sherman M, Blendis L: Transjugular intrahepatic portosystemic stent shunt: effects on hemodynamics and sodium homeostasis in cirrhosis and refractory ascites. Ann Intern Med 1995;122:816–822.

14 Umgelter A, Reindl W, Geisler F, Saugel B, Huber W, Berger H, Schmid RM: Effects of TIPS on global end-diastolic volume and cardiac output and renal resistive index in ICU patients with advanced alcoholic cirrhosis. Ann Hepatol 2010;9:40–45.

15 Wong F, Sniderman K, Liu P, Blendis L: The mechanism of the initial natriuresis after transjugular intrahepatic portosystemic shunt. Gastroenterology 1997;112:899–907.

16 Guevara M, Ginès P, Bandi JC, Gilabert R, Sort P, Jiménez W, Garcia-Pagan JC, Bosch J, Arroyo V, Rodés J: Transjugular intrahepatic portosystemic shunt in hepatorenal syndrome: effects on renal function and vasoactive systems. Hepatology 1998; 28:416–422.

17 Solis-Herruzo JA, Duran A, Favela V, Castellano G, Madrid JL, Muñoz-Yagüe MT, Morillas JD, Estenoz J: Effects of lumbar sympathetic block on kidney function in cirrhotic patients with hepatorenal syndrome. J Hepatol 1987;5:167–173.

18 Brensing KA, Textor J, Perz J, Schiedermaier P, Raab P, Strunk H, Klehr HU, Kramer HJ, Spengler U, Schild H, Sauerbruch T: Long term outcome after transjugular intrahepatic portosystemic stent-shunt in non-transplant cirrhotics with hepatorenal syndrome: a phase II study. Gut 2000;47:288–295.

19 Wong F, Pantea L, Sniderman K: Midodrine, octreotide, albumin, and TIPS in selected patients with cirrhosis and type 1 hepatorenal syndrome. Hepatology. 2004;40:55–64.

20 Rabie RN, Cazzaniga M, Salerno F, Wong F: The use of E/A ratio as a predictor of outcome in cirrhotic patients treated with transjugular intrahepatic portosystemic shunt. Am J Gastroenterol. 2009;104: 2458–2466.

21 Malinchoc M, Kamath PS, Gordon FD, Peine CJ, Rank J, ter Borg PC: A model to predict poor survival in patients undergoing transjugular intrahepatic portosystemic shunts. Hepatology 2000;31: 864–871.

22 Rouillard SS, Bass NM, Roberts JP, Doherty CA, Gee L, Bacchetti P, Somberg KA: Severe hyperbilirubinemia after creation of transjugular intrahepatic portosystemic shunts: natural history and predictors of outcome. Ann Intern Med 1998;128:374–377.

23 Appenrodt B, Zielinski J, Brensing KA, Heller J, Sauerbruch T, Schepke M: Degree of hepatic dysfunction and improvement of renal function predict survival in patients with HRS type 1: a retrospective analysis. Eur J Gastroenterol Hepatol 2009;21:1428–1432.

24 Testino G, Ferro C, Sumberaz A, Messa P, Morelli N, Guadagni B, Ardizzone G, Valente U: Type-2 hepatorenal syndrome and refractory ascites: role of transjugular intrahepatic portosystemic stent-shunt in eighteen patients with advanced cirrhosis awaiting orthotopic liver transplantation. Hepatogastroenterology 2003;50:1753–1755.

Prof. Dr. med. Tilman Sauerbruch
Medizinische Klinik und Poliklinik I, Allgemeine Innere Medizin
Sigmund-Freud-Strasse 25
DE–53105 Bonn (Germany)
Tel. +49 228 287 15255, Fax +49 228 287 14322, E-Mail sauerbruch@uni-bonn.de

Gerbes AL (ed): Ascites, Hyponatremia and Hepatorenal Syndrome: Progress in Treatment.
Front Gastrointest Res. Basel, Karger, 2011, vol 28, pp 149–162

Vasoconstrictor Therapy for Hepatorenal Syndrome

Chong-Meng Yeo[a] · Guadalupe Garcia-Tsao[a,b]

[a]Digestive Diseases Section, Yale University School of Medicine, New Haven, Conn., and [b]Digestive Diseases Section, VA-CT Healthcare System, West Haven, Conn., USA

Abstract

Hepatorenal syndrome (HRS) is a potentially reversible form of kidney injury in cirrhotic patients. Marked splanchnic and systemic vasodilatation is the main pathogenic mechanism. Various vasoconstrictors have been used to treat HRS, with the intention of ameliorating vasodilatation to improve effective arterial blood volume, attenuate the neurohormonal system activation, thereby reducing renal vasoconstriction and increasing renal perfusion. Three main classes of vasoconstrictors have been used: vasopressin receptor agonists (vasopressin, ornipressin, terlipressin), alpha adrenergic receptor agonists (midodrine, noradrenaline) and octreotide. Vasoconstrictors have always been used in conjunction with intravenous albumin. Terlipressin is the only vasoconstrictor of proven efficacy in HRS based on randomized clinical trials and is considered first line therapy, where available. Vasoconstrictors other than terlipressin are comparable to terlipressin regarding hemodyamic, neurohumoral and renal function effects. However, clinical trials with these vasoconstrictors are limited by small sample sizes and suboptimal study design. Only two small randomized trials compare noradrenaline to terlipressin with equivalent results. In countries where terlipressin is unavailable, such as the USA, noradrenaline could be utilized. Even though the evidence is less strong for the combination of oral midodrine plus subcutaneous octreotide, it is the preferred alternative therapy given its ease of administration and safety profile. No definite recommendation can be made for type 2 HRS in view of scanty data available. Vasoconstrictors, including terlipressin, should be used cautiously as they can be associated with cardiovascular and ischemic adverse events. Mortality is still high in patients who develop HRS and therefore vasoconstrictors should be considered as a bridge to the definitive therapy, liver transplantation.

Hepatorenal syndrome (HRS) is a potentially reversible form of kidney injury in patients with cirrhosis and ascites. It is a functional type of pre-renal kidney injury [1] characterized by intense renal vasoconstriction with very low renal perfusion and glomerular filtration rate (GFR) [2]. The incidence of HRS in cirrhotic patients with ascites is 18% after 1 year, and rises up to 39% after 5 years [3]. Progressive splanchnic and systemic vasodilatation, its main pathogenic mechanism, is a consequence of portal hypertension and is attributable mostly to nitric oxide overproduction, though other vasodilatory substances also participate in this complex process [4, 5]. HRS represents the final phase of cirrhosis, with extreme vasodilatation that results in marked decrease in effective arterial blood volume which in turn leads to maximal activation of vasoconstrictive systems, specifically the renin-angiotensin-aldosterone axis and the sympathetic nervous system and, thereby, renal vasoconstriction (fig. 1). The prognosis is very poor and is somewhat ameliorated with therapeutic interventions. Therapies for HRS include pharmacological therapies, mainly with vasoconstrictors.

Pathophysiological Bases of Pharmacological Therapy in Hepatorenal Syndrome

Since vasodilatation leading to a decreased arterial blood volume is the main mechanism in the pathogenesis of HRS, it follows that pharmacological treatment would be directed towards the use of vasoconstrictors (to overcome vasodilatation) and albumin (to replenish the intravascular volume) (fig. 1).

Vasoconstrictors

Various vasoconstrictors have been used to treat HRS, with the intention of ameliorating vasodilatation. This will improve effective arterial blood volume, attenuate activation of the renin-angiotensin-aldosterone and sympathetic nervous systems, thereby ameliorating renal vasoconstriction, increasing renal perfusion and improving GFR (fig. 1).

Three main classes of vasoconstrictors have been used in the treatment of HRS:

1 Vasopressin receptor agonists like vasopressin and its analogues, ornipressin and terlipressin, that bind to V_1 receptors on vascular smooth muscle to cause vasoconstriction via the IP3 signal transduction pathway. They have greatest vasoconstrictive effects on the splanchnic, muscular and cutaneous vessels.

2 Alpha-adrenergic receptor agonists such as noradrenaline and midodrine that cause vasoconstriction by binding predominantly to α_1-adrenergic receptors that leads to increased intracellular calcium resulting in smooth muscle contraction. Given intravenously to healthy dogs at 0.2–0.4 μg/kg/min, noradrenaline has also been shown to have a renal vasodilatory effect [6].

3 The vasoconstrictive effect of octreotide, a somatostatin analogue, is mediated by inhibition of the release of glucagon and other vasodilating peptides, but that has also been shown to have a direct vasoconstrictive effect [7] not only in the splanchnic but also in the systemic circulation [8].

The first proof-of-concept study used a continuous infusion of ornipressin over a 4-hour period in 11 patients with decompensated cirrhosis and deteriorating renal

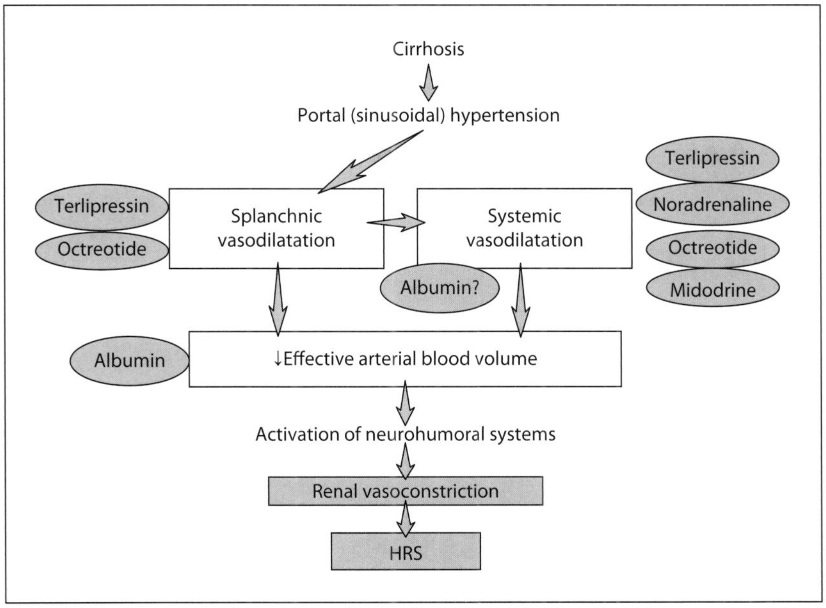

Fig. 1. Pathogenesis of HRS and site of action of different vasoconstrictors and albumin.

function [9]. Ornipressin led to an improvement in renal clearance parameters, an increase in systemic vascular resistance and a decrease in renin and aldosterone plasma levels [9]. In a subsequent study performed in 16 patients with HRS, ornipressin was associated with intravenous albumin and administered for 3 or 15 days [10]. The 3-day course was associated with a normalization of the renin-angiotensin and sympathetic nervous systems, but with only a slight improvement in renal function. However, when ornipressin and albumin were administered for 15 days, a significant improvement in renal function was observed, with normalization of serum creatinine, a marked increase in renal plasma flow and GFR, and a persistent suppression in the activity of vasoconstrictor systems. Notably, of 8 patients that were to receive the 15-day course of ornipressin, only 4 could complete the course because of the development of severe side effects (ischemic colitis, tongue ischemia and ventricular extrasystoles).

After this, other uncontrolled small studies also performed as proof-of-concept have confirmed that other vasoconstrictors, prominently terlipressin [11–14] but also octreotide plus midodrine [15] and noradrenaline [16], administered for periods greater than 3 days lead to an increase in mean arterial pressure (MAP) and GFR and to decreases in serum creatinine and plasma renin activity (table 1), thereby providing evidence in favor of the vasodilatation concept as the driving force behind HRS. One of these studies also confirmed a high rate of ischemic side effects with ornipressin [17]. In contrast, study of the combination of octreotide

Table 1. Significant changes in MAP, parameters of renal function and plasma renin activity in prospective studies of vasoconstrictors + albumin administered for >3 days

Author, year	Vasoconstrictor	n	MAP	Serum creatinine	GFR	Urine output	Plasma renin activity
Guevara, 1998 [10]	ornipressin	4	↑ 20%	↓ 77%	↑ 356%	↑ 207%	↓ 96%
Gulberg, 1999 [17]	ornipressin	7	↑ 20%	–	↑ 153%	↑ 112%	–
Angeli, 1999 [15]	ocreotide + midodrine	5	↑ 28%	↓ 64%	↑ 343%	↑ 126%	↓ 77%
Uriz, 2001 [11]	terlipressin	9	↑ 18%	↓ 62%	↑ 200%	↑ 57%	↓ 85%
Mulkay, 2001 [12]	terlipressin	12	↑ 14%	↓ 53%	↑ 200%	↑ 132%	–
Ortega, 2002 [13]	terlipressin	13	↑ 13%	↓ 58%	↑ 200%	↑ 85%	↓ 80%
Duvoux, 2002 [16]	noradrenaline	12	↑ 12%	↓ 59%	↑ 187%	↑ 211%	↓ 71%
Pomier, 2003 [18]	octreotide alone	9[1]	↑ 13%*	↓ 7%*	↑ 43%*	–	↓ 58%*
Solanki, 2003 [14]	terlipressin	12	↑28%	↓ 59%	↑ 255%	↑ 134%	ND

*Not significantly different from baseline.
All other changes in the table were statistically significant compared to baseline.
[1]Only patients who received octreotide first.

(administered orally) and midodrine (administered subcutaneously) that included only 5 patients reported no adverse events [15]. Notably, in this study, the dose of vasoconstrictors was adjusted based on a MAP increase of at least 15 mm Hg. This is a rational approach as a low MAP is the clinical hallmark of systemic vasodilatation and an increase in MAP would indicate improvement of this pathogenic mechanism. Importantly, in a study of octreotide alone (administered in a continuous intravenous infusion), and even though the changes were in the correct direction, the effect was mild and did not achieve statistical significance [18] (table 1). This suggests that the combination octreotide/midodrine is better than the use of octreotide alone.

The effect of vasoconstrictors on the systemic or splanchnic circulation can help determine which vascular bed, if any, plays a more important role in the vasodilatation leading to HRS. In animal models of endotoxin-induced vasodilatation, both vasopressin and norepinephrine increase systemic arterial pressure but only vasopressin reduces portal flow (indicating splanchnic vasoconstriction) while norepinephrine has no effect or may even increase portal flow [19]. The fact that a noradrenaline infusion has the same effect as ornipressin or terlipressin in patients with HRS (table 1) indicates that systemic vasodilatation plays an important role in the genesis of HRS.

Key Messages: Box 1

- HRS is a potentially reversible form of kidney injury which is characterized by an intense renal vasoconstriction.
- Progressive splanchnic and systemic vasodilatation is the main pathogenic mechanism in HRS.
- Various vasoconstrictors have been used to treat HRS, with the intention of ameliorating splanchnic and systemic vasodilatation.
- Three main classes of vasoconstrictors have been used in the treatment of HRS – vasopressin receptor agonists, α-adrenergic receptor agonists and octreotide.
- Vasoconstrictors have always been used in conjunction with intravenous albumin in the treatment of HRS.
- Terlipressin is the only agent proven effective in several randomized, controlled trials.

Albumin

Vasoconstrictors have generally been used in conjunction with intravenous albumin. A recent study suggests that the beneficial effect of albumin on circulatory and renal function in patients with HRS is related not only to the expansion of the plasma volume but also to a direct vasoconstrictive effect on the peripheral arterial circulation [20]. It is conceivable that an improvement of renal function in HRS patients treated with vasoconstrictors and albumin is attributable to the additive effects of both compounds in producing vasoconstriction (fig. 1). Alternatively, albumin may also have important under-recognized antioxidant or vascular properties, such as nitric oxide trapping that can improve renal function [21]. The need for albumin in addition to vasoconstrictors in HRS has only been examined in a nonrandomized small study that showed that treatment with terlipressin and albumin was associated with a significant decrease in serum creatinine and an increase in MAP, changes that were not observed in a non-concurrent group of patients treated with terlipressin alone [22].

In the most recent consensus from the International Ascites Club, albumin was the recommended volume expander over 0.9% sodium chloride therapy for the diagnosis and management of HRS. The recommended albumin dosage in the initial management of HRS is 1 g/kg/day (up to a maximum 100 g/day) [23]. The maintenance dose of albumin, once the diagnosis of HRS is established and vasoconstrictors are initiated, is of 25–50 g/day. Albumin may be discontinued if serum albumin concentration

Table 2. Vasoconstrictors other than terlipressin in HRS: doses used, titration and adverse events

Vasoconstrictor	Doses used and titration	Observed adverse events
Vasopressin [32]	initial dose: i.v. infusion of 0.01 U/min. titrate dose up to a maximum of 0.8 U/min to achieve a 10 mm Hg increase in MAP from baseline or MAP >70 mm Hg	none reported[1]
Ornipressin [10, 17]	initial dose: i.v. infusion of 2 IU/h on 1st day, increase to 4 IU/h on 2nd day and 6 IU/h on 3rd day	abdominal cramps, intestinal ischemia ± bleeding (13%), tongue ischemia (13%), ventricular arrhythmias (13%)
Midodrine + octreotide [15, 36, 37]	initial dose: oral midodrine 5–10 mg t.i.d. plus subcutaneous octreotide 100 μg t.i.d. If no increase in MAP by 15 mm Hg: increase the doses every 24 h – midodrine up to 15 mg t.i.d. and octreotide up to 200 μg t.i.d. (octreotide can also be given intravenously 25 μg/h after a bolus injection of 25 μg)	diarrhea, tingling, goosebumps, hypertensive urgency (1.3%)
Noradrenaline [16, 33, 34]	initial dose: continuous i.v. infusion, 0.5 mg/h. If no increase in MAP by 10 mm Hg: increase the dose by 0.5 mg/h every 4 h up to a maximum of 3.0 mg/h	ventricular arrhythmia } (7%), myocardial hypokinesia (5%)

[1]Ischemic and cardiovascular adverse events have been reported in a study used for vasodilatory shock at a dose of 0.04 U/min and in studies of variceal hemorrhage in patients with cirrhosis.

is greater than 4.5 g/dl and should be immediately withdrawn in case of pulmonary edema. As this pulmonary complication is uncommon, monitoring of central venous pressure is not mandatory; however, careful monitoring of the cardiopulmonary function is recommended [23].

Clinical Use of Vasoconstrictors in Hepatorenal Syndrome Type 1

Terlipressin has been the most widely investigated vasoconstrictor in the treatment of HRS not only in uncontrolled clinical trials [11–13, 24–27] but also in controlled randomized trials [14, 28–30]. A recent Cochrane meta-analysis of the latter shows that

Table 3. Clinical outcomes of HRS-1 patients treated with vasopressin receptor agonists (other than terlipressin) plus intravenous albumin

Author, year	n (n HRS-2)	Vasoconstrictor	Definition of CR	CR	Days to CR	HRS recurrence	Median survival
Guevara, 1998 [10]	8 (?)	omipressin	sCr <1.5 mg/dl	6 (75%)	7 (4–15)[a]	2 (33%)	60 days
Gulberg, 1999 [17]	7 (0)	omipressin	2-fold increased in CrCl to > 40ml/min	4 (57%)	14 (8–27)[a]	2 (50%)	90 days
Kiser, 2005 [32]	19 (1)	vasopressin + octreotide	sCr ≤1.5 mg/dl without dialysis	8 (42%)[b]	7[c]	NA	NA
	8 (2)	vasopressin	sCr ≤1.5 mg/dl without dialysis	3 (38%)[b]	6[c]	NA	NA
Total	42			21 (50%)	7	4/15 (27%)	

CR = Complete response; sCr = serum creatinine; CrCl = creatinine clearance; NA = not available.
[a]Median (range).
[b]Percentages refer to HRS-1.
[c]Mean.

terlipressin has a greater efficacy than placebo in reversing renal dysfunction in HRS with an improvement in survival [31]. Terlipressin is the most common vasoconstrictor used in Europe and Asia for the treatment of HRS type 1 (HRS-1). However, this agent is still not available or approved for use in many countries including the United States. In these countries, vasoconstrictors other than terlipressin, such as vasopressin, midodrine plus octreotide or noradrenaline play an important role. The use of terlipressin will be reviewed in detail in other chapters in this book. Therefore, the remainder of this chapter will discuss the clinical use of vasoconstrictors other than terlipressin. The doses used in different studies and the observed adverse events are shown in table 2.

Vasopressin Receptor Agonists Other than Terlipressin

Clinical outcomes of 4 uncontrolled series (2 ornipressin, 2 vasopressin) including 42 patients mostly with HRS-1 are summarized in table 3 [10, 17, 32]. Complete response (mostly defined as a decrease in serum creatinine to <1.5 mg/dl) was observed in 50%

(21/42) of the cases in a median of 7 days. HRS recurred in only 27% of patients that had a complete response.

Ornipressin has been administered in a continuous intravenous infusion, starting at 2 IU/h on the first day and increase by 2 IU/day to a maximum dose of 6 IU/h on the third day [10] (table 2). The most common adverse event is abdominal cramps which are usually self-limited; but severe adverse events leading to treatment discontinuation such as intestinal ischemia with or without bleeding (13%), tongue ischemia (13%) and ventricular arrhythmias (13%) have been reported. Because of them, ornipressin is not recommended for use in patients with HRS.

Vasopressin has been administered as continuous intravenous infusion with initial starting dose of 0.01 U/min, titrated up to 0.8 U/min to achieve a 10 mm Hg increase in MAP from baseline or a MAP greater than 70 mm Hg (table 2). The mean vasopressin dose required to achieve these goals in the only study investigating vasopressin was 0.23 U/min which was significantly higher than doses normally used in critically ill patients [32]. Although no adverse effects were reported in the study, cardiac arrest, ischemic digits/extremities, myocardial infarction have been associated with vasopressin doses of 0.04 U/min in the treatment of vasodilatory shock and in patients with cirrhosis and variceal hemorrhage. Extreme caution and careful monitoring of ischemic complications is recommended in patients receiving doses greater than 0.1 U/min [32].

Noradrenaline

The result of the first uncontrolled pilot study using noradrenaline showed a promising result, with 83% reversal in 12 patients with HRS-1 [16] (table 4). Similar results were shown in two subsequent studies [33, 34] for an overall complete response rate of 64% (23/36) in a median of 6.5 days. HRS recurrence is very low at 8% (table 4).

The two more recent studies were a part of small prospective open-label randomized studies of noradrenaline versus terlipressin that found both vasoconstrictors to be equally effective in the treatment of HRS-1 with a similar rate of side effects [33, 34]. No firm conclusions can be drawn from these studies given the very small sample sizes (9 and 40, respectively) that did not define noninferiority or equivalence margins in their calculation [31].

Noradrenaline has been used as a continuous intravenous infusion at an initial dose of 0.5 mg/h, adjusted to achieve an increase in MAP of at least 10 mm Hg or an increase in 4-hour urine output to more than 200 ml. If these goals are not reached, the dose can be increased every 4 h in steps of 0.5 mg/h, up to the maximum dose of 3 mg/h [16, 34] (table 2). In this setting and at doses of 1.5 mg/h, noradrenaline has been associated with ventricular arrhythmias (7%) and myocardial hypokinesia (5%), both having reversed with dose reduction. Given the much lower cost and wider availability of noradrenaline, it can be considered a reasonable alternative treatment for HRS-1, especially in the countries where terlipressin is not available and cost is a major concern.

Table 4. Clinical outcomes of HRS-1 patients treated with noradrenaline plus intravenous albumin

Author, Year	n (n HRS-2)	Vasoconstrictor	Definition of CR	CR	Days to CR[a]	HRS recurrence	Median survival
Duvoux, 2002 [16]	12 (0)	noradrenaline	sCr <1.5 mg/dl or increased CrCl to >40 ml/min	10 (83%)	7 (5–10)	0 (0)	median survival 60 days
Alessandria, 2007 [33]	4 (6)	noradrenaline	decrease of sCr of ≥30% to ≤1.5 mg/dl	3 (75%)	5 (2–10)	1 (33%)	all bridged for liver transplantation
Sharma, 2008 [34]	20 (0)	noradrenaline	sCr <1.5 mg/dl	10 (50%)	6.5 (4–15)	not available	not available
Total	36			23 (64%)	6.5	1/13 (8%)	

CR = Complete response; sCr = serum creatinine; CrCl = creatinine clearance.
[a]Median (range).

Octreotide plus Midodrine

In two clinical trials, octreotide monotherapy was proven to be no more effective than placebo in reversing HRS [32] or the abnormalities that lead to it [18] (table 1). In experimental studies it has been shown that octreotide exerts a local vasoconstrictive effect on vascular smooth muscle of the superior mesenteric arterial bed, but only in the presence of vasoconstrictors that activate protein kinase C [7]. Midodrine, as an alpha-1 adrenergic receptor agonist is one of such vasoconstrictors and it is therefore logical that the combination would be more effective than octreotide alone and will probably be more effective than midodrine alone, although this has not been investigated. The combination of midodrine and octreotide has been used for treatment of HRS-1 in three studies totaling 79 patients [35–37] (table 5) HRS reversal was observed in 49% of patients in a median of approximately 17 days (longer than with other vasoconstrictors).

Midodrine has been administered orally at an initial dose of 5–10 mg three times daily and octreotide subcutaneously at an initial dose of 100 μg three times daily. If there is no increase in MAP of 15 mm Hg, the dose of midodrine can be increased up to 15 mg three times daily and octreotide up to 200 mcg three times daily every 24 h (table 2). The dose of midodrine has been found to be important in determining the

Table 5. Clinical outcomes of HRS-1 patients treated with octreotide plus midodrine

Author, year	n	Vasoconstrictor	Definition of CR	CR	Days to CR	HRS recurrence	Median survival
Angeli, 1999 [15]	5	midodrine + octreotide	sCr ≤2 mg/dl	5 (100%)	20 (5–20)[a]	0 (0)	60% survived >6 months
Wong, 2004 [36]	14	midodrine + octreotide	sCr <1.5 mg/dl for 3 consecutive days	10 (71%)	16[b]	0 (0)	not available
Esrailian, 2007 [37]	60	midodrine + octreotide[1]	sCr ≤1.5 mg/dl	40% had a sustained reduction in sCr at 30 days	16.8[b]	not available	43% in treatment group had died at 30 days
Total	79			39/79 (49%)	17	0/15	

CR = Complete response; sCr = serum creatinine.
[a]Median (range).
[b]Mean.
[1]Without concurrent albumin.

reduction in serum creatinine. While 88% of patients that received midodrine at a dose of 15 mg three times daily had a reduction in serum creatinine to ≤1.5 mg/dl, this reduction only occurred in 33% of those receiving ≤12.5 mg TID [37]. With regards to the adverse events, use of midodrine and octreotide has been associated with mild side effects such as diarrhea, tingling and goosebumps which are usually self-limited. No other serious ischemic or cardiovascular complication have been observed except one case of hypertensive urgency reported which was resolved with dose reduction (table 2). Given the additional advantage of oral and subcutaneous administration, the combination of midodrine and octreotide offers an appealing alternative for the treatment of HRS-1 especially in countries where terlipressin is not available. Randomized controlled trials of octreotide and midodrine versus terlipressin are necessary.

Clinical use of Vasoconstrictors in Hepatorenal Syndrome Type 2

The data on vasoconstrictors in the treatment of HRS type 2 (HRS-2) are scarce. Some of the studies using different vasoconstrictors have included patients with HRS-2 (tables 3, 4); however, the numbers are very small and data specific for HRS-2 cannot be abstracted. A randomized pilot study comparing terlipressin versus noradrenaline in the treatment of HRS included 6 patients with HRS-2 randomized to noradrenaline [33]. HRS reversal occurred in 4 (67%) of them and recurred in 1 (25%), which is identical to a 67% reversal rate in HRS-2 observed with terlipressin in a randomized controlled trial of terlipressin plus albumin vs. albumin alone [30]. In this study reversal rate was higher in HRS-2 compared to HRS-1 (35%); however, recurrence also seems to be higher in HRS-2 (~90%) [38].

The combination of octreotide/midodrine, by not requiring intravenous administration, is appealing in patients with HRS-2, the majority of which are treated in an outpatient setting. A retrospective study showed that patients with HRS-1 and HRS-2 who received octreotide/midodrine and albumin had a better survival than a historical control group [39] and showed that in 26 patients with HRS-2, treatment was associated with a trend towards an improvement in GFR and a median survival greater than 12 months. In another small case-control study, 10 patients with HRS-2 that had been successfully treated with terlipressin and then with midodrine (7.5–12.5 mg TID) were compared to 10 historical responders to terlipressin that did not receive midodrine [38]. HRS recurrence was 90% in both groups and there were no differences in serum creatinine, creatinine clearance and plasma renin activity after terlipressin withdrawal.

It is clear that more studies are required to further evaluate and characterize the effect of vasoconstrictors in patients with HRS-2.

Key Messages: Box 2

- In countries where terlipressin is not available, noradrenaline infusion or the combination of oral midodrine and subcutaneous octreotide is recommended as an alternative treatment for HRS-1.
- No definite treatment recommendation can be made for HRS-2 in view of the limited data available.
- The optimal dose and duration of non-terlipressin vasoconstrictors remain to be determined.
- Vasoconstrictor therapy is not recommended in patients with certain cardiac and vascular diseases.

Conclusions

Clinical studies have shown that vasoconstrictors (both splanchnic and/or systemic) are useful in reversing the hemodynamic and neurohumoral abnormalities that lead to HRS and are therefore useful in reverting HRS in a significant proportion of patients. These studies prove that vasodilatation (both splanchnic and systemic) is the major pathogenic mechanism in HRS.

The bulk of evidence for the treatment of HRS-1 supports the use of terlipressin which should be considered first-line medical therapy for HRS. Where not available, evidence points towards the use of noradrenaline since two recent small open-label randomized trials showed that noradrenaline is as effective as terlipressin. In clinical practice, at least in the United States, the combination octreotide/midodrine is preferred given its good safety profile and the possibility of administration outside an intensive care unit. However, if a MAP response is not observed with maximal doses, the patient should be transferred to an intensive care unit where a noradrenaline infusion should be initiated. With any of these vasoconstrictors, extreme caution should be exercised for the development of cardiovascular and ischemic complications and patients should be closely monitored. Although higher doses have been associated to a higher rate of HRS reversal [37], they will also be associated with a higher rate of adverse events [21]. In view of the potential associated cardiovascular and ischemic complications, vasoconstrictors are generally not recommended in patient with coronary artery disease, cardiomyopathy, cardiac arrhythmias, cardiac failure, arterial hypertension, cerebrovascular disease and peripheral vascular disease.

No firm recommendation regarding the use of vasoconstrictors can be made for HRS-2.

Key Messages

- The main pathogenic mechanism in HRS is splanchnic and systemic vasodilatation.
- Vasoconstrictors (both splanchnic and/or systemic) ameliorate vasodilatation and reverse the abnormalities that lead to HRS.
- Terlipressin (splanchnic and systemic vasoconstrictor) is the most investigated vasoconstrictor and is the first-line pharmacological treatment in HRS.
- Alternatives to terlipressin are noradrenaline (systemic vasoconstrictor) and the combination octreotide/midodrine (systemic and splanchnic vasoconstrictors). The latter is preferred given its ease of administration but has not been compared to terlipressin.
- Albumin acts by increasing arterial volume but may also have a vasoconstrictive effect. It is always administered with a vasoconstrictor, although its need has not been assessed prospectively.
- Most of the evidence is on HRS-1. More studies are needed in HRS-2. The rate of HRS-2 reversal with vasoconstrictors appears to be higher but recurrence is also higher.

References

1 Garcia-Tsao G, Parikh CR, Viola A: Acute kidney injury in cirrhosis. Hepatology 2008;48:2064–2077.

2 Gines P, Schrier RW: Renal failure in cirrhosis. N Engl J Med 2009;361:1279–1290.

3 Gines A, Escorsell A, Gines P, et al: Incidence, predictive factors, and prognosis of the hepatorenal syndrome in cirrhosis with ascites. Gastroenterology 1993;105:229–236.

4 Martin PY, Gines P, Schrier RW: Nitric oxide as a mediator of hemodynamic abnormalities and sodium and water retention in cirrhosis. N Engl J Med 1998;339:533–541.

5 Iwakiri Y, Groszmann RJ: The hyperdynamic circulation of chronic liver diseases: from the patient to the molecule. Hepatology 2006;43:S121–S131.

6 Anderson WP, Korner PI, Selig SE: Mechanisms involved in the renal responses to intravenous and renal artery infusions of noradrenaline in conscious dogs. J Physiol 1981;321:21–30.

7 Wiest R, Tsai M-H, Groszmann RJ: Octreotide potentiates PKC-dependent vasoconstrictors in portal-hypertensive and control rats. Gastroenterology 2000;120:975–983.

8 Chatila R, Ferayorni L, Gupta TK, et al: Local arterial vasoconstriction induced by octreotide in patients with cirrhosis. Hepatology 2000;31:572–576.

9 Lenz K, Hortnagel H, Druml W, et al: Ornipressin in the treatment of functional renal failure in decompensated liver cirrhosis: effects on renal haemodynamics and atrial natriuretic factor. Gastroenterology 1991;101:1060–1067.

10 Guevara M, Gines P, Fernandez-Esparrach G, et al: Reversibility of hepatorenal syndrome by prolonged administration of ornipressin and plasma volume expansion. Hepatology 1998;27:35–41.

11 Uriz J, Gines P, Cardenas A, et al: Terlipressin plus albumin infusion: an effective and safe therapy of hepatorenal syndrome. J Hepatol 2001;33:43–48.

12 Mulkay JP, Louis H, Donckier V, et al: Long-term terlipressin administration improves renal function in cirrhotic patients with type I hepatorenal syndrome: a pilot study. Acta Gastroenterol Belg 2001; 64:15–19.

13 Ortega R, Gines P, Uriz J, et al: Terlipressin therapy with and without albumin for patients with hepatorenal syndrome: results of a prospective, nonrandomized study. Hepatology 2002;36:941–948.

14 Solanki P, Chawla A, Garg R, et al: Beneficial effects of terlipressin in hepatorenal syndrome: a prospective, randomized placebo-controlled clinical trial. J Gastroenterol Hepatol 2003;18:152–156.

15 Angeli P, Volpin R, Gerunda G, et al: Reversal of type 1 hepatorenal syndrome with the administration of midodrine and octreotide. Hepatology 1999; 29:1690–1697.

16 Duvoux C, Zanditenas D, Hezode C, et al: Effects of noradrenalin and albumin in patients with type I hepatorenal syndrome: a pilot study. Hepatology 2002;36:374–380.

17 Gulberg V, Bilzer M, Gerbes AL: Long-term therapy and retreatment of hepatorenal syndrome type I with ornipressin and dopamine. Hepatology 1999;30 870–875.

18 Pomier-Layrargues G, Paquin SC, Hassoun Z, et al: Octreotide in hepatorenal syndrome: a randomized, double-blind, placebo-controlled, crossover study. Hepatology 2003;38:238–243.

19 Martikainen TJ, Tenhunen JJ, Uusaro A, et al: The effects of vasopressin on systemic and splanchnic hemodynamics and metabolism in endotoxin shock. Anesth Analg 2003;97:1756–1763.

20 Fernandez J, Navasa M, Garcia-Pagan JC, et al: Effect of intravenous albumin on systemic and hepatic hemodynamics and vasoactive neurohormonal systems in patients with cirrhosis and spontaneous bacterial peritonitis. J Hepatol 2004;41: 384–390.

21 Lim JK, Groszmann RJ: Vasoconstrictor therapy for the hepatorenal syndrome. Gastroenterology 2008; 134:1608–1611.

22 Ortega R, Gines P, Uriz J, et al: Terlipressin therapy with and without albumin for patients with hepatorenal syndrome: results of a prospective, non-randomized study. Hepatology 2002;36:941–948

23 Salerno F, Gerbes A, Gines P, et al: Diagnosis, prevention and treatment of the hepatorenal syndrome in cirrhosis: a consensus workshop of the international ascites club. Gut 2007;56:1310–1318.

24 Hadengue A, Gadano A, Moreau R, et al: Beneficial effects of the 2-day administration of terlipressin in patients with cirrhosis and hepatorenal syndrome. J Hepatol 1998;29:565–570.

25 Moreau R, Durand F, Poynard T, et al: Terlipressin in patients with cirrhosis and type I hepatorenal syndrome: a retrospective multicenter study. Gastroenterology 2002;122:923–930.

26 Colle I, Durand F, Pessione F, et al: Clinical course, predictive factors and prognosis in patients with cirrhosis and type 1 hepatorenal syndrome treated with Terlipressin: a retrospective analysis. J Gastroenterol Hepatol 2002;17:882–888.

27 Halimi C, Bonnard P, Bernard B, et al: Effect of terlipressin (Glypressin) on hepatorenal syndrome in cirrhotic patients: results of a multicentre pilot study. Eur J Gastroenterol Hepatol 2002;14:153–158.

28 Neri S, Pulvirenti D, Malaguarnera M, et al: Terlipressin and albumin in patients with cirrhosis and type I hepatorenal syndrome. Dig Dis Sci 2008; 53:830–835.

29 Sanyal AJ, Boyer T, Garcia-Tsao G, et al: A randomized, prospective, double-blind, placebo-controlled trial of terlipressin for type 1 hepatorenal syndrome. Gastroenterology 2008;134:1360–1368.

30 Martin-Llahi M, Pepin M N, Guevara M, et al: Terlipressin and albumin vs albumin in patients with cirrhosis and hepatorenal syndrome: a randomized study. Gastroenterology 2008;134:1352–1359.

31 Gluud LL, Christensen K, Christensen E, et al: Systematic review of randomized trials on vasoconstrictor drugs for hepatorenal syndrome. Hepatology 2010;51:576–584.
32 Kiser TH, Fish DN, Obritsch MD, et al: Vasopressin, not octreotide, may be beneficial in the treatment of hepatorenal syndrome: a retrospective study. Nephrol Dial Transplant 2005;20:1813–1820.
33 Alessandria C, Ottobrelli A, Debernardi-Venon W, et al: Noradrenalin vs terlipressin in patients with hepatorenal syndrome: a prospective, randomized, unblinded, pilot study. J Hepatol 2007;47:499–505.
34 Sharma P, Kumar A, Shrama BC, et al: An open label, pilot, randomized controlled trial of noradrenaline versus terlipressin in the treatment of type 1 hepatorenal syndrome and predictors of response. Am J Gastroenterol 2008;103:1689–1697.
35 Angeli P, Volpin R, Piovan D, et al: Acute effects of the oral administration of midodrine, an a-adrenergic agonist, on renal hemodynamics and renal function in cirrhotic patients with ascites. Hepatology 1998;28:937–943.
36 Wong F, Pantea L, Sniderman K: Midodrine, octreotide, albumin, and TIPS in selected patients with cirrhosis and type 1 hepatorenal syndrome. Hepatology 2004;40:55–64.
37 Esrailian E, Pantangco ER, Kyulo NL, et al: Octreotide/Midodrine therapy significantly improves renal function and 30-day survival in patients with type 1 hepatorenal syndrome. Dig Dis Sci 2007;52:742–748.
38 Alessandria C, Debernardi-Venon W, Carello M, et al: Midodrine in the prevention of hepatorenal syndrome type 2 recurrence: a case-control study. Dig Liver Dis 2009;41:298–302.
39 Skagen C, Einstein M, Lucey MR, et al: Combination treatment with octreotide, midodrine, and albumin improves survival in patients with type 1 and type 2 hepatorenal syndrome. J Clin Gastroenterol 2009;43: 680–685.

Guadalupe Garcia-Tsao, MD
333 Cedar Street-1080 LMP
New Haven, CT 06520 (USA)
Tel. +1 203 737 6063, Fax +1 203 785 7273
E-Mail guadalupe.garcia-tsao@yale.edu

Gerbes AL (ed): Ascites, Hyponatremia and Hepatorenal Syndrome: Progress in Treatment.
Front Gastrointest Res. Basel, Karger, 2011, vol 28, pp 163–171

Terlipressin for Hepatorenal Syndrome: The US Experience

Apollo K. Musana · Arun J. Sanyal

Division of Gastroenterology, Hepatology and Nutrition, Department of Internal Medicine, Virginia Commonwealth University School of Medicine, Richmond, Va., USA

Abstract

Hepatorenal syndrome (HRS) is characterized by the development of renal insufficiency without morphologic evidence of renal disease in subjects with advanced liver failure. Typically, it develops in subjects with cirrhosis and ascites and may be either steadily progressive (type 1) or follow a subacute course (type 2). The use of vasoconstrictor therapy has resulted in a reversal of HRS in many of these patients. In this chapter, we review the rationale for the use of vasoconstrictor therapy for HRS and discuss the United States experience with the use of terlipressin for the treatment of type 1 HRS.

Hepatorenal syndrome (HRS) is characterized by the development of renal insufficiency without morphologic evidence of renal disease in subjects with advanced liver failure. Typically, it develops in subjects with cirrhosis and ascites and may be either steadily progressive (type 1) or follow a subacute course (type 2) [1]. The onset of renal insufficiency in a patient with cirrhosis is an ominous finding; when the renal failure is due to HRS, it is particularly significant because it is a harbinger of death [2]. However, in recent years, the use of vasoconstrictor therapy has provided hope for such patients and HRS can be reversed in many such patients. In this chapter, we will review the rationale for the use of vasoconstrictor therapy for HRS and the US experience with the use of terlipressin, a vasopressin analog, for the treatment of type 1 HRS.

Rationale for the Use of Terlipressin for Type 1 HRS

Progressive systemic arterial vasodilation is the principal driver of the progression of diuretic sensitive ascites to refractory ascites to HRS [3]. Arterial vasodilation is associated with cirrhosis and worsened by bouts of infection which occur frequently in this population [4]. Arterial vasodilation causes effective hypovolemia. Initially, a hyperdynamic circulation develops to compensate for this but eventually the onset of myocardial dysfunction leads to a critical drop in forward flow which, in turn, triggers renal sodium retentive mechanisms including renal vasoconstriction [5]. In the face of effective hypovolemia, renal perfusion is maintained by autoregulatory mechanisms in the kidney. When these autoregulatory mechanisms are overwhelmed by the severity of effective hypovolemia, the GFR declines and renal failure ensues [6].

Appreciation of the central role of arterial vasodilation in the pathogenesis of HRS has led to the use of arterial vasoconstrictors for the treatment of type 1 HRS. Initial uncontrolled pilot studies using a variety of vasoconstrictors including midodrine, octreotide, norepinephrine and terlipressin appeared promising [7–9]. Of these, terlipressin, a 12 amino acid synthetic analog of vasopressin, which functions both as a pro-drug and an agonist at V1 vasopressin receptors, has been reported to reverse type 1 HRS in up to 60% of subjects in uncontrolled studies [10, 11]. Also, in a small randomized study, terlipressin reversed HRS in 5/12 subjects compared to none of the control subjects [12]. While these data suggested that terlipressin could be an effective therapy for type 1 HRS, they were not conclusive. These data provided the rationale for the performance of a phase III randomized placebo-controlled trial of terlipressin for the treatment of type 1 HRS [13]. This study was performed in 30 centers across the United States and 5 centers in Europe and represents the US experience with terlipressin for the treatment of HRS. Below, we will summarize the study design and the key findings of this study and the lesions learned from it.

Summary of the Study Design

Study Population

The study population were adult subjects (age >18 years) with type 1 HRS. Type 1 HRS was defined strictly according to the International Ascites Club criteria [1]. The exclusion criteria included absolute hypovolemia, intrinsic renal disease, factors that would affect renal function independent of the HRS, factors that would preclude use of terlipressin, and refusal to consent. Hypovolemia was diagnosed by clinical evaluation and responsiveness to a volume challenge with 1.5 liters of saline with or without additional albumin administration. The principal renal diseases excluded were acute tubular necrosis, glomerular diseases, interstitial nephritis and urinary obstruction. Subjects who had received aminoglycosides or nonsteroidal anti-inflammatory drugs or other known nephrotoxins were excluded. Active sepsis, as defined by fever, leukocytosis and positive blood cultures with or without focal signs of infection, could independently affect renal function and was an exclusion criteria. Similarly, the presence of recent gastrointestinal bleeding or established multiorgan failure and expected survival of less than 7 days were exclusion criteria. The safety of terlipressin in those with severe heart failure or known coronary artery disease was not well known and these conditions were exclusion criteria as well.

Study Design

This study was a prospective randomized controlled phase III clinical trial in which eligible subjects were randomized to receive either terlipressin or placebo in a 1:1 ratio stratified for the presence of alcoholic hepatitis. Following randomization, subjects received either terlipressin at a dose of 1 mg every 6 h or placebo. Terlipressin was administered by slow intravenous push in all cases. Concomitantly, fluids were administered to replace renal and insensible losses. Albumin was administered intravenously to all subjects for the first 3–5 days unless clinical evidence of volume overload was apparent. In those subjects where HRS was precipitated by infection, antibiotics were continued for up to 10–14 days. Hepatic encephalopathy was managed according to standard of care. All subjects who were transplant candidates were kept on the active transplant waiting list according to local standards of care.

The study drug was continued up to 14 days or if the subject met criteria for treatment success. Treatment success was defined by a decrease in serum creatinine to less than 1.5 mg/dl on two occasions at least 48 h apart without the need for dialysis or liver transplantation. If the serum creatinine decreased by less than 30% of baseline values by day 3, the dose was escalated to 2 mg every 6 h by slow intravenous push. Within the 14-day study period, the drug was stopped and the subject removed from the study if they received a liver transplant, dialysis or died. Also, subjects were considered to have failed therapy if the serum creatinine on day 7 was equal to or higher than values seen at baseline. Those who met the failure criteria were also censored and removed from the study. Finally, subjects who chose to withdraw from the study were taken off the study drug and followed for survival data only. Subjects who survived to the end of the active treatment period (day 14 or treatment success) were followed according to standard of care to document survival data.

Outcomes with Terlipressin Treatment

In total, 56 subjects were enrolled in each arm of this trial. Of these 112 subjects, 92 were followed without a liver transplant for at least 14 days. 89% and 88% of subjects on terlipressin and placebo, respectively, received intravenous albumin infusions in the first 5 days after randomization. The two groups were comparable with respect to age, distribution of etiologies for cirrhosis and the severity of liver failure as well as the number of cases precipitated by infection. The mean serum creatinine levels were 4 and 3.9 mg/dl in the terlipressin and placebo arms, respectively, at the time of randomization. There were, however, 6 subjects with serum creatinine levels greater than 7 mg/dl. These subjects, who had the most severe HRS, were all randomly assigned to the terlipressin treatment arm. While there were a greater number of subjects with hepatocellular cancer in those randomized to terlipressin (11 vs. 7), this did not reach significance.

Primary Endpoint

The primary endpoint was rigorously defined as a live subject on day 14 with persistent normalization of serum creatinine to values less than 1.5 mg/dl, as defined by two values obtained at least 48 h apart, without a liver transplant, dialysis or relapse of HRS following initial treatment success. By intention-to-treat analysis, 15 versus 7 subjects (27 vs. 13%) on terlipressin and placebo respectively reached the primary endpoint ($p < 0.059$). It is, however, noteworthy that in one subject receiving terlipressin, the serum creatinine decreased below 1.5 mg/dl on day 14 for the first time thereby precluding them from meeting the primary endpoint even though they experienced persistent reversal of HRS. In another subject receiving terlipressin, the serum creatinine decreased to 1.5 mg/dl and then stabilized at 1.6 mg/dl thus also precluding them from meeting the primary endpoint despite persistent improvement in renal function. There was also one case each of a subject on terlipressin who relapsed after initially achieving treatment success on day 11 and another who decided to withdraw from the study despite normalization of the creatinine. The patient who relapsed was successfully retreated with the same drug and had persistent decrease of the serum creatinine below 1.5 mg/dl. Thus, although by the strict definitions used, the pre-specified primary endpoint was not met; however, this under-represents the number of subjects who responded to terlipressin.

Impact on Renal Function

The serum creatinine increased compared to baseline values in those receiving placebo ($p < 0.9$) while it decreased significantly in those receiving terlipressin ($p < 0.001$) (fig. 1). Compared to placebo, terlipressin produced a significant improvement in serum creatinine ($p < 0.009$). Terlipressin also produced a highly significant improvement in the mean MELD score compared to placebo (–4.1 vs. –1.7, $p < 0.008$) by day 14.

When the traditional endpoint of HRS reversal, defined by a decrease in creatinine to values <1.5 mg/dl at anytime during treatment, terlipressin was significantly superior to placebo with 19 (34%) versus 7 (13%) subjects, respectively, meeting this

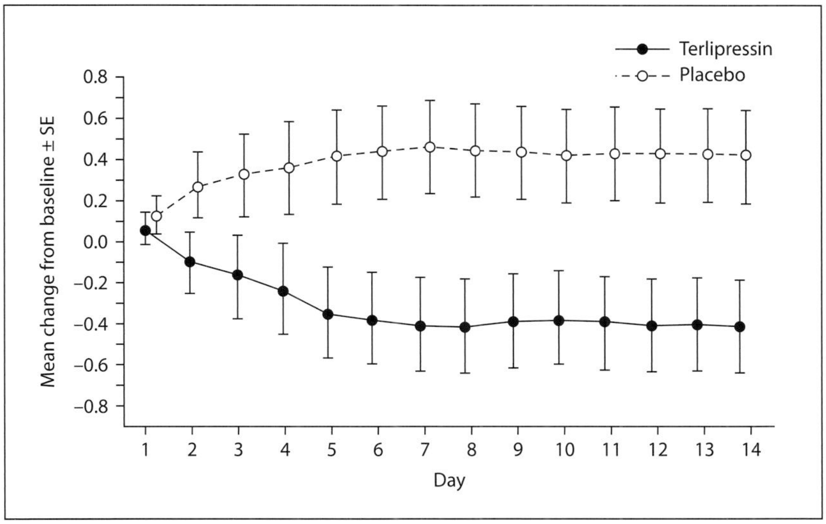

Fig. 1. Mean change from baseline in SCr (mg/dl) to end of treatment. Changes in serum creatinine from baseline over time during the study. Whereas the creatinine trended upward in those on placebo, there was a decline in those receiving terlipressin. These differences were highly significant ($p < 0.009$). Reproduced with permission from Sanyal et al. [13].

endpoint ($p < 0.008$). The relative risk of HRS reversal on terlipressin was 2.7 (95% CI 1.2–5.9) and the number needed to treat to reverse HRS in 1 patient was 4.7. This highly significant improvement in HRS can be reconciled against the failure to show a statistically significant improvement for the primary endpoint by the 4 subjects discussed above who reversed their HRS but could not be included in the analysis for the primary endpoint.

Time Course of Changes in Renal Function

In subjects receiving placebo, renal function either continued to worsen or level off in most cases (fig. 2). In the minority of subjects who demonstrated improvement in renal function while receiving placebo and albumin, the improvement occurred invariably within the first 72 h without any additional subjects demonstrating improvement after this time period. On the other hand, two patterns of response to terlipressin were seen. While some subjects improved over the first 72 h, others did not demonstrate substantial improvement until later in the course of treatment. These latter subjects, however, had all shown an at least 30% drop in creatinine from pre-treatment values over the first 72 h. Importantly, if the creatinine did not show an at least 30% drop after 72 h of treatment, reversal of HRS was not seen in any cases.

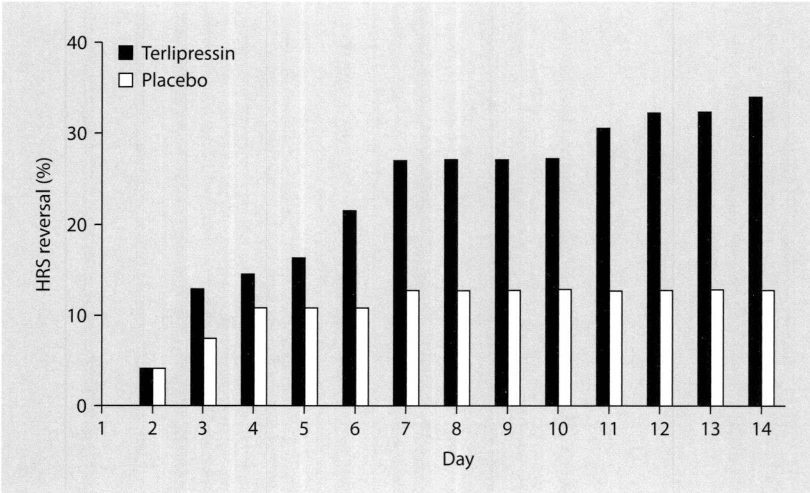

Fig. 2. Reversal of type 1 HRS. Cumulative incidence of HRS reversal over time. Some subjects receiving placebo and albumin reversed their HRS within the first 72 h. However, subjects on terlipressin showed continued increase in the number of subjects with HRS reversal until days 10–11 after initiation of treatment. Reproduced with permission from Sanyal et al. [13].

Factors Predictive of Response to Terlipressin

Several factors have been identified to be predictive of the response to terlipressin. First, in all subjects with a creatinine >6 mg/dl, there was no response. This indicates that the window for therapeutic benefit is open when the renal failure is not severe and that treatment should not be delayed once a diagnosis of HRS has been made. Also, in no cases was there reversal of HRS when treatment was provided for less than 72 h. This also appears to be rational because it is difficult for a drug to provide benefit if it is not given. Unfortunately, in the context of this trial, a number of subjects in either arm were withdrawn from the trial within the first 48 h because of a perception of futility of treatment. It is therefore strongly recommended that a decision regarding futility not be made until at least 72 h of treatment have been provided unless the subject develops multiorgan failure which is invariably fatal in this population.

Since the rationale for the use of terlipressin was an increase in splanchnic vasoconstriction, it was anticipated that this would be reflected in the mean arterial pressure (MAP). The acute MAP response was similar in those receiving terlipressin who were either responders or nonresponders. However, whereas the MAP, averaged over the day, remained relatively unchanged in terlipressin responders, it increased in terlipressin responders. Unfortunately, the number of subjects involved does not permit meaningful statistical analysis to identify a threshold value which is required to see a response to terlipressin.

Impact on Survival

Using intention-to-treat analysis, there were no differences in either overall survival or transplant-free survival in the two study arms. The overall survival at 60 days was 48 and 46% for those on terlipressin and placebo, respectively, while the transplant-free survival was 38 and 34%, respectively. The principal cause of death was liver failure with progression to multi-organ failure. In contrast to the lack of improvement in survival based on intent to treat analysis, those who reversed their HRS had a markedly improved overall survival regardless of which treatment arm they were in ($p < 0.009$ log-rank analysis). This improvement was also reflected in the transplant-free survival.

These data corroborate other studies on the outcomes of HRS [14]. Given the differences in rates of improvement in HRS between terlipressin and placebo, it is estimated that about 900 subjects would be required to show a survival difference. Conducting such a study is impractical given the logistic challenges and costs involved in a study of this magnitude in this extremely sick population. Given the superiority of terlipressin over placebo for HRS reversal, it is implied but not proven that if enough subjects are treated with terlipressin, a survival advantage would become apparent.

Impact on Liver Transplantation

Thirty-five patients received a liver transplant. There were no dual liver/kidney transplants. The mean time to transplant was 31 days for the terlipressin group compared to 21 days for placebo ($p > 0.05$). As expected, those who received a liver transplant had a significantly better survival at 6 months (the duration up to which data were collected). The benefits of transplant were present regardless of whether the subject received terlipressin or placebo. It has been suggested that pretransplant reversal of type 1 HRS improves post-transplant outcomes [15]. Given the small number of subjects to analyze, it is not possible to tell with certainty whether reversal of HRS with terlipressin or placebo prior to the transplant affected post-transplant outcomes. These data suggest that terlipressin should be considered as a bridge to transplant by increasing the likelihood of reversing HRS and thus increasing pre-transplant survival probability and the ability to get the patient to transplant. The US experience does not suggest a major impact of terlipressin on post-transplant outcomes.

Conclusion

The principal experience with terlipressin within the US has been in the context of the pivotal trial of terlipressin for type 1 HRS. The data suggest that the drug is effective in improving renal function and reversal of HRS. However, in the context of the trial, no effect on survival was seen. Those who responded however had a significantly improved survival. Failure to provide treatment for at least 72 h and a baseline creatinine >6 mg/dl were risk factors for failure of treatment. Liver transplantation remains the definitive treatment of type 1 HRS.

Key Messages

Rationale for the Use of Terlipressin for Type 1 HRS

- Progressive systemic arterial vasodilation is the principal driver for the development of HRS.
- Infection can potentiate the development of HRS.
- The use of arterial vasoconstrictors for the treatment of type 1 HRS targets the pathophysiologic mechanisms.
- Terlipressin, a synthetic analog of vasopressin, has been reported to reverse type 1 HRS in up to 60% of subjects in uncontrolled studies.

Terlipressin for the Treatment of Type 1 HRS

- Compared to placebo, terlipressin produced a significant improvement in serum creatinine (SCr).
- Terlipressin produced a highly significant improvement in the mean MELD score compared to placebo.
- Terlipressin was significantly superior to placebo in the reversal of HRS (SCr <1.5 mg/dl).
- No differences in either overall survival or transplant-free survival in the two study arms.

References

1 Salerno F, Gerbes A, Ginès P, Wong F, Arroyo V: Diagnosis, prevention and treatment of hepatorenal syndrome in cirrhosis. Gut 2007;56:1310–1318.

2 Arroyo V, Guevara M, Ginès P: Hepatorenal syndrome in cirrhosis: pathogenesis and treatment. Gastroenterology 2002;122:1658–1676.

3 Arroyo V, Terra C, Ginès P: Advances in the pathogenesis and treatment of type-1 and type-2 hepatorenal syndrome. J Hepatol 2007;46:935–946.

4 Fernández J, Navasa M, Planas R, Montoliu S, Monfort D, Soriano G, Vila C, Pardo A, Quintero E, Vargas V, Such J, Ginès P, Arroyo V: Primary prophylaxis of spontaneous bacterial peritonitis delays hepatorenal syndrome and improves survival in cirrhosis. Gastroenterology 2007;133:818–824.

5 Ruiz-del-Arbol L, Monescillo A, Arocena C, Valer P, Ginès P, Moreira V, Milicua JM, Jiménez W, Arroyo V: Circulatory function and hepatorenal syndrome in cirrhosis. Hepatology 2005;42:439–447.

6 Arroyo V, Fernandez J, Gines P: Pathogenesis and treatment of hepatorenal syndrome. Seminars in liver disease 2008;28:81–95.

7 Angeli P, Volpin R, Gerunda G, Craighero R, Roner P, Merenda R, Amodio P, Sticca A, Caragero L, Maffei-Faccioli A, Gatta A: Reversal of type 1 hepatorenal syndrome with the administration of midodrine and octreotide. Hepatology 1999;29:1690–1697.

8 Guevara M, Ginès P, Fernández-Esparrach G, Sort P, Salmerón JM, Jiménez W, Arroyo V, Rodés J: Reversibility of hepatorenal syndrome by prolonged administration of ornipressin and plasma volume expansion. Hepatology 1998;27:35–41.

9 Sharma P, Kumar A, Shrama BC, Sarin SK: An open label, pilot, randomized controlled trial of noradrenaline versus terlipressin in the treatment of type 1 hepatorenal syndrome and predictors of response. Am J Gastroenterol 2008;103:1689–1697.

10 Nazar A, Pereira GH, Guevara M, Martib-Llahi M, Pepin MN, Marinelli M, Solá E, Baccaro ME, Terra C, Arroyo V, Ginès P: Predictors of response to therapy with terlipressin and albumin in patients with cirrhosis and type 1 hepatorenal syndrome. Hepatology 2010;51:219–226.

11 Ortega R, Ginès P, Uriz J, Cárdenas A, Calahorra B, De Las Heras D, Guevara M, Bataller R, Jiménez W, Arroyo V, Rodés J: Terlipressin therapy with and without albumin for patients with hepatorenal syndrome: results of a prospective, nonrandomized study. Hepatology 2002;36:941–948.
12 Solanki P, Chawla A, Garg R, Gupta R, Jain M, Sarin SK: Beneficial effects of terlipressin in hepatorenal syndrome: a prospective, randomized placebo-controlled clinical trial. J Gastroenterol Hepatol 2003;18:152–156.
13 Sanyal AJ, Boyer T, Garcia-Tsao G, Regenstein F, Rossaro L, Appenrodt B, Blei A, Gülberg V, Sigal S, Teuber P, Terlipressin Study Group: A randomized, prospective, double-blind, placebo-controlled trial of terlipressin for type 1 hepatorenal syndrome. Gastroenterology 2008;134:1360–1368.
14 Alessandria C, Ozdogan O, Guevara M, Restuccia T, Jiménez W, Arroyo V, Rodés J, Ginès P: MELD score and clinical type predict prognosis in hepatorenal syndrome: relevance to liver transplantation. Hepatology 2005;41:1282–1289.
15 Restuccia T, Ortega R, Guevara M, et al: Effects of treatment of hepatorenal syndrome before transplantation on post-transplantation outcome: a case-control study. J Hepatol 2004;40:140–146.

Arun J. Sanyal, MD
Professor of Medicine, Pharmacology and Molecular
MCV Box 980342
Richmond, VA 23298–0342 (USA)
Tel. +1 804 828 6314, Fax +1 804 828 2992, E-Mail asanyal@mcvh-vcu.edu

Gerbes AL (ed): Ascites, Hyponatremia and Hepatorenal Syndrome: Progress in Treatment.
Front Gastrointest Res. Basel, Karger, 2011, vol 28, pp 172–177

Terlipressin for Hepatorenal Syndrome: Predictors of Response

Andrés Cárdenas[a] · Pere Ginès[b]

[a]GI Unit and [b]Liver Unit, Institut Clinic de Malalties Digestives i Metaboliques, Hospital Clinic, and University of Barcelona, Institut d'Investigacions Biomèdiques August Pi-Sunyer (IDIBAPS), Ciber de Enfermedades Hepáticas y Digestivas (CIBEREHD), Barcelona, Spain

Abstract

Hepatorenal syndrome (HRS) is a reversible cause of renal impairment that occurs in patients with cirrhosis and ascites. The best available therapy for HRS, other than liver transplantation, is the use of intravenous terlipressin (splanchnic vasoconstrictor) and intravenous albumin. Response rates in patients with type 1 HRS range between 40 and 50%. In patients that do not respond, terlipressin does not improve renal function and the available data on why these patients do not respond is limited. In this regard, it is crucial to identify non-responder patients early in order to plan alternative therapies. There are limited data regarding predictors of response to terlipressin therapy. However, the available data indicates that patients with high baseline serum bilirubin (≥10 mg/dl) and creatinine (>5.6 mg/dl) and those without a change or increase in mean arterial pressure or reduction in serum creatinine at day 3 after treatment, respond poorly to terlipressin. This article will review the data on terlipressin therapy for HRS as well as the predictors of response to terlipressin in this condition. Finally, we will discuss further areas of research that may help identify patients with HRS that will and will not respond to terlipressin.

Hepatorenal syndrome (HRS) is a reversible cause of renal impairment that occurs in patients with cirrhosis and ascites, as well as in patients with acute liver failure or alcoholic hepatitis [1, 2]. HRS is characterized by impaired renal function, marked alterations in cardiovascular function and over-activity of the sympathetic nervous and renin-angiotensin systems that lead to severe renal vasoconstriction with significant decrease of the glomerular filtration rate (GFR) [1, 2]. There are two types of HRS. In type 1 HRS renal function deteriorates rapidly with an increase in serum creatinine (SCr) to a level >2.5 mg/dl in less than 2 weeks. This type of HRS is associated with a very poor prognosis without treatment, with a median survival time of only 2 weeks. In type 2 HRS there is a steady impairment of renal function and SCr levels usually range between 1.5 and 2.5 mg/dl. Patients with type 2 HRS have a median survival time of 6 months if they do not receive a transplant. Patients with type 2 HRS may go on to develop type 1, either due to progression of disease or triggering factors such as bacterial infections. The most important aspect of providing care to patients with HRS is assessment of candidacy for orthotopic liver transplantation. Current available therapies other than liver transplantation for HRS include the use vasoconstrictors such as terlipressin and albumin. In this chapter we will discuss the role of terlipressin in the treatment of HRS, the predictors of response to treatment and HRS reversal.

Terlipressin for Hepatorenal Syndrome

Terlipressin has been successfully used in the past decade and randomized and non-randomized studies indicate that it reverses renal failure in HRS [3–13]. Most of the available information relates to patients with type 1 HRS. There is limited data on the role of terlipressin or other vasoconstrictors in type 2 HRS [10, 12]. Albumin (20–40 g/day) is concomitantly used with terlipressin in order to help improve effective arterial blood volume. In non-randomized studies, the use of terlipressin and intravenous albumin improved renal function in approximately 60–75% of patients with type 1 HRS [3–10]. However, results from recent randomized controlled studies comparing terlipressin and albumin versus albumin and placebo indicate that treatment with terlipressin and albumin is associated with HRS reversal (defined as a decrease in SCr level to ≤1.5 mg/dl) in approximately 40% of patients [11, 12]. The recommended doses of terlipressin are 1 mg/4–6 h i.v. bolus, with a dose increase up to a maximum of 2 mg/4–6 h after 2–3 days if there is no response to therapy (defined as a reduction of SCr >25% of pretreatment values). Response to therapy is associated with a marked increase in urine volume and improvement of hyponatremia, a condition almost constantly present in these patients. The incidence of ischemic side effects during terlipressin therapy, which are usually reversible after discontinuation of treatment, is approximately 10% [11, 12].

Predictors of Response

A recent systematic review and two meta-analyses indicate that terlipressin plus albumin improves renal function in 46–52% of patients with type 1 HRS [13–15]. However, in non-responder patients, terlipressin does not alter renal function and the available data on why these patients do not respond is limited. It is important to identify non-responder patients early in the management of HRS in order to plan alternative therapies. This is particularly necessary for those awaiting liver transplantation, who should be given high priority on the liver transplant list. The predictors of response were recently investigated in a study of 39 consecutive patients with cirrhosis

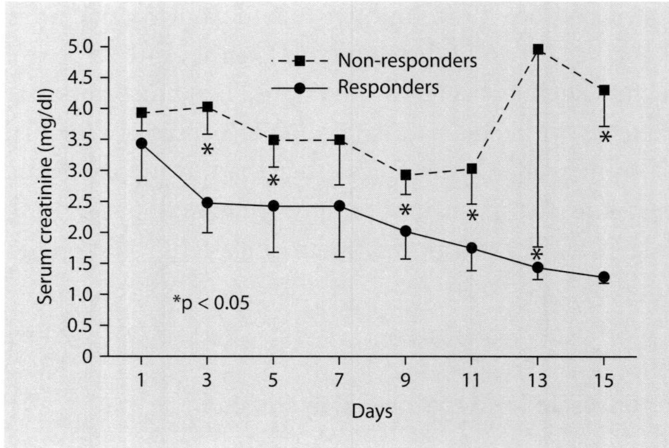

Fig. 1. Serum creatinine concentration (mean and SD) during treatment with terlipressin and albumin in responders and nonresponders. Reprinted with permission from Nazar et al. [16].

and type 1 HRS treated with terlipressin (dose of 0.5–1 mg/4 h as i.v. bolus for 3 days with an increase up to 2 mg/4 h in those whose values did not decrease by at least 25% of the pretreatment values) plus albumin (1 g/kg BW. during the first 24 h, followed by 40 g/day) given for a maximum of 2 weeks [16]. In the study, 18 (46%) patients responded to treatment and 21 (54%) patients did not meet the criteria of response to treatment (fig. 1). In those that responded, there was an increase in arterial pressure with marked suppression in the activity of the renin-angiotensin-aldosterone system and sympathetic nervous system. However, arterial pressure did not increase in those that did not respond to terlipressin therapy. Other variables associated with response to treatment were serum transaminases, Model for End-Stage Liver Disease (MELD) score, urine volume, leukocyte count, and serum bilirubin. Multivariate analysis showed that a serum bilirubin level that best predicted response to treatment was 10 mg/dl. Response rates in patients divided according to baseline serum bilirubin ≥10 mg/dl or <10 mg/dl were 13% (2/15) and 67% (16/24), respectively (p = 0.001).

Although baseline arterial pressure was not a predictive factor of response, early changes of mean arterial pressure within the first days of treatment predicted response. In the study, patients with an increase in mean arterial pressure equal to or greater than 5 mm Hg at day 3 of treatment had a response rate at the end of therapy of 73% (8/11) compared with 36% (10/28) in patients with minimal increases in mean arterial pressure (<5 mm Hg) or a decrease in mean arterial pressure [16]. When this increase in arterial pressure of 5 mm Hg or more at day 3 was included in the multivariate analysis with the baseline variables, the predictive factors of response to therapy were the baseline serum bilirubin level and the increase in mean arterial pressure ≥5 mm Hg at day 3 (fig. 2). In the analysis, 1 of 4 patients (25%) responded if there was an increase in MAP ≥5mm Hg in those with baseline serum bilirubin level ≥10 mg/dl, compared to a response in 1 of 11 (9%) in those with a change in MAP <5 mm Hg with baseline serum bilirubin level ≥10 mg/dl (fig. 2). The early reduction

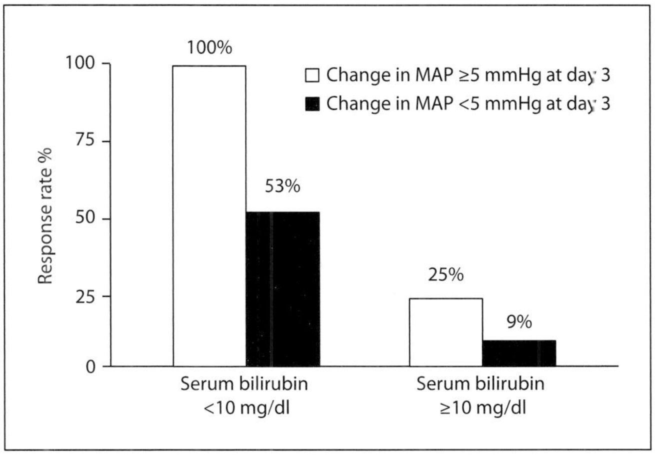

Fig. 2. Response rate according to change in mean arterial pressure (MAP) at day 3 and its relationship to serum bilirubin at baseline. Adapted with permission from Nazar et al. [16].

in serum creatinine during treatment was also a predictor of response to therapy. Response to treatment was observed in 13 of the 17 patients (76%) in whom serum creatinine decreased by at least 0.5 mg/dl at day 3, compared with only 5 of the 22 patients (23%) in whom serum creatinine did not decrease 0.5 mg/dl or increased at day 3 compared with baseline ($p = 0.001$). The value of the reduction in serum creatinine at day 3 as a predictor of response to therapy was also confirmed in a multivariate analysis [16].

Another analysis from a multicenter study investigated the baseline patient characteristics of 112 patients with type 1 HRS enrolled in a randomized, double-blind, placebo-controlled trial of terlipressin for HRS [17]. The baseline variables evaluated included treatment (terlipressin/placebo), age (>65/<65 years), gender, race (non-white/white), alcoholic hepatitis (absent/present), MELD score (per 1 point increase), Child-Pugh score, and SCr concentration. Baseline SCr concentration, baseline MELD score and treatment with terlipressin were found to be significant predictors of HRS response. Lower baseline SCr levels, lower baseline MELD scores and terlipressin therapy were found to be predictive of HRS reversal. In fact, the probability of HRS reversal decreased by 39% for each 1 mg/dl increase in SCr, while the probability for HRS reversal improved 271% with terlipressin treatment. In this analysis only patients with baseline SCr <5.6 mg/dl and receiving more than 3 days of therapy achieved HRS reversal. This indicates that less severe renal failure (i.e. lower SCr) is associated with a good probability of HRS reversal for those treated with terlipressin for more than 3 days.

The available data on predictors of response to therapy indicate that there is a clear relationship between the presence of an early increase in mean arterial pressure and the renal response to terlipressin. This shows the importance of improving systemic hemodynamics in order to achieve reversal of type 1 HRS. However, not all patients showing an early increase in arterial pressure improved renal function. On the other hand, about 30% of patients without an early hemodynamic response had an improvement of renal function at the end of therapy, which means that terlipressin should not be stopped after day 3 if there is no improvement in arterial pressure. The predictive value of serum bilirubin level as a predictor of response cannot be explained on the basis of hemodynamic changes during therapy; however, it could be explained on the basis of advanced hepatic failure that leads to a suboptimal response to therapy. Finally, the relationship of response with Scr levels at baseline and during therapy also indicates less-severe renal impairment and an early drop in Scr levels after initiation of therapy is a good predictor of response.

Although the currently accepted treatment for HRS is terlipressin with albumin, there is a suboptimal response to therapy with over 50% of patients not responding to this treatment. It is therefore of paramount importance that we continue to investigate and search not only for prognostic factors but also adequate predictors of response before starting therapy or early afterwards. Further studies specifically looking at dosing, type of administration (bolus vs. infusion), side effects, prognostic factors and early predictors of response will help identify those patients who will be likely or unlikely to respond to therapy. These data will undoubtedly enable the treating physician to plan ahead for other treatments. Advances in pharmacological therapy for implementation in clinical practice are only accepted if they are based on the results of large randomized controlled trials. Since HRS is not an overly prevalent condition, most centers end up treating a small number of patients every year. Therefore, adequately sized randomized controlled trials are likely possible only if a significant number of centers collaborate as a consortium or a working group. Studies conducted by such groups will likely help answer many of the concerns raised above.

Key Messages

- Terlipressin is the most accepted pharmacological therapy for patients with cirrhosis and type 1 hepatorenal syndrome, with response rates around 40–50%.
- The identification of those patients that will and will not respond to therapy is of key importance in planning treatment, particularly for those awaiting liver transplantation.
- Recent data indicate that patients with high baseline serum bilirubin and creatinine and those without a change in mean arterial pressure or reduction in serum creatinine at day 3 after treatment respond poorly to terlipressin.
- Further studies are needed to confirm these findings, taking into account the dose, type of administration (bolus vs. infusion) and side effects, in addition to the above-mentioned predictors of response.

References

1 Arroyo V, Ginès P, Gerbes A, et al: Definition and diagnostic criteria of refractory ascites and hepatorenal syndrome in cirrhosis. Hepatology 1996;23:164–176.

2 Salerno F, Gerbes A, Wong F, et al: Diagnosis, prevention and treatment of the hepatorenal syndrome in cirrhosis: a consensus workshop of the international ascites club. Gut 2007;56:1310–1318.

3 Uriz J, Ginès P, Cardenas A, et al: Terlipressin plus albumin infusion: an effective and safe therapy of hepatorenal syndrome. J Hepatol 2000;33:43–48.

4 Moreau R, Durand F, Poynard T, et al: Terlipressin in patients with cirrhosis and type 1 hepatorenal syndrome: a retrospective multicenter study. Gastroenterology 2002;122:923–930.

5 Ortega R, Ginès P, Uriz J, et al: Terlipressin therapy with and without albumin for patients with hepatorenal syndrome: efficacy and outcome. Hepatology 2002;36:941–948.

6 Solanki P, Chawla A, Garg R, et al: Beneficial effects of terlipressin in hepatorenal syndrome: a prospective, randomized placebo-controlled clinical trial. J Gastroenterol Hepatol 2003;18:152–156.

7 Halimi C, Bonnard P, Bernard B: Effect of terlipressin (Glypressin) on hepatorenal syndrome in cirrhotic patients: results of a multicentre pilot study. Eur J Gastroenterol Hepatol 2002;14:153–158.

8 Neri S, Pulvirenti D, Malaguarnera M, et al: Terlipressin and albumin in patients with cirrhosis and type I hepatorenal syndrome. Dig Dis Sci 2008;53:830–835.

9 Triantos CK, Samonakis D, Thalheimer U, et al: Terlipressin therapy for renal failure in cirrhosis. Eur J Gastroenterol Hepatol 2010;22:481–486.

10 Alessandria C, Ottobrelli A, Debernardi-Venon W, et al: Noradrenalin vs. terlipressin in patients with hepatorenal syndrome: a prospective, randomized, unblinded, pilot study. J Hepatol 2007;47:499–505.

11 Sanyal A, Boyer T, Garcia-Tsao G, et al: A prospective, randomized, double blind, placebo-controlled trial of terlipressin for type 1 hepatorenal syndrome (HRS). Gastroenterology 2008;134:1360–1368.

12 Martin-Llahi M, Pepin MN, Guevara G, et al: Terlipressin and albumin vs. albumin in patients with cirrhosis and hepatorenal syndrome: a randomized study. Gastroenterology 2008;134:1352–1359.

13 Gluud LL, Christensen K, Christensen E, Krag A: Systematic review of randomized trials on vasoconstrictor drugs for hepatorenal syndrome. Hepatology 2010;51:576–584.

14 Fabrizi F, Dixit V, Martin P: Meta-analysis: terlipressin therapy for the hepatorenal syndrome. Aliment Pharmacol Ther 2006;24:935–944.

15 Sagi SV, Mittal S, Kasturi KS, Sood GK: Terlipressin therapy for reversal of type 1 hepatorenal syndrome: a meta-analysis of randomized controlled trials. J Gastroenterol Hepatol 2010;25:880–885.

16 Nazar A, Pereira GH, Guevara M, et al: Predictors of response to therapy with terlipressin and albumin in patients with cirrhosis and type 1 hepatorenal syndrome. Hepatology 2010;51:219–226.

17 Sanyal AJ, Boyer T, Teuber P: Prognostic factors for hepatorenal syndrome (HRS) reversal in patients with type 1 HRS enrolled in a randomized, double-blind, placebo-controlled trial. Hepatology 2007;46:737A.

Pere Ginès, MD
Liver Unit – Hospital Clinic
Villarroel 170
ES–08036 Barcelona (Spain)
Tel. +34 93 227 1713, Fax +34 93 451 5522, E-Mail pgines@clinic.ub.es

Gerbes AL (ed): Ascites, Hyponatremia and Hepatorenal Syndrome: Progress in Treatment.
Front Gastrointest Res. Basel, Karger, 2011, vol 28, pp 178–188

Safety of Terlipressin for Hepatorenal Syndrome

Aleksander Krag[a] · Søren Møller[b]

Departments of [a]Medical Gastroenterology, and [b]Clinical Physiology and Nuclear Medicine, Hvidovre Hospital, Faculty of Health Sciences, University of Copenhagen, Hvidovre, Denmark

Abstract

Terlipressin has affinity with vasopressin 1 and 2 receptors (V receptors), which reflects its pharmacological effects and safety profile. V1 receptor-related side effects occur when vasoconstriction is too intense and they are usually ischemic. V2 receptor-related side effects are mainly hyponatremia and, potentially, hypokalemia. No deaths due to adverse events have been reported so far in randomized clinical trials but withdrawal of terlipressin owing to adverse events was necessary in 4% of patients in the published trials. Mild adverse events occurred in about 30% of the patients. However, the number of side effects may be considerably higher in unselected patients. Before therapy is started absolute and relative contraindications should be assessed. Terlipressin is contraindicated or should be used with extreme caution in patients with severe atherosclerotic cardiovascular disease. On initiation and during therapy, patients should be monitored with ECG, blood pressure, daily electrolytes and clinically for peripheral ischemia. There is no specific antidote to terlipressin and prevention and handling of side effects include careful selection of patients, close surveillance, daily consideration of dose and duration of therapy.

Terlipressin has proven to be effective in the treatment of the hepatorenal syndrome (HRS) and may also improve survival [1]. It is a potent drug and has a number of potential side effects, both mild and severe, which should be taken into account before and during treatment. Terlipressin has an affinity with vasopressin 1 and 2 receptors (V receptors), which mediates its pharmacological effects and reflects the safety profile. This chapter discusses the adverse events reported in trials on HRS and summarizes case reports. However, it should be borne in mind that patients selected for clinical trials may differ from the population at large.

Pharmacokinetics and Receptor Affinity

Terlipressin is a synthetic 12-amino acid peptide (1-triglycyl-8-lysine-vasopressin) derived from the natural hormone, lysine vasopressin. 1-Triglycyl-8-lysine- vasopressin is rapidly converted to the biologically active lysine vasopressin, which reaches its peak concentration after 60–120 min. The half-life of terlipressin is about 50 min, with a metabolic clearance of 9 ml/kg/min. Terlipressin has affinity with vasopressin receptors (V receptors), especially V1. V1 receptors are mainly found on vascular smooth muscle cells in the splanchnic circulation as well as in the systemic circulation, the kidneys, aorta and heart [2]. The effects of V1 receptors are mediated by an increase in intracellular calcium from the sarcoplasmic reticulum, thereby causing vasoconstriction. Adverse events related to V1 receptors occur when vasoconstriction is too intense and are usually ischemic. V2 receptors are located on the basolateral membrane of the principal cells in collecting ducts in the kidneys and their stimulation mediates transport of water in the renal collecting ducts by forming water channels of aquaporin 2 (AQP2) in the apical plasma membrane [3]. This increases water permeability and allows the osmotically driven movement of water from the tubule lumen into the interstitium, thereby decreasing plasma osmolality [3]. V2 receptor-related adverse events are hyponatremia and possibly also hypokalemia.

Adverse Events Reported in Trials on the Hepatorenal Syndrome

Table 1 gives a list of the adverse events reported in randomized clinical trials on HRS. No deaths were considered to be related to terlipressin in the 149 patients treated for HRS, but it was withdrawn in 6 patients (4%) because of side effects. Overall, adverse events considered to be related to terlipressin were seen in 30% of the patients, with some experiencing more than one. Two recent randomized clinical trials showed no overall difference in adverse events the between terlipressin and the placebo groups (table 1) [4, 5]. However, without reaching statistical significance, more cardiovascular adverse events were observed in the terlipressin groups versus placebo groups: 10 vs. 4 and 5 vs. 1 in the Spanish and the American studies, respectively. In a recent systematic review and meta-analyses of randomized trials on terlipressin for HRS, we looked at the number of side effects reported [1]. Three trials [4–6] reported the number of withdrawals due to adverse events (6/105 (6%) vs. 0/105; RR = 4.81; 95% CI = 0.84–27.56). The number of adverse events was reported in four trials with 117 patients in the treatment and control groups. These trials compared terlipressin given alone or in combination with albumin versus no intervention or albumin. A meta-analysis showed that the treatment group had an increased risk of cardiovascular adverse events, such as cardiac arrhythmia, myocardial infarction, suspected intestinal or peripheral ischemia, and arterial hypertension (14% vs. 0%; RR = 9.00; 95% CI = 2.14–37.85). Twenty-one percent in the treatment group and 2% in the control

Table 1. Adverse events of terlipressin in randomized trials on hepatorenal syndrome

Study, year (number of patients in terlipressin group)	AE: n (%) Death: n (%)	Withdrawal due to AE	Cardiac
Sanyal, 2008 [5] (n = 56) number of patients with AE given	related SEAs terlipressin: 5 (8.9%) placebo: 1 (1.8%) deaths=0 AE: up to 7 days posttreatment: all: terlipressin: 52 (92.9%) placebo: 49 (89.1%) related: terlipressin: 18 (32.1%) placebo: 12 (21.8%)	related AEs terlipressin 3 (5.4%) nonfatal MI 1, livido reticularis 1, cyanosis of fingers 1 placebo: 0 (0%)	terlipressin: MI 1, supraventricular tachycardia 1, atrial fibrillation 1 placebo: arrhythmia: 1 (placebo)
Martín-Llahí, 2008 [4] (n = 23) number of AEs given	number of AEs during treatment: terlipressin: 50 placebo: 40 deaths=0	terlipressin: high blood pressure 1 placebo: 0	terlipressin: MI 1, transient bardycardia 1, transient, transient ventricular extrasystolia 1, arterial hypertension 1 (terli) Placebo: 0
Neri, 2008 [6] (n = 26)	AE 9 (17%) deaths=0	2	tachycardia 2 , chest pain 1
Solanki, 2003 [7] (n = 12) number of AEs given	5 (22%) deaths=0	N/A	arrhythmia: 3 (occasional supraventricular and ventricular ectopics)
Alessandria, 2007 [8] (n = 12)	N/A	N/A	N/A

Pulmonary	Ischemia and skin	GI	Other
terlipressin: respiratory distress 2, respiratory acidosis 1 placebo: 0	terlipressin: livido reticularis 1, cyanosis of fingers 1 placebo: 0	N/A	N/A
terlipressin: respiratory failure 2, placebo: 0	terlipressin: signs of intestinal ischemia 3	terlipressin: gastrointestinal bleeding 4, transient abdominal pain and diarrhea 4 placebo: abdominal pain 1, gastrointestinal bleeding 6	terlipressin: circulatory overload 7, HE 16, bacterial infection 9 other 1 placebo: circulatory overload 4, HE 16, bacterial infection 12, anemia 1
bronchspasm 1	peripheral. ischemia 1, suspected abdominal ischemia 1	abdominal pain 1, diarrhea 3	N/A
N/A	N/A	abdominal pain and diarrhea 2	N/A
N/A	N/A	abdominal pain and diarrhea: 'most patients'	N/A

Table 1. Continued

Study, year (number of patients in terlipressin group)	AE: n (%) Death: n (%)	Withdrawal due to AE	Cardiac
Sharma, 2008 [9] (n = 20)	AE 5 (25%)	N/A	ST segment depression 1
Overall (n = 149)	deaths 0 (0%) overall related 37 (30%)	6 (4%)	nonfatal MI 2 (1.4%) arrhythmia 10 (7%) overall cardiac 14 (9%)

AE = Adverse events; SAE = serious adverse events; N/A = not available/none mentioned; MI = myocardial infarction; HE = hepatic encephalopathy.

group experienced abdominal pain and diarrhea (RR = 6.82; 95% CI = 0.79–59.15). There were no differences between the treatment and the control groups in any of the remaining adverse events: hepatic encephalopathy (70%), bacterial infections (46%), circulatory overload (24%), gastrointestinal bleeding (9%), respiratory distress or acidosis (3%), chest pain (5%), and livedo reticularis (1%).

Cardiac and Pulmonary Adverse Events

Cardiac side effects of terlipressin are fewer and less severe than those of vasopressin [10]. Table 1 list the various cardiac adverse events reported in clinical trials. The studies in the table, which cover 149 patients treated with terlipressin for HRS, describe 2 cases of nonfatal myocardial infarction (1.4%). In two case reports, myocardial infarction occurred during terlipressin treatment in patients with bleeding esophageal varices (BOV) [11, 12]. Arrhythmias are reported in 7% of the patients: 13 cases of bradycardia, 6 cases of tachycardia and 10 other or nonspecified types of arrhythmias. The literature describes only 1 case of torsades de pointes arrhythmia during terlipressin treatment and this was converted by DC shock and was not sustained [13]. Terlipressin is safer than vasopressin, which carries a rather high risk of development of malignant arrhythmia including torsades de pointes arrhythmia [14]. This is supported by an animal study, which showed that terlipressin, unlike vasopressin only affected coronary blood flow in supratherapeutic levels [15]. A recent study by Wu et al. [16] investigated the relation and risk factors of myocardial injury in patients with upper gastrointestinal bleeding. A total of 155 patients, 25 of whom had BOV, had their ECG recorded and cardiac enzymes followed during the bleeding episode. Cirrhosis with more than three cardiac risk factors comprised a high-risk group for myocardial

Pulmonary	Ischemia and skin	GI	Other
N/A	N/A	abdominal pain and diarrhea 4	N/A
6 (4%)	7 (5%)	abdominal pain and diarrhea 24 (16%)	

injury. Conversely, vasopressin and terlipressin administrations were not significant predictors of myocardial injury in that study. Recently, we investigated myocardial perfusion during terlipressin therapy in patients with no history of coronary artery disease [unpubl. data]. After 2 mg of terlipressin, we performed a gated myocardial scintigraphy with single photon emission computed tomography and could not detect any change in myocardial perfusion. This supports the observations that only patients with cardiac risk factors have an increased risk of cardiac side effects. Special caution should be shown in patients with ischemic heart disease, impaired peripheral circulation, diabetes, and in obese patients. Terlipressin is contraindicated in patients with manifest cardiovascular disease or should be administered with extreme caution.

Pulmonary adverse events such as respiratory failure and bronchospasm have been described. In the randomized trials, 4% of the patients were found to have pulmonary complications (table 1). In a retrospective study, Halimi et al. [17] reported a case of bronchospasm leading to death during terlipressin therapy. Asthma and chronic obstructive pulmonary disease are relative contraindications to terlipressin therapy.

Skin Ischemia

Peripheral ischemia with cyanosis of fingers, ischemia of the extremities, livido reticularis or cutaneous necrosis are reported in 5% of patients treated with terlipressin (table 1). The largest study on HRS reports only 2 cases of peripheral ischemia (livedo reticularis and cyanosis of fingers) among the 56 patients treated with terlipressin (table 1) [5]. There are 4 case reports, comprising 7 patients who experienced skin reactions during terlipressin treatment [18–20]. Vaccaro et al. [21] report a case of HRS-1 after spontaneous bacterial peritonitis. After 10 boluses of 0.5 mg of terlipressin at

4-hour intervals, the patient developed ischemic skin complications of the abdomen, lower limbs, scrotum and penis. The second report describes a 41-year-old man who developed gangrene in his toes and necrosis at the infusion site after treatment with terlipressin for HRS [20]. Donnellan et al. [19] reported 3 cases of death during terlipressin treatment and the occurrence of ischemic skin complications. A 47-year-old man received terlipressin at a dose of 0.5 mg four times a day for treatment of HRS; 48 h later he developed bullous hemorrhagic lesions on his legs. Skin biopsy revealed the lesion to be epidermal skin necrosis. The second case was a 53-year-old woman who had extensive bruising and large exudative blistering of the skin of the abdominal wall and upper thighs after 5 days of terlipressin 0.5 mg four times a day for HRS. The third case was a 56-year-old man who after 3 days of treatment with terlipressin 1 mg four times a day developed large areas of ecchymosis and blistering of the skin of the right groin and flank. Di Micoli et al. [18] reported the case of a 65-year-old woman with HRS who developed extensive bilateral cyanosis of the breast skin on the fourth day of terlipressin treatment when the dose was increased to 9 mg/day. A recent report from Korea describes a 71-year-old man who, after 36 h of treatment with terlipressin 1 mg/6 h for BOV, developed skin blistering and ecchymosis on his upper thigh, scrotal area and trunk [22]. Recently, we studied the effects of terlipressin on transcutaneous oxygen pressure ($TcPO_2$) [23]. The mean whole body $TcPO_2$ decreased after 2 mg of terlipressin by 34%, and was most pronounced in the lower extremities: above knee –33% (50 vs. 33 mm Hg, $p = 0.01$) and below knee –52% (52 vs. 26 mm Hg, $p = 0.001$). Levels below 30 mm Hg, which is considered critical, were found in 60% of the patients after terlipressin, compared to 0% in the placebo group [23]. However, the relation between development of $TcPO_2$ and clinical ischemic events remains to be established. During terlipressin therapy, the skin, especially on the fingers and toes, must be inspected frequently for ischemia and necroses. Contraindications with particular focus on obliterative arterial disease of the lower limbs, diabetes, and the presence of skin wounds are important, and the skin, especially at the periphery, should be inspected frequently in order to prevent ischemic lesions

Gastrointestinal Adverse Events

The most common adverse events of terlipressin are abdominal cramps and diarrhea. These are reported in most terlipressin studies ranging from 2 to 23% of the patients, with a mean of 16%. They are usually mild and transient and do not seems to prompt in discontinuation of treatment. There are 3 case reports on intestinal ischemia. One describes segmental ischemic necrosis of the cecum in a patient with suspected BOV [24]. The second describes a 57-year-old man treated with terlipressin 2 mg/4 h for suspected BOV [25]. This patient developed a transient intestinal ischemia, which was verified during surgery. The third report refers to a patient who developed ischemic colitis probably due to terlipressin treatment [26].

Hyponatremia and Hypokalemia

Terlipressin improves renal function and induces natriuresis, but decreases the excretion of solute-free water, which can induce hyponatremia and possibly hypokalemia [27, 28]. A recent study found that during 5 days of treatment with terlipressin 1 mg/4 h, serum sodium decreased from 138 ± 5 to 130 ± 9 mmol/l, and in the 10-day treatment group, serum sodium decreased from 135 ± 7 to 121 ± 8 mmol/l [29]. Hyponatremia has been reported in two trials on BOV, Escorsell's group observed 4 cases in 105 (4%) treated with terlipressin compared with none in the sclerotherapy group, and Feu and coworkers observed 5 (6%) among 80 in the terlipressin group compared with 3 of 81 treated with somatostatin. There are 2 case reports on hyponatremia during terlipressin treatment, one of which developed a tonic-clonic seizure after a decrease in serum sodium from 132 to 115 mmol/l. Among 62 patients with BOV, who were treated in our department with high-dose, short-term terlipressin 2 mg/4 h for a mean of 1.7 days (range 1–6 days) serum sodium decreased from 136 ± 6 to 130 ± 7 mmol/l [30]. A confounding factor could be blood transfusions. However, there was no difference in the number of transfusions given when the group with post-treatment serum sodium below 130 mmol/l was compared to that with sodium levels above 130 mmol/l (3.8 vs. 3.5, $p = 0.83$). Hypokalemia is often seen in the clinic during terlipressin treatment. Possible mechanisms are the dilutional affects of antidiuresis and a V2 receptor-mediated increase in potassium excretion [31]. However, little is known about the relation to the use of terlipressin in cirrhosis and only a single report of 2 cases has described terlipressin-exacerbated hypokalemia [32].

These observations emphasize the importance of monitoring sodium and potassium levels during terlipressin treatment. Potassium can be replaced, but in the presence of HRS and ascites terlipressin may cause or worsen hyponatremia and discontinuation or a dose reduction should be considered, as saline is not an option.

Contraindications to Terlipressin and Prevention of Side Effects

Trials with terlipressin showed the drug to be generally well tolerated, probably because significant efforts were made to separate out patients with contraindications, that is patients with cardiovascular diseases were excluded in most of the studies. More side effects are to be expected in the daily clinical setting, therefore, before initiating therapy, absolute and relative contraindications must be carefully assessed (table 2). Terlipressin is either contraindicated or should be given with extreme caution to patients with severe atherosclerotic cardiovascular disease. On initiation and during therapy, patients should be monitored with ECG, blood pressure, daily electrolytes and clinically for skin ischemia to detect adverse events at an early stage. Table 2

Table 2. Contraindications to terlipressin

Contraindications
Coronary artery disease
Dilated and nondilated cardiomyopathies
Uncontrolled cardiac arrhythmias
Obliterative arterial disease of the limbs
Arterial hypertension
Asthma and chronic obstructive pulmonary disease

All mentioned contraindications are to be considered absolute if the comorbidity is severe. In less-severe cases, the contraindications are relative.

lists some contraindications. All those mentioned are to be considered absolute if the co-morbidity is severe, and in less-severe cases the contraindications are relative. Contraindications must be carefully evaluated in each patient and the possible benefit of treatment weighed against the risk of harm.

Dealing with Side Effects

There is no specific antidote to terlipressin. Prevention and handling of side effects requires careful selection of patients, close surveillance, daily consideration of dose and duration of therapy.

Close surveillance of side effects during terlipressin therapy for hepatorenal syndrome is mandatory for their early detection and management and to prevent deaths, serious adverse events and withdrawals due to adverse events. Myocardial infarctions and malignant arrhythmias are absolute contraindications to continued therapy. Less-severe side effects, such as skin cyanosis without necrosis, can usually be managed by reducing the dose and oxygen supply, or changing to continuous infusion therapy. Abdominal pain and loose stools are the most common side effects and are usually self-limiting. In patients at increased risk, i.e. patients with mild-to-moderate atherosclerotic cardiovascular disease, terlipressin treatment can be instituted at a low dose or as continuous infusion with careful titration and monitoring. Efficacy in HRS has been established in studies with a bolus infusion [1], but continuous infusion may have fewer side effects and be as effective as a bolus [33]. Continuous low-dose infusion can therefore, until further data document its noninferiority to bolus infusion, only be recommended in patients with a significantly higher risk of adverse events or as an alternative in the case of moderate adverse effects.

Conclusions

The safety profile of terlipressin is favorable when considering clinical efficacy and the high mortality of untreated HRS. Adverse events are mostly cardiovascular and related to vasoconstriction. Mortality due to adverse events has not been reported in randomized clinical trials on HRS and terlipressin was withdrawn in 4% of patients because of adverse events. Mild adverse events related to terlipressin occur in 30% of the patients. If possible, patients should be informed about the most common side effects such as pallor, abdominal pain or cramps and loose stools. This is important if the demands for informed consent to treatment are to be met and to prepare the patient to be aware of side effects. There is no specific antidote to terlipressin. Prevention and handling of side effects include careful selection of patients, close surveillance, daily assessment of dose, and duration of therapy.

Key Messages

- 30% of patients treated with terlipressin for the hepatorenal syndrome develop side effects.
- Prevention and management of side effects include careful selection of patients, close surveillance, daily assessment of dose, and duration of therapy.

References

1 Gluud LL, Christensen K, Christensen E, Krag A: Systematic review of randomized trials on vasoconstrictor drugs for hepatorenal syndrome. Hepatology 2010;51:576–584.

2 Hirasawa A, Shibata K, Kotosai K, Tsujimoto G: Cloning, functional expression and tissue distribution of human cDNA for the vascular-type vasopressin receptor. Biochem Biophys Res Commun 1994;203:72–79.

3 Nielsen S, Frokiaer J, Marples D, Kwon TH, Agre P, Knepper MA: Aquaporins in the kidney: from molecules to medicine. Physiol Rev 2002;82:205–244.

4 Martin-Llahi M, Pepin MN, Guevara M, Diaz F, Torre A, Monescillo A, Soriano G, Terra C, Fabrega E, Arroyo V, Rodes J, Gines P: Terlipressin and albumin vs albumin in patients with cirrhosis and hepatorenal syndrome: a randomized study. Gastroenterology 2008;134:1352–1359.

5 Sanyal AJ, Boyer T, Garcia-Tsao G, Regenstein F, Rossaro L, Appenrodt B, Blei A, Gulberg V, Sigal S, Teuber P: A randomized, prospective, double-blind, placebo-controlled trial of terlipressin for type 1 hepatorenal syndrome. Gastroenterology 2008;134:1360–1368.

6 Neri S, Pulvirenti D, Malaguarnera M, Cosimo BM, Bertino G, Ignaccolo L, Siringo S, Castellino P: Terlipressin and albumin in patients with cirrhosis and type I hepatorenal syndrome. Dig Dis Sci 2008;53:830–835.

7 Alessandria C, Ottobrelli A, Bernardi-Venon W, Todros L, Cerenzia MT, Martini S, et al.: Noradrenalin vs terlipressin in patients with hepatorenal syndrome: a prospective, randomized, unblinded, pilot study. J Hepatol 2007;47:499–505.

8 Solanki P, Chawla A, Garg R, Gupta R, Jain M, Sarin SK: Beneficial effects of terlipressin in hepatorenal syndrome: a prospective, randomized placebo-controlled clinical trial. J Gastroenterol Hepatol 2003;18:152–156.

9 Sharma P, Kumar A, Shrama BC, Sarin SK: An open label, pilot, randomized controlled trial of noradrenaline versus terlipressin in the treatment of type 1 hepatorenal syndrome and predictors of response. Am J Gastroenterol 2008;103:1689–1697.

10 Freeman JG, Cobden I, Lishman AH, Record CO: Controlled trial of terlipressin ('Glypressin') versus vasopressin in the early treatment of oesophageal varices. Lancet 1982;ii:66–68.

11 Lee MY, Chu CS, Lee KT, Lee HC, Su HM, Cheng KH, Sheu SH, Lai WT: Terlipressin-related acute myocardial infarction: a case report and literature review. Kaohsiung J Med Sci 2004;20:604–608.
12 Rosario R, Lalanne B, Lebre P, Lepesan D, Martelet JP, Dupont M, Camatte R, Lambot G, Bourliere M: Myocardial infarction after injection of terlipressin for digestive hemorrhage. Gastroenterol Clin Biol 1996;20:712–713.
13 Urge J, Sincl F, Prochazka V, Urbanek K: Terlipressin-induced ventricular arrhythmia. Scand J Gastroenterol 2008:1–4.
14 Kelly KJ, Stang JM, Mekhjian HS: Vasopressin provocation of ventricular dysrhythmia. Ann Intern Med 1980;92:205–206.
15 Ouattara A, Landi M, Le MY, Lecomte P, Leguen M, Boccara G, Coriat P, Riou B: Comparative cardiac effects of terlipressin, vasopressin, and norepinephrine on an isolated perfused rabbit heart. Anesthesiology 2005;102:85–92.
16 Wu IC, Yu FJ, Chou JJ, Lin TJ, Chen HW, Lee CS, Wu DC: Predictive risk factors for upper gastrointestinal bleeding with simultaneous myocardial injury. Kaohsiung J Med Sci 2007;23:8–16.
17 Halimi C, Bonnard P, Bernard B, Mathurin P, Mofredj A, di Martino V, Demontis R, Henry-Biabaud E, Fievet P, Opolon P, Poynard T, Cadranel JF. Effect of terlipressin (Glypressin) on hepatorenal syndrome in cirrhotic patients: results of a multicentre pilot study: Eur J Gastroenterol Hepatol 2002; 14:153–158.
18 Di Micoli A, Bracci E, Cappa FM, Casadio R, Zambruni A, Fontana K, Bernardi M, Trevisani F: Terlipressin infusion induces ischemia of breast skin in a cirrhotic patient with hepatorenal syndrome. Dig Liver Dis 2008;40:304–305.
19 Donnellan F, Cullen G, Hegarty JE, McCormick PA: Ischaemic complications of Glypressin in liver disease: a case series. Br J Clin Pharmacol 2007;64:550–552.
20 Lee JS, Lee HS, Jung SW, Han WS, Kim MJ, Lee SW, Choi JH, Kim CD, Ryu HS, Hyun JH: A case of peripheral ischemic complication after terlipressin therapy. Korean J Gastroenterol 2006;47:454–457.
21 Vaccaro F, Giorgi A, Riggio O, De SA, Laviano A, Rossi-Fanelli F: Is spontaneous bacterial peritonitis an inducer of vasopressin analogue side-effects? A case report. Dig Liver Dis 2003;35:503–506.
22 Oh JE, Ha JS, Cho DH, Yu GJ, Shim SG: A case of ischemic skin necrosis after glypressin therapy in liver cirrhosis. Korean J Gastroenterol 2008;51:381–384.
23 Krag A, Møller S, Henriksen JH, Bendtsen F: Effects of a single dose of terlipressin on transcutaneous oxygen pressures. Scand J Gastroenterol 2010;in press.
24 Willems MG, Schoenemann J, Rey C, Schafer H, Lindecken KD: Ischemia of the cecum caused by glycylpressin. Leber Magen Darm 1985;15:165–168.
25 Hansen M, Bjerg J, Gilsaa T: Terlipressin and reversible intestinal ischaemia. Ugeskr Laeger 2007;169: 1802–1803.
26 Schmitt W, Wagner-Thiessen E, Lux G: Ischaemic colitis in a patient treated with glypressin for bleeding oesophageal varices. Hepatogastroenterology 1987;34:134–136.
27 Krag A, Møller S, Henriksen JH, Holstein-Rathlou NH, Larsen FS, Bendtsen F: Terlipressin improves renal function in patients with cirrhosis and ascites without hepatorenal syndrome. Hepatology 2007;46: 1863–1871.
28 Krag A, Bendtsen F, Pedersen EB, Holstein-Rathlou NH, Møller S: Effects of terlipressin on the aquaretic system: evidence of antidiuretic effects. Am J Physiol Renal Physiol 2008;295:F1295–F1300.
29 Bruha R, Marecek Z, Prochazka V, Lata J, Spicak J, Ehrmann J, Kroupa R, Petrtyl J, Dolina J, Taimr P, Drastich P, Urbanek P, Vrzalova D: Double-blind randomized multicenter study comparing the efficacy and safety of 10-day to 5-day terlipressin treatment of bleeding esophageal varices. Hepatogastroenterology 2009;56:390–394.
30 Krag A, Hobolth L, Møller S, Bendtsen F: Hyponatraemia during terlipressin therapy. Gut 2010;59:417–418.
31 Nadvornikova H, Schuck O: The influence of a single dose of vasopressin analogs on human renal potassium excretion. Int J Clin Pharmacol Ther Toxicol 1982;20:155–158.
32 Stephan F, Paillard F: Terlipressin-exacerbated hypokalaemia. Lancet 1998;351:1249–1250.
33 Gerbes AL, Huber E, Gulberg V: Terlipressin for hepatorenal syndrome: continuous infusion as an alternative to i.v. bolus administration. Gastroenterology 2009;137:1179–1181.

Aleksander Krag, MD, PhD
Department of Medical Gastroenterology 439
Copenhagen University Hospital, Hvidovre
Kettegaard Alle 30, DK–2650 Hvidovre (Denmark)
Tel. +45 3632 3182, Fax +45 3632 3750, E-Mail aleksander.krag@hvh.regionh.dk

Gerbes AL (ed): Ascites, Hyponatremia and Hepatorenal Syndrome: Progress in Treatment.
Front Gastrointest Res. Basel, Karger, 2011, vol 28, pp 189–197

Terlipressin for Hepatorenal Syndrome: Novel Strategies and Future Perspectives

P. Angeli

Department of Clinical and Experimental Medicine, University of Padova, Padova, Italy

Abstract

Type 1 hepatorenal syndrome (HRS) is a functional renal failure that often occurs in patients with cirrhosis and ascites. Type 1 HRS develops as the consequence of a severe reduction of effective circulating volume due to both extreme splanchnic arterial vasodilatation and reduction of cardiac output. Several pilot studies and two randomized control studies have shown that terlipressin plus albumin improves renal function in patients with type 1 HRS. Terlipressin plus albumin can also improve short-term survival in these patients. Terlipressin was most commonly given in intravenous boluses starting from an initial dose of 0.5–1 mg every 4 h to 3 mg every 4 h in case of nonresponse. While there is evidence that terlipressin alone may be less effective than terlipressin combined with intravenous albumin in improving renal function in patients with type 1 HRS, the best way to use terlipressin in these patients is still under evaluation. In particular, some preliminary data show that terlipressin given via continuous intravenous infusion is better tolerated than when given in intravenous boluses. Future randomized studies should confirm this difference and outline the best way to use this drug in the treatment of type 1 HRS. In any case, the available data are sufficient to state that use of terlipressin plus albumin has really changed the management of type 1 HRS in patients with advanced cirrhosis. Finally, there is some preliminary evidence suggesting that terlipressin may also be a novel therapeutic approach targeting splanchnic arterial vasodilation involved in the pathophysiology of type 2 HRS, septic shock and paracentesis-induced circulatory dysfunction, but further studies are needed in these clinical scenarios.

Novel Strategies

Terlipressin for the Treatment of Type 1 Hepatorenal Syndrome

The administration of vasoconstrictors and albumin in patients with type 1 hepatorenal syndrome (HRS) is based on the current knowledge of the pathophysiology of this severe complication. A marked renal arterial vasoconstriction, which is the extreme renal functional abnormality that can occur in patients with cirrhosis and ascites, represents the pathophysiological basis of HRS [1]. It develops in the context of a marked reduction of effective circulating volume, which is related to splanchnic arterial vasodilation and inadequate cardiac output [1–3] and implies an extreme overactivation of the endogenous systemic vasoconstrictors systems, namely the renin-angiotensin system, the sympathetic nervous system, and the nonosmotic release of vasopressin [1]. Splanchnic arterial vasodilatation is thought to be mainly the consequence of an increased release of endogenous vasodilators due to portal hypertension and/or hepatic failure [1]. The inadequate cardiac output can be an extreme manifestation of systolic dysfunction which represents one of the components of cirrhotic cardiomyopathy [4]. Thus, the rationale of the use of vasoconscrictors in the treatment of type 1 HRS is to counteract the splanchnic arterial vasodilation in order to improve effective circulating volume and reduce portal pressure. In this way, the final aim of this therapeutic approach is to reduce severe renal arterial vasoconstriction [5].

In small pilot perspective and retrospective studies, it has been demonstrated that the prolonged use of a vasoconstrictor derived from vasopressin, ornipressin [6, 7] or terlipressin [8–19] or of an α-agonist vasoconstrictor (midodrine plus octreotide or noradrenaline alone) [20–25] in association with human albumin is capable of recovering renal function in patients with type 1 HRS. These studies have shown that a vasoconstrictor plus albumin can recover renal function in 40–60% of the cases. In most cases, dilutional hyponatremia associated with HRS also improves during treatment. Recurrence of HRS after treatment withdrawal (a sharp increase in serum creatinine within few days) occurs in approximately 20% of patients, but retreatment is often effective.

Among vasoconstrictors, to this day, terlipressin is the most widely used in the treatment of type 1 HRS [8–19, 26]. Terlipressin has been used in more than 200 patients, either as an intravenous bolus starting from an initial dose of 0.5 mg every 4–6 h, or continuous intravenous infusion starting from an initial dose of 2 mg/day. In patients without response (no significant reduction of serum creatinine within 3 days), the initial dose of terlipressin was doubled. The maximal doses of terlipressin used in the treatment of type 1 HRS were 2 mg every 4–6 h by intravenous boluses, or 12 mg/day by continuous intravenous infusion. Complete reversal (defined by a decrease OD serum creatinine with a final value <1.5 mg/dl) or partial reversal (defined with a decrease of serum creatinine >50% with a final value ≥1.5 mg/dl) of type 1 HRS was observed in almost 59% of the patients [26]. In most studies, terlipressin has been used together with albumin starting with a priming dose of 1 g/kg BW followed by 20–40 g/day, monitoring central venous pressure. In two studies in which terlipressin was given also alone [13, 16], reversal of renal failure was lower than in the studies in which terlipressin was associated with albumin. The decrease in serum creatinine as a result of the administration of vasoconstrictors and albumin takes several days. Therefore, the length of treatment is usually 10–15 days. Despite the normalization of serum creatinine, GFR, when measured specifically [20], remains below the normal values in most responders to treatment. Up to now, two randomized controlled clinical trials comparing terlipressin and albumin with albumin alone

Table 1. Terlipressin and albumin vs. albumin in cirrhotic patients with ascites and type 1 HRS: results of two controlled trials

	Spanish trial (n = 45)		American trial (n = 112)	
	terlipressin and albumin	albumin	terlipressin and albumin	placebo and albumin
Response	43.5%*	8.7%	34%#	13%
	at 3 months		at 6 months	
Survival	27%	19%	13%	9%

* $p < 0.025$, # $p < 0.01$.
Data for the Spanish trial are from Martin-Llahi et al. [28] and those for the American trial are from Sanyal et al. [27].

have been published. While both trials confirm the effectiveness of terlipressin in recovering renal function in patients with type 1 HRS, they fail in improving survival [27, 28] (table 1). Nonetheless, a systematic review of all the randomized controlled clinical trials has more recently shown that terlipressin plus albumin may prolong 15-day survival in patients with type 1 HRS [29]. This evidence stresses the meaning of the use of terlipressin and albumin as a bridge treatment towards liver transplantation (LT). In this perspective, it has been shown that this therapeutic option increases the number of patients with type 1 HRS reaching LT [26, 30], and, after LT, reduces the need for renal replacement therapy (RRT), thus improving survival [31]. Nonetheless, it appears more and more evident that in clinical practice this treatment is often used in patients with type 1 HRS who are not candidates for LT [26, 30].

The small effect of terlipressin and albumin on survival needs some further observation. First, it should be taken into account that the prognosis in these patients is not only related to a recovery of renal function but also to the degree of liver failure. A marked impairment of liver function represents a poor predictor for the response to treatment with terlipressin and albumin [16, 17] but, overall, a poor predictor for their survival [16, 17]. In particular, a Child-Pugh score >11, predicts a poor survival [13, 16, 17]. More recently, it has been shown that a serum total bilirubin ≥10 mg/dl is also a predictor of nonresponse as is an increase in arterial pressure <5 mm Hg at day 3 of treatment [32]. Thus, the severity of liver failure in patients with type 1 HRS can contribute to explain why the efficacy of terlipressin plus albumin in type 1 HRS was found to be less than 50% in patients with type 1 HRS. In addition, terlipressin is targeted on splanchnic arterial vasodilation but it has no effect on the impaired cardiac output in these patients, which has been shown to play an important role in the pathophysiology of type 1 HRS. Thus, the only effect on cardiac output of this therapeutic approach is associated with the albumin infusion. Consequently, albumin

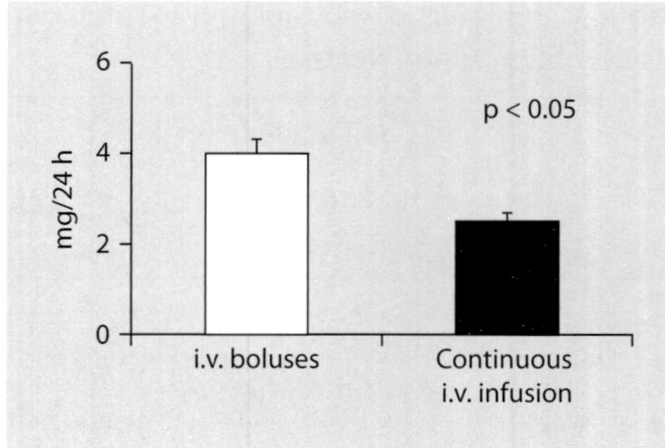

Fig. 1. Mean effective daily dose of terlipressin. Comparison between terlipressin given by intravenous boluses and terlipressin given as continuous intravenous infusion. Data from Angeli et al. [35].

infusion plays an important role in the effectiveness of this new therapeutic approach to type 1 HRS. It has been shown in patients with cirrhosis and spontaneous bacterial peritonitis [33] as well in an experimental model of sepsis [34] that albumin infusion can improve not only cardiac function but also the reactivity of the arterial wall to vasoconstrictors as a result of an albumin-related reduced availability of nitric oxide. These observations can lead to another main comment. The effect of terlipressin and albumin on survival in patients with cirrhosis and type 1 HRS could have been limited by comparing this approach to albumin infusion and not to a placebo. It is too easy to hypothesize today that in the future some more complex therapeutic approaches should be tested including, for example, an inotropic agent.

Finally, it should be stressed that terlipressin can induce side effects in up to 40% of patients and that severe side effects – including myocardial infarction, arrhythmia and intestinal infarction – require discontinuation of treatment in up to 10% of patients [26]. There is some preliminary evidence showing that when terlipressin has been given as a continuous intravenous infusion, it was effective at a lower dose than when it was given as an intravenous bolus, and, as a consequence, it was much better tolerated [19]. These observations have recently been confirmed by the preliminary data of a controlled clinical study in which terlipressin given as an intravenous bolus was compared to terlipressin given as a continuous intravenous infusion in the treatment of type 1 HRS in patients with cirrhosis [35]. Despite a similar efficacy, the daily effective dose of terlipressin was lower in patients who were treated with terlipressin given by continuous intravenous infusion (fig. 1). In this context it should be underlined that 10 of 14 full responders to terlipressin given as a continuous intravenous infusion responded at the initial dose of the provided schedule (2 mg/24 h). As a consequence, severe adverse effects to treatment were more frequent in patients who received terlipressin given by intravenous boluses than in those who received terlipressin via continuous intravenous infusion (fig. 2). The higher efficacy of terlipressin given as a continuous intravenous infusion as compared to terlipressin given by intravenous boluses can be explained by phamacodynamic data on the effect of the drug on portal pressure in cirrhosis. In fact, it has been observed that continuous intravenous

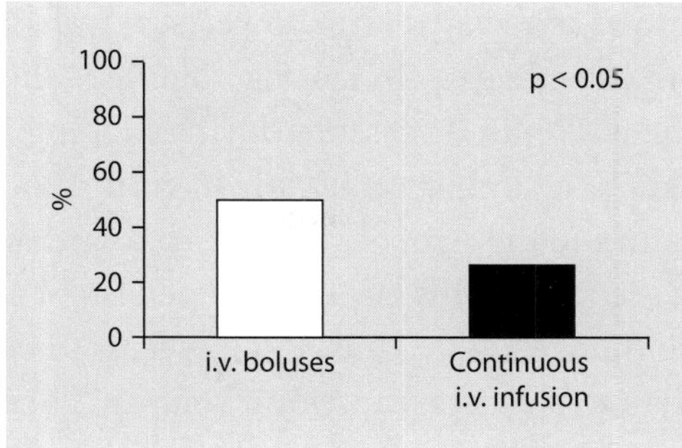

Fig. 2. Number of patients with adverse effects. Comparison between terlipressin given by intravenous boluses and terlipressin given as continuous intravenous infusion. Data from Angeli et al. [35].

infusion of terlipressin assures a more steady profile of the lowering effect of the drug on portal pressure in patients with cirrhosis [36].

Future Perspectives

Terlipressin for Treatment of Type 2 HRS

Type 2 HRS is a more stable impairment of renal function in patients with cirrhosis and ascites. Thus, patients with type 2 HRS do not present with acute renal failure, but rather refractory ascites. As a consequence, these patients have been investigated for the treatment of refractory ascites comparing paracentesis and transjugular intrahepatic portosystemic shunt, rather than for the recovery of renal function. As a consequence, the effects of vasoconstrictors and albumin in type 2 HRS treatment have not been investigated extensively. Nevertheless, because the pathophysiology of type 2 HRS seems to be similar to that of type 1 HRS at least as far as splanchnic arterial vasodilation is concerned, terlipressin has been used in some pilot studies also in patients with type 2 HRS. Nonrandomized studies that enrolled a small number of patients with type 2 HRS have shown that the percentage of response to treatment in terms of recovered renal function does not, however, seem to be different from that observed in patients with type 1 HRS [37, 38], while survival appears longer (100% at 3 months).

Terlipressin for the Treatment of Post-Paracentesis Circulatory Dysfunction

Therapeutic paracentesis is the first-line treatment of both massive and refractory ascites [39]. The mobilization of tense ascites by paracentesis is not always safe since it can provoke further deterioration of circulatory function, namely post-paracentesis circulatory dysfunction (PPCD) [39]. The incidence of PPCD, which is defined as an increase ≥50% of plasma renin activity 1 week after the procedure, is irreversible and is associated with lower survival [40]. The mechanism by which paracentesis affects effective circulating volume is thought to be related to the rapid reduction of the abdominal pressure during tapping. The reduction in intra-abdominal pressure causes a similar reduction in intra-thoracic pressure with increased venous blood return to the right heart, increased cardiac output and decreased peripheral resistance. It seems that this last effect is persistent and favors a reduction of effective circulating volume [41, 42]. Thus, PPCD seems to be due to increased arterial compliance rather than to a decrease of blood volume. These observations represent the potential rationale for the use of vasoconstrictors in this clinical context. Preliminary data showed the possibility of preventing PPCD by methods other than volume expansion, e.g. administration of vasoconstrictors [43–45]. In particular, it has been shown that the administration of terlipressin (1 mg i.v. bolus just before and 1 mg i.v. bolus 8 and 16 h after paracentesis) resulted in a proportion of PPCD similar to that obtained with the albumin administration. A good tolerance to terlipressin was also noted [43]. Large randomized studies should be performed to evaluate the effects of terlipressin as well as other vasoconstrictors in patients with cirrhosis who need therapeutic paracentesis for the control of ascites.

Septic Shock

Vasopressin or vasopressin analogues [46, 47] are used in patients without cirrhosis but with septic shock, since these patients have marked decreases in the plasma concentrations of endogenous vasopressin. Moreover, in patients with arterial hypotension refractory to exogenous catecholamine administration, the intravenous administration of vasopressin has been shown to be capable of increasing arterial pressure [4]. In patients with cirrhosis with septic shock, the plasma concentrations of endogenous vasopressin have not yet been measured, and the effects of vasopressin or vasopressin analogues are unknown. Nevertheless, it has been shown that in rats with cirrhosis challenged with LPS, a Gram-negative bacteria product, terlipressin administration improves LPS-induced arterial hypotension through, at least in part, an inhibitory effect on the LPS-induced over-expression and over-activity of inducible nitric oxide synthase [48]. Taking into account that a similar effect on the arterial wall was observed as a consequence of albumin infusion in an experimental model of septic shock [34], it can be hypothesized that terlipressin and albumin may also be a novel approach in the treatment of patients with cirrhosis and septic shock.

Conclusions

The use of terlipressin and albumin in the treatment of type 1 HRS represents a landmark in the treatment of complications in patients with advanced cirrhosis. Its rationale is closely related to our current knowledge of the pathophysiology of type 1 HRS. The use of terlipressin and albumin was proved to be effective in recovering renal function and it has also increased short-term survival in responders, making it possible to increase the number of patients who undergo LT. In addition, it has changed the outcome of LT in these patients since it reduced the post-LT need for RRT and increased post-LT survival. These results appear to be quite an encouraging development for an effective treatment of type 1 HRS. Nevertheless, it is important to recognize that recovery of renal function can be achieved in less than 50% of patients with type 1 HRS and that the recovery of renal function may be partial even in patients who are defined as full responders. This is not surprising, taking into account the complexity of the pathophysiology of type 1 HRS and the need to understand how to best use the existing approach, particularly how to best use terlipressin. Thus, in the future, a shift is needed in the treatment of type 1 HRS moving from 'a predomin ant vasoconstrictor therapy' toward a combine therapy including, for example, an inotropic agent. In addition, ongoing randomized controlled clinical trials on different modalities of the use of terlipressin in the treatment of type 1 HRS should be completed and other trials on this important issue should be planned and performed. Finally, studies should be performed in order to clarify the potential role of terlipressin and other vasoconstrictors in the treatment of type 2 HRS and septic shock as well as in the prevention of PPCD in patients with cirrhosis.

Key Messages

- The use of terlipressin and albumin is effective in recovering renal function in patients with type 1 HRS and it also increases short-term survival in responders.
- The use of terlipressin and albumin has increased the number of patients with type 1 HRS who undergo OLT and it has changed the outcome of OLT in these patients since it has reduced the post-OLT need for RRT and increased post-OLT survival.
- At the time of writing, the best way to use terlipressin in patients with type 1 HRS was still under evaluation. Preliminary data seem to suggest that terlipressin given as continuous intravenous infusion is better tolerated and cheaper than its administration as intravenous boluses.
- There are some preliminary data suggesting that terlipressin and albumin may also be a novel therapeutic approach for type 2 HRS, septic shock and paracentesis-induced circulatory dysfunction in patients with cirrhosis.

References

1 Schrier RW, Arroyo V, Bernardi M, et al: Peripheral arteriolar vasodilation hypothesis: a proposal for the initiation of renal sodium and water retention in cirrhosis. Hepatology 1988;8:1151–1157.

2 Ruiz del Arbor L, Urman J, Fernandez J, et al: Systemic, renal and hepatic haemodynamic derangement in cirrhotic patients with spontaneous bacterial peritonitis. Hepatology 2003;38:1210–1218.

3 Ruiz del Arbor W, Urman J, Fernandez J: Systemic, renal, and hepatic hemodynamic derangement in cirrhotic patients with spontaneous bacterial peritonitis. Hepatology 2003;38:1210–1218.
4 Alqahtani SA, Fouad TR, Lee SS: Cirrhotic cardiomyopathy. Semin Liver Dis 2008;28:59–69.
5 Narahara Y, Kanazawa H, Taki Y, et al: Effects of terlipressin on systemic, hepatic and renal hemodynamics in patients with cirrhosis. J Gastroenterol Hepatol 2009;24:1791–1797.
6 Guevara M, Gines P, Fernandez-Esparrach G, et al: Reversibility of hepatorenal syndrome by prolonged administration of ornipressin and plasma volume expansion. Hepatology 1998;27:35–41.
7 Gülberg V, Bilzer M, Gerbes AL: Long-term therapy and retreatment of hepatorenal syndrome type 1 with ornipressin and albumin. Hepatology 1999;30: 870–875.
8 Ganne-Carrie N, Hadegue A, Mathurin P, et al: Hepatorenal syndrome: long-term tretament with terlipressin as bridge to liver transplantation. Dig Dis Sci 1996;41:1054–1056.
9 Le Moine O, El Nawar A, Jagodzinski R, et al: Treatment with terlipressin as a bridge to translantation in a patient with hepatorenal syndrome. Acta Gastroenterol Belg 1998;61;268–270.
10 Duhamel C, Mauillon J, Berkelmans J, Bourienne A, Tranvuez JL: Hepatorenal syndrome in cirrhotic patients: terlipressin is a safe and efficient treatment; propoanolol and digitalic treatment: precipitating and preventing factors? Am J Gastroenterol 2000;95: 2984–2985.
11 Halimi C, Bonnard P, Bernard B. et al: Effect of terlipressin (Glypressin) on hepatorenal syndrome in cirrhotic patients: results of a multicenter pilot study. Eur J Gastroenterol Hepatol 2002;14:153–158.
12 Mulkay JP, Louis H, Donckier V, et al; Long-term terlipressin administration improves renal function in cirrhotic patients with type 1 hepatorenal syndrome: a pilot study. Acta Gastroelerol Belg 2001;64: 15–19.
13 Uriz J, Gines P, Cardenas A, et al: Terlipressin plus albumin infusion: an effective and safe therapy of hepatorenal syndrome. J Hepatol 2000;33:43–48.
14 Ortega R, Giniss P, Uriz J, et al: Terlipressin therapy with and without albumin for patients with hepatorenal syndrome: results of a prospective, nonrandomized study. Hepatology 2002;36:941–948.
15 Solanki P, Chawala A, Garg R, et al: Beneficial effects of terlipressin in hepatorenal sindrome: a prospective, randomized placebo-controlled clinical trial. J Gastroenterol Hepatol 2003;18:152–156.
16 Moreau R, Durand F, Poynard T, et al: Terlipressin in patients with cirrhosis and type 1 hepatorenal syndrome: a retrospective multicenter study. Gastroenterology 2002;122:923–930.
17 Colle I, Durand F, Pessione F, et al: Clinical course, predictive factors and prognosis in patients with cirrhosis and type 1 hepatorenal syndrome treated with terlipressin: a retrospective analysis. J Gastroenterol Hepatol 2002;17:882–888.
18 Angeli P, Guarda S, Fasolato S, et al: Switch therapy with ciprofloxacin versus intravenous ceftazidime in the treatment of spontaneous bacterial peritonitis in patients with cirrhosis: similar efficacy at lower cost. Aliment Pharmacol Ther 2006;23:75–84.
19 Gerbes AL, Huber E, Gülberg V: Terlipressin for hepatorenal syndrome: continuous infusion as an alternative to i.v. bolus administration. Gastroenterology 2009;137:1179.
20 Angeli P, Volpin R, Gerunda G, et al: Reversal of type 1 hepatorenal syndrome (HRS) with the combined administration of midodrine and octreotide. Hepatology 1999;29:1690–1697.
21 Wong F, Pantea L, Sniderman K. Midodrine, octreotide, albumin, and TIPS in selected patients with cirrhosis and type 1 hepatorenal syndrome. Hepatology 2004;40:55–64.
22 Esrailian E, Pantageo ER, Kyulo NL, Hu KQ, Runyon BA: Octretide/midodrine therapy significantly improves renal function and 30-day survival in patients with type 1 hepatorenal syndrome. Dig Dis Sci 2007;52:742–748.
23 Skagen C, Einstein M, Lucey MR, Said A: Combination treatment with ocreotide, midodrine, and albumin improves survival in patients with type 1 and type 2 hepatorenal syndrome. J Clin Gastroenterol 2009;43:680–685.
24 Devoux C, Zanditenas D, Hezode C, et al: Effects of noradrenalin and albumin in patients with type 1 hepatorenal syndrome: a pilot study. Hepatology 2002;36:374–380.
25 Sharma P, Kumar A, Sharma BC, Sarin SK: An open label, pilot, randomized controlled trial of noradrenaline versus terlipressin in the treatment of type 1 hepatorenal syndrome and predictors of response. Am J Gastroenterol 2008;103:1689–1697.
26 Gines P, Schier RW: Renal failure in cirrhosis. N Engl J Med 2009;361:1279–1290.
27 Sanyal A, Boyer T, Garcia-Tsao G, et al: A randomized, prospective, double blind placebo-controlled trial of terlipressin for type 1 hepatorenal syndrome. Gastroenterology 2008;134:1360–1368.
28 Martin-Llahi MM, Pepin MN, Guevara M, et al: Terlipressin and albumin versus albumin in patients with cirrhosis and hepatorenal syndrome: a randomized study. Gastroenterology 2008;134:1352–1359.

29 Gluud LL, Christensen K, Krag A: Systematic review of randomized trials on vasoconstrictor drugs for hepatorenal syndrome. Hepatology 2010;51:576–584.
30 Angeli P: Review article: prognosis of hepatorenal syndrome – has it changed with current practice? Aliment Pharmacol Ther 2004;20(suppl 3):1–4.
31 Restuccia T, Ortega R, Guevara M, et al: Effects of treatment of hepatorenal syndrome before transplantation on post-transplantation outcome: a case control study. Liver Transpl 2004;40:140–146.
32 Nezar A, Pereira GH, Guevara M, et al: Predictors of response to therapy with terlipressin and albumin in patients with cirrhosis and type 1 hepatorenal syndrome. Hepatology 2010;51:219–226.
33 Fernandez J, Navasa M, Garcia-Pagan JC, et al: Effect of intravenous albumin on systemic and hepatic hemodynamics and vasoactive neurohormonal systems in patients with cirrhosis and spontaneous bacterial peritonitis. J Hepatol 2004;41: 384–390.
34 Meziani F, Kremer H, Tesse A, et al: Human serum albumin improves arterial dysfunction during early resuscitation in mouse endotoxic model via reduced oxidative and nitrosative stresses. Am J Pathol 2007; 171:1753–1761.
35 Angeli P, Fasolato S, Cavallin M, et al: Terlipressin given as continuous intravenous infusion is the more suitable schedule for the treatment of type 1 heptorenal syndrome (HRS) in patients with cirrhosis: results of a controlled clinical study (abstract). Hepatology 2008;48(suppl):378A.
36 Escorsell A, Bandi JC, Moitinho E, Feu F, García-Pagan JC, Bosch J, Rodés J: Time profile of the haemodynamic effects of terlipressin in portal hypertension. J Hepatol 1997;26:621–627.
37 Testino G, Ferro C, Sumberaz A, et al: Type-2 hepatorenal syndrome and refractory ascites: role of transjugular intrahepatic portosystemic stent-shunt in eighteen patients with advanced cirrhosis awaiting orthotopic liver transplantation. Hepatogastroenterology 2003;50:1753–1755.
38 Alessandria C, Venon WD, Marzano A, Barletti C, Fadda M, Rizzetto M: Renal failure in cirrhotic patients: role of terlipressin in clinical approach to hepatorenal syndrome type 2. Eur J Gastroenterol Hepatol 2002;14:1363–1368.
39 Moore KP, Wong F, Gines P, et al: The management of ascites in cirrhosis: report on the consensus conference of the International Ascites Club. Hepatology 2003;38:258–266.
40 Gines A, Fernandez-Esparrach G, Monescillo A, et al: Randomized controlled trial comparing albumin, dextran-70 and polygelin in cirrhotic patients with ascites treated by paracentesis. Gastroenterology 1996;111:1002–1010.
41 Ruiz del Arbor L, Monescillo A, Jimenez W, et al: Paracentesis-induced circulatory dysfunction: mechanism and effect on hepatic hemodynamics in cirrhosis. Gastroenterology 1997;113:579–586.
42 Vila MC, Solà R, Molina L, et al: Haemodynamic changes in patients developing effective hypovolemia after total paracentesis. J Hepatol 1998;28:639–645.
43 Moreau R, Asselah T, Condat B, et al: Comparison of the effect of terlipressin and albumin on arterial volume in patients with cirrhosis and tense ascites treated by paracentesis: a randomized pilot study. Gut 2002;50:90–94.
44 Singh V, Dheerendra PC, Singh B, et al: Midodrine versus albumin in the prevention of paracentesis-induced circulatory dysfunction in cirrhotics: a randomized pilot study. Am J Gastroenterol 2008;103: 1399–1405.
45 Appenrodt B, Wolf A, Grünhage F, et al: Prevention of paracentesis-induced circulatory dysfunction: midodrine vs albumin. A randomized pilot study. Liver Int 2008;28:1019–1025.
46 Russell JA, Walley KR, Singer J, et al: Vasopressin versus norepinephrine infusion in patients with septic shock. N Engl J Med 2008;358:877–887.
47 Morelli A, Ertmer C, Rehberg S, et al: Continuous terlipressin versus vasopressin infusion in septic shock (TERLIVAP): a randomized, controlled pilot study. Crit Care 2009;13:R130.
48 Moreau R, Barrière E, Tazi KA, et al: Terlipressin inhibits in vivo aortic iNOS expression induced by lipopolysaccharide in rats with biliary cirrhosis. Hepatology 2002;36:1070–1078.

Paolo Angeli, MD, PhD
Department of Clinical and Experimental Medicine, University of Padova
Via Giustiniani 2
IT–35100, Padova (Italy)
Tel. +39 0498212204, Fax +39 0498218676, E-Mail pangeli@unipd.it

Gerbes AL (ed): Ascites, Hyponatremia and Hepatorenal Syndrome: Progress in Treatment.
Front Gastrointest Res. Basel, Karger, 2011, vol 28, pp 198–207

Hepatorenal Syndrome and Liver Transplantation

Thomas A. Gonwa

Mayo Clinic College of Medicine, Department of Transplantation, Mayo Clinic in Florida, Jacksonville, Fla., USA

Abstract

Patients with end-stage liver disease often present with hepatorenal syndrome (HRS). Prior to the introduction of liver transplant this was a fatal complication. However, these patients can now undergo successful liver transplantation. HRS, however, leads to increased mortality on the waiting list, difficult intraoperative and postoperative challenges and decreased survival compared to non-HRS patients. These include renal replacement support, fluid and electrolyte shifts, and post-operative immunosuppression. HRS patients have longer ICU stays, hospital length of stay, decreased long-term renal function and a higher incidence of end-stage renal disease following liver transplantation. Despite this, the 5-year survival can exceed 65%. There has been a recent trend in increasing liver kidney transplantation. Efforts are underway to develop criteria for patients who would benefit from combined liver kidney transplantation, and these are reviewed. Recent research has indicated that reversing HRS preoperatively may improve long-term survival postoperatively and this area of research needs to be expanded.

Prior to the successful introduction of orthotopic liver transplantation into clinical practice, the diagnosis of hepatorenal syndrome (HRS) was a uniformly fatal one. However, early experience in patients with HRS who underwent liver transplant demonstrated recovery of renal function [1]. The normal status of kidneys in HRS was further demonstrated by the successful use of kidneys from patients dying with HRS in successful deceased donor kidney transplantation [2]. This early experience demonstrated that the presence of HRS was not a contraindication to liver transplant. Over the years, however, more experience has demonstrated that the presence of HRS and decreased renal function have profound impacts on the patient awaiting liver transplant and on the outcome following successful transplant. These can be grouped into several areas and will be the focus of this chapter. First, the impact of HRS and renal dysfunction on survival of patients awaiting liver transplantation will be explored. Secondly, support for the HRS patient on the waiting list will be discussed. Third, ramifications of HRS on the actual liver transplant procedure will be reviewed. Finally, the impact of HRS on patient survival and long-term prognosis will be reviewed.

Patients with renal dysfunction awaiting liver transplant often suffer from HRS. The effect of HRS on morbidity and mortality of patients awaiting liver transplantation has not been specifically studied. However, the effect of renal dysfunction and dialysis has been investigated. The development of the Model for End-Stage Liver Disease (MELD) was spurred by a desire to predict mortality of patients with this condition. It has been adopted in the USA and by Eurotransplant as the primary method to determine allocation of livers for transplantation after fulminant cases in the USA and fulminant and combined cases in Eurotransplant. It is based on the premise that sicker patients benefit more from liver transplantation in terms of life years gained [3–5]. One of the primary determinants of the MELD score is serum creatinine. Furthermore, any patient on renal replacement therapy (RRT) is given a value of 4 mg/dl for creatinine, which automatically gives a MELD score of 20. Thus, renal dysfunction, whether it is from HRS or another etiology, pushes patients toward the top of the list. This has clearly been demonstrated in the USA where the percentage of patients with renal dysfunction awaiting liver transplant increased after the introduction of MELD for allocation [6]. Furthermore, there has been an increase in patients receiving combined liver kidney transplantation during the MELD era. Although there has been an increase in transplantation in these patients, there is no evidence that the overall survival of patients after liver transplantation in the USA has been compromised [6]. However, patients with HRS and those requiring RRT do have a higher mortality on the waiting list, are more difficult to care for, and have worse outcomes.

Patients suffering from cirrhosis with renal dysfunction and those on dialysis have a higher mortality. This was demonstrated by Fraley et al. [7] in 1998 when they examined the mortality in patients referred for liver transplantation who had acute renal failure. Most of these patients were labeled as HRS. In the 186 patients who were not selected for liver transplant, 66 had acute renal failure requiring RRT. The ones receiving hemodialysis (HD) had a mortality of 64% while those receiving continuous renal replacement therapy (CRRT) had a mortality of 98%. The mortality of these patients when they are awaiting liver transplant has been examined by two consensus conferences in the USA [8, 9]. Both of these conferences examined the waiting list mortality and found it to be elevated compared to patients without renal dysfunction. The one-year mortality of patients on the waiting list with a serum creatinine >1.5 mg/dl was about 30%, compared to 10% in patients with serum creatinine less than that. If the patients had a serum creatinine >2 mg/dl or required RRT, the 1-year mortality on the waiting list rose to 40–50%. Furthermore, a study by Alessandria et al. [10] reported that patients with HRS may be disadvantaged by use of the MELD syndrome. Their analysis of HRS patients compared to matched controls indicated that HRS patients had worse outcomes for any given MELD score. They suggested that HRS patients should have a different allocation formula.

Caring for these patients is difficult and when they require RRT providing it and choosing the right type is sometimes problematical. Patients with advanced renal failure suffer from hypotension, coagulopathy, and encephalopathy which make it difficult to deliver effective RRT. There is no consensus or evidence on the best method to deliver RRT. CRRT appears to be better tolerated than intermittent HD because of cardiovascular stability and gradual corrections of hyponatremia. Furthermore, intracranial pressure is better controlled with CRRT and most clinicians prefer this method for the comatose liver failure patient requiring RRT [11, 12]. Despite this preference there are no convincing studies that have demonstrated a superiority of CRRT to HD. In fact, most studies demonstrate that patients treated with CRRT may fare worse than others. However, none of these studies were randomized and suffer from comparing different populations of patients. Witzke et al. [13] studied 30 HRS patients waiting for liver transplant. In this study, patients were placed on CRRT if they were mechanically ventilated, and on HD if they were not. The 30-day survival was 53% for the HD patients and 0% for the CRRT patients. A more recent study by Wong et al. [14] examined the outcome of 102 patients with cirrhosis and acute renal failure requiring RRT. HRS was the diagnosis in 48% of the patients. Mortality in this study was 78% for CRRT and 50% for HD. Thus, the presence of HRS or renal dysfunction in patients with cirrhosis leads to increased mortality whether or not the patient is waiting for liver transplantation. Its presence in the liver transplant candidate increases mortality on the waiting list, and conventional therapies may support patients until they receive a liver transplant but there continues to be excessive mortality. Differences in survival comparing HD to CRRT most likely represent the severity of the underlying liver disease and not the modality of RRT. Although one can control the uremia of these patients, the underlying pathophysiology or the ability to survive to liver transplant determines survival.

Once a patient survives to receive a liver transplant a new set of problems arises. Early experience demonstrated that clamping of the inferior vena cava and the portal vein prior to removing the diseased liver resulted in a 20–30% fall in cardiac output. Furthermore, engorgement of the vascular bed leads to hyperkalemia and acidosis once circulation is restored. Use of venovenous bypass prevents most of these changes and preserves adequate renal hemodynamics during liver transplantation [15, 16]. The introduction of the piggyback technique of liver transplant allowed side clamping of the inferior vena cava which allows blood from the lower extremities to return to the heart. This leads to minimal changes in cardiac output and better stability during the procedure. However, the portal vein is still clamped and the release of the portal vein clamps at the end of the anastomosis leads to release of a large amount of desaturated blood containing high concentrations of potassium and lactic acid into the circulation [17]. In addition, large volumes of blood products may be utilized during the procedure. Patients with good renal function can tolerate these changes but the patient with HRS or decreased renal function may not. Intraoperative concerns in the patient with renal dysfunction were recently reviewed at an international consensus conference [18].

These issues have prompted clinicians to consider intraoperative RRT to deal with these issues. Although there appear to be good reasons to consider the use of CRRT in this situation, there is a general lack of data. A few case reports were published in the 1990s [19–21]. Recently, Townsend et al. [22] reviewed their experience in utilizing intraoperative CRRT during liver transplantation. They utilized CRRT in 6.4% of 636 liver transplant recipients. Common indications for CRRT included patients already receiving RRT (63.4%), dysnatremia (22%), lactic acidosis (17%), and hyperkalemia (12.1%). There were no complications during the procedure and the 1-year survival was 75%. All patients who survived were dialysis independent at 1 year. We follow a similar approach in Florida. Patients with HRS or renal dysfunction are considered for intraoperative CRRT if they are currently on RRT, have oliguria with ascites, hyperkalemia, or serum creatinine >1.6 mg/dl. We are currently analyzing our experience in over 90 patients. It should be pointed out that the 1-year survival following liver transplant in patients with serum creatinine at the time of transplant >2 mg/dl or those on RRT reported from the United Network for Organ Sharing (UNOS) data is about 75% [6]. Thus, the actual role of intraoperative RRT in liver transplantation is yet to be decided.

Renal function prior to liver transplantation in patients with and without HRS is an independent predictor of both short- and long-term patient and graft survival [6, 23, 24]. The group from Baylor Dallas investigated the outcome of liver transplantation in patients with HRS, compared to non-HRS, over a decade [25–27]. These studies demonstrated the clinical behavior of HRS patients after liver transplant. Compared to non-HRS patients, patients with HRS are more likely to be in hospital or in the ICU pretransplant (91 vs. 29%), more likely to require pre- and post-transplant dialysis, require longer ICU stays and have a longer length of stay in the hospital. Renal function recovered in most cases but dialysis was necessary in 33.8% of the HRS patients in the first six weeks after transplant [27]. The measured GFR in HRS patients was significantly lower posttransplant than in non-HRS patients who underwent liver transplant (HRS patients 44 ± 21, 39 ± 17 and 45 ± 12 ml/min compared to 59 ± 25, 59 ± 26, and 57 ± 31 ml/min in the non-HRS patients at 1, 2, and 4 years, $p < 0.03$) [26]. Although HRS patients can safely undergo liver transplant, their long-term survival at 3 and 5 years is significantly less than that observed in patients without HRS (table 1). In the Baylor experience, the 3- and 5-year patient survival was 60% and 60% in the HRS patients compared to 71% and 68% in the non-HRS patients [26]. By the end of the 1990s, the 5-year survival in HRS patients who received a liver only was 67.1% at Baylor compared to 70.1% in patients undergoing liver transplant alone who had a preoperative creatinine <2 mg/dl [27]. The lower GFR at time of transplantation and the worse outcome led to a higher incidence of end-stage renal disease (ESRD) in HRS patients. In the Baylor series, patients were followed over a 10-year period. Of the 720 patients without HRS who underwent transplantation, 4.4% had progressed to ESRD by 10 years, compared to 13/114 patients (11.4%) of the HRS patients [28]. Although not specifically looking

Table 1. Comparison of patient and graft survival in HRS and non-HRS patients

	HRS (n = 59)		Non-HRS (n = 513)	
	graft[a]	patient[b]	graft	patient
3 months	77%	83%	86%	90%
1 year	62%	71% (38)	75%	83% (352)
2 years	56%	65% (30)	69%	76% (264)
3 years	51%	60% (25)	66%	73% (190)
4 years	51%	60% (15)	64%	71% (136)
5 years	51%	60% (8)	61%	68% (78)

Figures in parentheses are numbers of patients.
[a] $p < 0.02$ (Wilcoxon) HRS vs. non-HRS; [b] $p < 0.03$ (Wilcoxon) HRS vs. non-HRS.
Adapted with permission from Gonwa et al. [26].

at HRS patients, a more recent study examined long-term outcome in patients with significant pre-transplant renal dysfunction (defined as a serum creatinine >1.5 mg/dl for at least 2 weeks prior to transplant) [24]. In this study, only 8/60 (13%) had an eGFR <20 ml/min after a median duration of 36 months, and 6 required institution of hemodialysis. Recently published data would seem to indicate that the outcome of HRS patients following liver transplant has not improved despite newer immunosuppressive strategies including induction therapy. A recent study from Pittsburgh estimated the posttransplant reversal of HRS to be only 58% [29]. Part of the explanation may be that waiting time for transplants has increased over the last 10 years. The length of time that renal insufficiency exists prior to transplantation may impact the recovery of renal function posttransplantation [24]. An examination of the UNOS database compared survival after liver transplant in groups with different levels of renal function [6]. In this study, there were over 3,000 patients who received a liver transplant alone who had a pre-transplantation creatinine >2 mg/dl or were on pretransplantation RRT. The 3- and 5-year survival in these groups were 70 and 64%, compared to 84 and 79% in patients who had a preoperative creatinine of <1 mg/dl (fig. 1). Although they were not classified as HRS, the patients with HRS would be expected to be in these groups, indicating that pre-operative renal dysfunction continues to be an indicator of worse outcome following liver transplantation. The fact that the outcomes have not improved over the last 10 years indicates the need for further research on the best way to approach these patients. One area of interest has been the use of induction therapy in patients with pre-operative renal dysfunction. The earlier studies from Dallas all utilized the monoclonal antibody OKT3 for induction in these patients. More recent studies have examined the

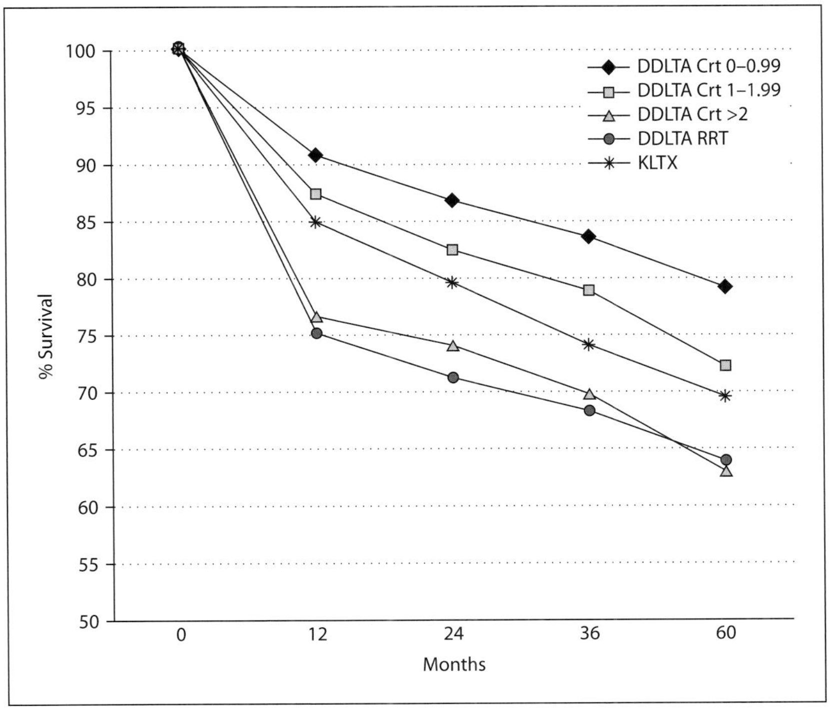

Fig. 1. Survival after liver transplant in the USA, stratified according to renal function at the time of transplant. DDLTA = Deceased donor liver transplant alone; KLTX = combined kidney liver transplant; Crt = serum creatinine (mg/dl); RRT = renal replacement therapy. Reprinted with permission from Gonwa et al. [6].

use of monoclonal antibodies against IL-2r (basiliximab and daclizumab) as well as polyclonal induction with antithymocyte globulin to protect renal function in these patients prior to exposure to Calcineurin agents. These were reviewed at a recent consensus conference. Although these studies are small and nonrandomized, many clinicians recommend their use [18].

As noted above, the introduction of the MELD system and the general increase in waiting time has increased the number of patients with renal dysfunction who present for transplant [6]. This has led to a marked increase in combined liver kidney transplants [6, 8, 9]. This trend has prompted at least three consensus conferences to address the issue of who should be listed for combined liver kidney transplantation [8, 9, 18]. It has prompted UNOS to draft policy in an attempt to determine who should be listed for a combined transplant (table 2). These recommendations were based on identifying patients not likely to recover renal function following liver transplant. Clearly those with ESRD and end-stage liver disease and those with metabolic causes (oxaluria) are not controversial (A1 and C1 in table 2). Patients with decreased GFR (<30) who have signs of fixed renal disease (with proteinuria, for example) constitute category A2 in table 2. There is also some evidence that

Table 2. Proposed criteria for placing a patient on the list for a combined kidney liver transplant

Category			Dialysis required?	Duration	Documentation requirement
A	Chronic renal failure	A1	yes	none	documentation of the date of initiation of dialysis and the cause of ESRD
		A2	no	none	GFR ≤30 ml/min by MDRD6 or direct measurement (Iothalamate or iohexol) and proteinuria (>3 g protein/day with 24-hour protein measurement or urine protein/creatinine ratio >3.0)
B	Sustained acute renal failure	B1	yes	>6 weeks	documentation of dialysis at least twice a week
		B2	no	>6 weeks	GFR ≤5 ml/min by MDRD6, Iothalamate, or iohexol (test results reported every 7 days)
		B3	yes	>6 weeks	combination of B1 and B2 documentation for at least 6 weeks
C	Metabolic disease	C1	no	none	documentation from a nephrologist specifying the reason for kidney transplant

Adapted from the United Network for Organ Sharing.

performing renal biopsy on these patients will help identify those patients who would benefit from combined transplant [30, 31]. The growing evidence that length of time on dialysis influences renal recovery generates the criteria in category B [8, 9, 24]. Hepatorenal syndrome is after all a vasoconstrictive disease of the renal vasculature. It is not hard to imagine that prolonged vasospasm will lead to ischemia and fibrosis in the HRS kidney. These proposed criteria constitute a synthesis of the consensus conferences and will serve to better define when a combined liver kidney transplant should be done.

Despite all the problems outlined above, liver transplantation remains the only 'cure' for HRS. Future directions of research should be focused on reversing HRS pretransplantation. An intriguing study examined the effects of vasopressin analogue treatment of patients with HRS prior to transplant on the outcome of these patients. Although a small series, 9 patients who responded to therapy underwent transplantation. They had a 3-year patient survival of 100% compared to 83% in 27 matched controls without HRS who underwent transplantation [32]. This suggests that correcting the underlying pathophysiology of HRS rather than just treating the symptoms prior to transplantation may improve outcome. As seen in table 1 most of the excessive mortality in these patients following liver transplant occurs in the first year. Therefore, future research should be directed at improving survival during this time period. This would include reversing HRS pretransplantation, investigating better support systems including intra-operative RRT for the treatment of these patients, and further studies on appropriate immunosuppression.

Key Messages

- Patients with HRS have increased mortality on the waiting list and worse long-term survival.
- Patients with HRS have worse long-term renal function and higher incidence of ESRD.
- Patient with HRS can achieve 5-year survival of 65% following liver transplantation.
- Future research should be directed at reversing HRS prior to transplantation.
- The excessive post-transplantation mortality is in the first year, and better methods of immunosuppressive therapy and postoperative support are needed.
- Criteria for selection of patients for combined liver kidney transplant are being developed.

References

1 Iwatsuki S, Popovtzer MM, Corman JL, Ishikawa M, Putnam CW, Katz FH, Starzl TE: Recovery from 'hepatorenal syndrome' after orthotopic liver transplantation. N Engl J Med 1973;289:1155–1159.

2 Koppel MH, Coburn JW, Mims MM, Goldstein H, Boyle JD, Rubini ME: Transplantation of cadaveric kidneys from patients with hepatorenal syndrome. Evidence for the functional nature of renal failure in advanced liver disease. N Engl J Med 1969;280:1367–1371.

3 Kamath PS, Wiesner RH, Malinchoc M, Kremers W, Therneau TM, Kosberg CL, D'Amico G, Dickson ER, Kim WR: A model to predict survival in patients with end-stage liver disease. Hepatology 2001;33:464–470.

4 Wiesner RH: Evidence-based evolution of the MELD/PELD liver allocation policy. Liver Transpl 2005;11:261–263.

5 Desschans B, Van Gelder F, Van Hees D, de Rocy J, Monbaliu D, Aerts R, Coosemans W, Pirenne J: Evolution in allocation rules for renal, hepatic, pancreatic and intestinal grafts. Acta Chir Belg 2008;108:31–34.

6 Gonwa TA, McBride MA, Anderson K, Mai ML, Wadei H, Ahsan N: Continued influence of preoperative renal function on outcome of orthotopic liver transplant (OLTX) in the US: where will MELD lead us? Am J Transplant 2006;6:2651–2659.

7 Fraley DS, Burr R, Bernardini J, Angus D, Kramer DJ, Johnson JP: Impact of acute renal failure on mortality in end-stage liver disease with or without transplantation. Kidney Int 1998;54:518–524.

8 Davis CL, Feng S, Sung R, Wong F, Goodrich NP, Melton LB, Reddy KR, Guidinger MK, Wilkinson A, Lake J: Simultaneous liver-kidney transplantation: evaluation to decision making. Am J Transplant 2007;7:1702–1709.

9 Eason JD, Gonwa TA, Davis CL, Sung RS, Gerber D, Bloom RD: Proceedings of Consensus Conference on Simultaneous Liver Kidney Transplantation (SLK). Am J Transplant 2008;8:2243–2251.

10 Alessandria C, Ozdogan O, Guevara M, Restuccia T, Jimenez W, Arroyo V, Rodes J, Gines P: MELD score and clinical type predict prognosis in hepatorenal syndrome: relevance to liver transplantation. Hepatology 2005;41:1282–1289.

11 Davenport A: Renal replacement therapy in the patient with acute brain injury. Am J Kidney Dis 2001;37:457–466.

12 Davenport A, Will EJ, Davison AM: Effect of renal replacement therapy on patients with combined acute renal and fulminant hepatic failure. Kidney Int Suppl 1993;41:S245–S251.

13 Witzke O, Baumann M, Patschan D, Patschan S, Mitchell A, Treichel U, Gerken G, Philipp T, Kribben A: Which patients benefit from hemodialysis therapy in hepatorenal syndrome? J Gastroenterol Hepatol 2004;19:1369–1373.

14 Wong LP, Blackley MP, Andreoni KA, Chin H, Falk RJ, Klemmer PJ: Survival of liver transplant candidates with acute renal failure receiving renal replacement therapy. Kidney Int 2005;68:362–370.

15 Brown M, Gunning T, Roberts C, Swygert T, Klintmalm G, Ramsay MA, Gonwa TA: Biochemical markers of renal perfusion are preserved during liver transplantation with venovenous bypass. Transplant Proc 1991;23:1980–1981.

16 Gunning TC, Brown MR, Swygert TH, Goldstein R, Husberg BS, Klintmalm GB, DiBona G, Paulsen AW, Ramsay MA, Gonwa TA: Perioperative renal function in patients undergoing orthotopic liver transplantation: a randomized trial of the effects of verapamil. Transplantation 1991;51:422–427.

17 Wadei HM, Davis CL: Renal replacement therapy in the liver transplant candidate. Adv Chronic Kidney Dis 2009;16:250–255.

18 Charlton MR, Wall WJ, Ojo AO, Gines P, Textor S, Shihab FS, Marotta P, Cantarovich M, Eason JD, Wiesner RH, Ramsay MA, Garcia-Valdecasas JC, Neuberger JM, Feng S, Davis CL, Gonwa TA: Report of the first international liver transplantation society expert panel consensus conference on renal insufficiency in liver transplantation. Liver Transpl 2009;15:S1–S34.

19 Korbet SM, Casey C, Rodby RA, Williams W: The use of continuous arteriovenous hemofiltration in orthotopic liver transplantation. Clin Nephrol 1995; 43:134–136.

20 Salord F, Bailly MP, Gaussorgues P, Workineh S, Pouyet M, Robert D: Continuous arteriovenous haemodialysis during emergency hepatic retransplantation: two case reports. Intensive Care Med 1990;16:330–331.

21 Bellomo R, Harris C, Kang Y, Daniel E, Fung JJ, Bronsther O: Combined veno-venous bypass and high volume hemofiltration during orthotopic liver transplantation. ASAIO J 1993;39:954–956.

22 Townsend DR, Bagshaw SM, Jacka MJ, Bigam D, Cave D, Gibney RT: Intraoperative renal support during liver transplantation. Liver Transpl 2009;15: 73–78.

23 Nair S, Verma S, Thuluvath PJ: Pretransplant renal function predicts survival in patients undergoing orthotopic liver transplantation. Hepatology 2002; 35:1179–1185.

24 Bahirwani R, Campbell MS, Siropaides T, Markmann J, Olthoff K, Shaked A, Bloom RD, Reddy KR: Transplantation: impact of pretransplant renal insufficiency. Liver Transpl 2008;14:665–671.

25 Gonwa TA, Morris CA, Goldstein RM, Husberg BS, Klintmalm GB: Long-term survival and renal function following liver transplantation in patients with and without hepatorenal syndrome: experience in 300 patients. Transplantation 1991;51:428–430.

26 Gonwa TA, Klintmalm GB, Levy M, Jennings LS, Goldstein RM, Husberg BS: Impact of pretransplant renal function on survival after liver transplantation. Transplantation 1995;59:361–365.

27 Jeyarajah DR, Gonwa TA, McBride M, Testa G, Abbasoglu O, Husberg BS, Levy MF, Goldstein RM, Klintmalm GB: Hepatorenal syndrome: combined liver kidney transplants versus isolated liver transplant. Transplantation 1997;64:1760–1765.

28 Gonwa TA, Mai ML, Melton LB, Hays SR, Goldstein RM, Levy MF, Klintmalm GB: End-stage renal disease (ESRD) after orthotopic liver transplantation (OLTX) using calcineurin-based immunotherapy: risk of development and treatment. Transplantation 2001;72:1934–1939.

29 Marik PE, Wood K, Starzl TE: The course of type 1 hepato-renal syndrome post liver transplantation. Nephrol Dial Transplant 2006:21:478–482.

30 Tanriover B, Mejia A, Weinstein J, Foster SV, Ghalib R, Mubarak A, Cheng SS: Analysis of kidney function and biopsy results in liver failure patients with renal dysfunction: a new look to combined liver kidney allocation in the post-MELD era. Transplantation 2008;86:1548–1553.

31 Wadei HM, Geiger XJ, Cortese C, Mai ML, Kramer DJ, Rosser BG, Keaveny AP, Willingham DL, Ahsan N, Gonwa TA: Kidney allocation to liver transplant candidates with renal failure of undetermined etiology: role of percutaneous renal biopsy. Am J Transplant 2008;8:2618–2626.

32 Restuccia T, Ortega R, Guevara M, Gines P, Alessandria C, Ozdogan O, Navasa M, Rimola A, Garcia-Valdecasas JC, Arroyo V, Rodes J: Effects of treatment of hepatorenal syndrome before transplantation on posttransplantation outcome: a case-control study. J Hepatol 2004;40:140–146.

Thomas A. Gonwa, MD, FASN
Mayo Clinic College of Medicine, Department of Transplantation
Mayo Clinic in Florida, 4500 San Pablo Road
Jacksonville, FL 32224 (USA)
E-Mail Gonwa.thomas@mayo.edu

Author Index

Angeli, P. 189
Appenrodt, B. 1, 142
Arroyo, V. 122

Bajaj, J.S. 23
Bernardi, M. 11

Cárdenas, A. 172
Cazzaniga, M. 52

Davies, N.A. 40

Fernandez, J. 122

Garcia, R. 40
Garcia-Tsao, G. 65, 149
Gerbes, A.L. VII
Ginès, P. 172
Gonwa, T.A. 198
Gustot, T. 112

Heuman, D.M. 83

Jalan, R. 40

Krag, A. 102, 178

Møller, S. 102, 178
Moreau, R. 112
Musana, A.K. 163

Proven, A. 40

Salerno, F. 52
Sanyal, A.J. 23, 163
Sauerbruch, T. 142
Shaw, J. 23

Terg, R.A. 32

Wiest, R. 65, 130
Wong, F. 91

Yeo, C.-M. 149

Subject Index

Acute kidney injury (AKI)
  causes 113, 114
  definition 113, 127, 128
  diagnosis 114, 115
  management 117, 118
  prevention 118, 119
AKI, *see* Acute kidney injury
Albumin
  comparison with other plasma volume expanders 34–37
  dysfunction in liver disease 48, 49
  functions 40
  indications for infusion
    hepatorenal syndrome 153, 154, 191
    liver disease 42–46
    non-liver disease 46–48
  levels and mortality prediction 47, 48
  paracentesis-induced circulatory dysfunction prevention 42, 45, 46
  serum ascites albumin gradient for ascites diagnosis 5, 6, 27
  structure 40
Aldosterone antagonists
  amiloride 15
  canrenoate 14, 15
  decompensating cirrhosis management 17
  dosing 15
  mechanism of action 12, 13
  pharmacology 15
  safety 15
  spironolactone 12, 14, 15
  triamterine 15
Amiloride, ascites management 15
Amylase, ascites fluid analysis 7
ANP, *see* Atrial natriuretic peptide
Ascites
  cirrhosis association 91, 92
  diuretic therapy, *see* Diuretics; Vaptan diuretics
  etiology 1, 2, 7, 8
  evaluation
    fluid analysis
      amylase 7
      appearance 4
      bacterial DNA 8
      cell count 4, 5, 27, 28
      cholesterol 6
      cytology 5
      glucose 7
      lactate dehydrogenase 6
      lactoferrin 8
      protein 5
      serum ascites albumin gradient 5, 6, 27
      tumor markers 7
    history 3
    imaging 3
    paracentesis, *see* Paracentesis
    physical examination 3
  grading 23, 24
  refractory ascites 19, 20, 92
  transjugular intrahepatic portosystemic shunt, *see* Transjugular intrahepatic portosystemic shunt
Atrial natriuretic peptide (ANP), cirrhosis levels 105

Bacterial translocation, hepatorenal syndrome 134–136
Burn patients, albumin levels and mortality 47, 48

Canrenoate, ascites management 14, 15

Cardiac surgery, albumin levels and mortality 47
Cardiorenal syndrome, cirrhosis 106–110
Cholesterol, ascites fluid analysis 6
Chronic kidney disease (CKD)
  acute-on-chronic kidney injury 116, 117
  causes 116
  definition 115, 116
  diagnosis 116
  management 119
Cirrhosis
  ascites association 91, 92
  cardiac dysfunction 105, 106
  cardiorenal axis 106–109
  decompensating cirrhosis management with diuretics
    aldosterone antagonists 17
    negative fluid balance extent 17
    refractory ascites 19, 20
    sequential versus combined treatment 17, 18
    side effects 18–20
  hepatic decompensation and hemodynamic derangements 103–105
  hyponatremia, *see* Hyponatremia, cirrhosis
  renal failure 105
  spontaneous bacterial peritonitis, *see* Spontaneous bacterial peritonitis
CKD, *see* Chronic kidney disease
Computed tomography (CT), ascites diagnosis 3
CT, *see* Computed tomography

Dextran 40, plasma volume expansion for paracentesis 34, 35
Dextran 70, plasma volume expansion for paracentesis 34, 35
Diuretics, *see also* Vaptan diuretics
  aldosterone antagonists 12–15
  amiloride 15
  decompensating cirrhosis management
    aldosterone antagonists 17
    negative fluid balance extent 17
    refractory ascites 19, 20
    sequential versus combined treatment 17, 18
    side effects 18–20
  loop diuretics 16, 17
  triamterine 15

Ethacrynic acid, ototoxicity 16

Furosemide, dosing 16

Glucose, ascites fluid analysis 7

Hemaccel, plasma volume expansion for paracentesis 34, 35
Hepatic encephalopathy, prediction with transjugular intrahepatic portosystemic shunt 61
Hepatorenal syndrome (HRS)
  acute kidney injury 113–115, 117–119
  albumin infusion 42, 44, 153, 154, 191
  cardiac dysfunction in pathogenesis 102
  chronic kidney disease 115–117, 119
  classification 172, 173
  combined liver and kidney transplantation 119, 120
  concept 122, 123
  definition 126, 127, 142
  diagnosis
    caveats 124, 126
    criteria 125–127
  epidemiology in cirrhosis 149, 150
  infection, *see also* Spontaneous bacterial peritonitis
    assessment 136
    bacterial translocation 134–136
    epidemiology and prognosis 130–132
    hemodynamics and cardiac function 132, 133
    prophylaxis 137
    risk factors for renal dysfunction 131
    site of infection and renal dysfunction 131, 132
    spontaneous bacterial peritonitis versus other infections in precipitation 133
    treatment 136, 137
  liver transplantation
    combination liver and kidney transplantation 203, 204
    intraoperative renal replacement therapy 201
    morbidity and mortality of waiting list patients 199
    renal function outcomes 201–203
    renal replacement therapy for waiting list patients 200
    survival 204, 205
    technique 200

transjugular intrahepatic portosystemic shunt, *see* Transjugular intrahepatic portosystemic shunt
types 123, 124
vasoconstrictor therapy, *see also* Terlipressin
drug types 150–152
HRS-1 154–158
HRS-2 158, 159
rationale 150–153
HRS, *see* Hepatorenal syndrome
Hypokalemia, terlipressin induction 185
Hyponatremia, cirrhosis
chronic disease 87, 88
pathophysiology 83, 84
prognostic significance 84–86
terlipressin induction 185
treatment 86, 87, 93, 96, 97
Kidney transplantation, combined liver and kidney transplantation 119, 120, 203, 204
Lactate dehydrogenase (LDH), ascites fluid analysis 6
Lactoferrin, ascites fluid analysis 8
Large volume paracentesis, *see* Paracentesis
LDH, *see* Lactate dehydrogenase
Liver transplantation
combined liver and kidney transplantation 119, 120, 203, 204
hepatorenal syndrome
combination liver and kidney transplantation 203, 204
intraoperative renal replacement therapy 201
morbidity and mortality of waiting list patients 199
renal function outcomes 201–203
renal replacement therapy for waiting list patients 200
survival 204, 205
technique 200
terlipressin effects on outcome 169
hyponatremia prognostic significance 84–86
Lixivaptin, hyponatremia management in cirrhosis 96

M0002, ascites management in cirrhosis 98
MELD, *see* Model for End Stage Liver Disease
Midodrine
hepatorenal syndrome management 151, 152, 156–159
vasoconstriction for paracentesis 37
Model for End Stage Liver Disease (MELD) 85, 112

Noradrenaline, hepatorenal syndrome management 154–157

Octreotide, hepatorenal syndrome management 151, 152, 157–159
Ornipressin, hepatorenal syndrome management 150, 151

Paracentesis
ascites diagnosis 3–7
complications 28–30
contraindications 24, 25
indications 24
large volume paracentesis
overview 26, 27, 32, 33
plasma volume expansion
albumin comparison with other expanders 34–37
dextran 40 34, 35
dextran 70 34, 35
hemaccel 34, 35
rationale 33, 34
vasoconstrictors
midodrine 37
terlipressin 37
paracentesis-induced circulatory dysfunction 33, 35–37, 42, 45, 46, 193, 194
techniques 25, 26

Refractory ascites
definition and diagnosis 19, 20
management 92

SAAG, *see* Serum ascites albumin gradient
Satavaptan
ascites management in cirrhosis 97, 98
hyponatremia management in cirrhosis 88, 96, 97
SBP, *see* Spontaneous bacterial peritonitis
Septic shock, terlipressin management 194
Serum ascites albumin gradient (SAAG), ascites diagnosis 5, 6, 27
Spironolactone, ascites management 12, 14, 15
Spontaneous bacterial peritonitis (SBP)
albumin infusion 42, 43
ascites fluid analysis 5, 6, 8
diagnosis 65, 66